Massage Fusion

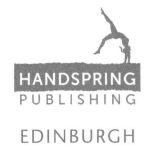

HANDSPRING
PUBLISHING

EDINBURGH

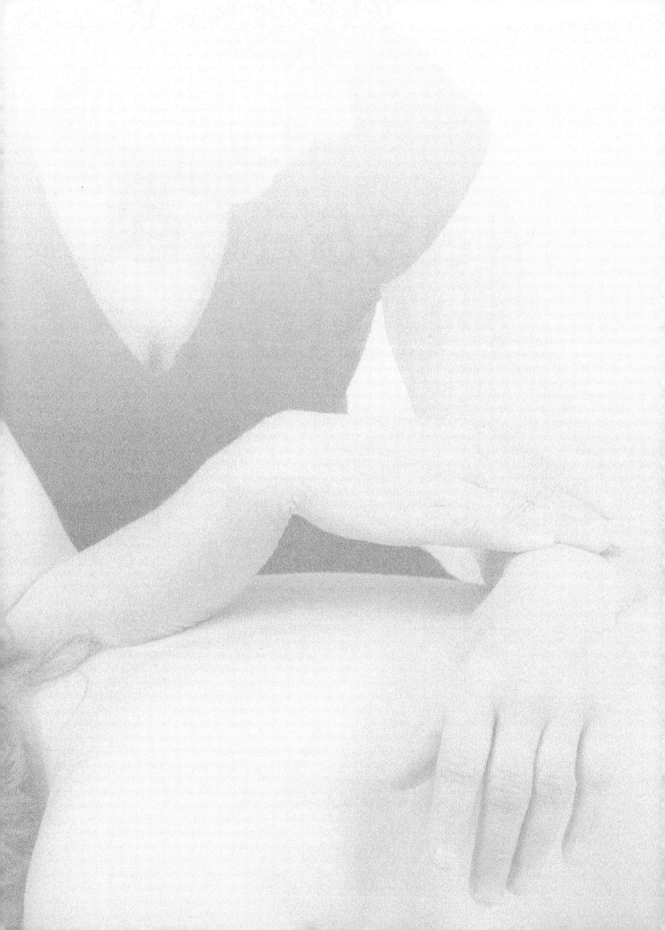

Massage Fusion

The Jing method for the treatment of chronic pain

Rachel Fairweather BA, LMT, AOS, CQSW

Meghan S. Mari MA, CHE, LMT

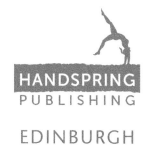

HANDSPRING
PUBLISHING

EDINBURGH

HANDSPRING PUBLISHING LIMITED
The Old Manse, Fountainhall,
Pencaitland, East Lothian
EH34 5EY, Scotland
Tel: +44 1875 341 859
Website: www.handspringpublishing.com

First published 2015 in the United Kingdom by Handspring Publishing
Reprinted 2016, 2021

3

ISBN 978-1-909141-23-0
British Library Cataloguing in Publication Data
A catalogue record for this book is available from the British Library

Library of Congress Cataloguing in Publication Data
A catalog record for this book is available from the Library of Congress

Commissioning Editor: Sarena Wolfaard
Project Manager: Joannah Duncan
Design Direction and Cover Design: Bruce Hogarth, kinesis-creative.com
Photographer: Anita Barratt
Index: Dr Laurence Errington
Typeset: DSM Soft
Printed: CPI Group (UK) Ltd, Croydon, CR0 4YY

The
Publisher's
policy is to use
paper manufactured
from sustainable forests

Foreword *vii*
Preface *ix*
Dedications and Acknowledgements *xi*
Self-Care Resources *xiii*

Section 1

Chapter 1   Massage fusion: the art and science of a multi-modal approach to massage therapy   3
Chapter 2   Back to basics: the art of advanced massage   9
Chapter 3   Working with emotions in bodywork   25
Chapter 4   Chronic pain: are the issues in the tissues or is the pain in the brain?   33

Section 2

Chapter 5   Clinical assessment   55
Chapter 6   The warm-up act: the power of hot and cold in advanced clinical massage   73
Chapter 7   Dedicated followers of fascia: the background and practice of fascial therapies   85
Chapter 8   Trigger happy! The art and science of trigger point therapy   115
Chapter 9   Meridian magic! Using meridians and acupressure points in massage   141
Chapter 10   Stretching the truth: what the new evidence tells us about stretching   157
Chapter 11   The importance of teaching self care   177

Section 3

Chapter 12   Low back pain protocol   201
Chapter 13   Neck and shoulder pain protocol   225
Chapter 14   Shoulder girdle pain protocol   247
Chapter 15   Forearm and wrist pain protocol   271
Chapter 16   Hip and pelvis pain protocol   291
Chapter 17   Leg, knee and foot pain protocol   317
Chapter 18   Temporomandibular joint pain protocol   345
Chapter 19   Stress and chronic pain protocol   355

Index 371

***Self-care resources* (available at uk.singingdragon.com/catalogue/
book/9781909141230)**

In your hands, you are holding nothing less than one of the most recent advances in our evolution as a species. For our 'handiness' is one of humans' most defining characteristics, and humans have surely been doing hands-on massage for just as long as we have had hands to do it with. This book, by fusing some of the most effective and highly evolved approaches to the very human art of massage, is a valuable addition to our collective advancement as a manual species.

The impulse to ease discomfort with touch is an instinctual one, whether the discomfort is physical, mental or emotional. This instinctual urge is likely connected to some of the deepest behaviours that define us and our kindred mammals – the touching, holding, grasping and physicality that literally connects us to one another, as baby and parent, as littermates, as lovers, as friend to friend, or as healer and healed. Touch has the power to comfort and calm; and this sets the stage for healing of all sorts, whether we are speaking biologically, psychologically, socially or spiritually.

Besides our very able human hands, our species' other defining feature is our outsized human brain. Naturally, as our brains have expanded, we have applied this growing mental capacity to developing and testing ever-more sophisticated explanations for how touch actually works. The pace of this learning and complexity is still accelerating. For example, though we have been identifiably human for between 100,000 to 200,000 years, almost all of Western anatomical knowledge has been developed in the last 500 years. Even more recently, the advent of detailed, real-time imaging has accelerated our learning to such an extent that massage and bodywork students who studied anatomy just 20 years ago have a far different visual narrative than those who have learned since the use of 3D modelling and graphics has become more commonplace.

Massage and bodywork's place in our species' body of knowledge is rapidly changing as well. Relatively recently in our evolutionary history (say, in the last 100 years or less), touch modalities have, probably for the first time, found themselves outside the medical mainstream. Biomedical innovation in the last century focused on technological and pharmaceutical interventions, which have had the advantage of often being very effective; easy to measure, study and distribute; and less labour intensive than hands-on work. This has led to the relative marginalisation of hands-on approaches, and at times, polarisation and estrangement between biomedicine and manual medicine. This gulf between mainstream medicine and manual therapies has at times reached absurd extremes, such as in 1967 when the American Medical Association told its members it was an ethical violation to professionally associate with, refer to, accept referrals from, or even to play golf with chiropractors and 'other unscientific' manual therapy practitioners (Lisa 1994).

But as successful as modern biomedical approaches have been, they have left many needs unaddressed, as evidenced by the vast sums people still elect to spend on 'alternative', 'complementary' or 'integrative' modalities, including massage therapy and hands-on bodywork. Partly as a result of people voting with their pocketbooks in this way, there are numerous examples of mixing and rapprochement between conventional and complementary approaches. And though many would say there is still a long way to go, 'integrative' medicine is becoming more common, where Western, Eastern, complementary and conventional approaches are combined.

In this spirit, this book provides massage students and therapists (as well as interested allied practitioners, such as chiropractors, osteopaths, physiotherapists, nurses, etc.) with a well-defined and compelling way forward. Its methods have been tested by many years of practice, not just by its able authors, but by thousands of practitioners from the diverse methods it draws together in its approach. And in an approach that emphasises the experiential alongside the intellectual, the enjoyment and passion of its authors for their craft clearly shines through, and inspires the reader to join them on the learning adventure this book represents.

By including careful attention to the therapeutic interaction between practitioner and client, its person-centred values give the Jing approach a clear place in the long humanistic and holistic health lineage it builds upon. And just as importantly, it updates the reader with a clear and comprehensible view into how the most recent research is informing massage and hands-on work, bringing together intellectual intelligence with manual intelligence, in a fusion that invites an evolutionary advance of not just our work, but of our innate humanity itself.

Til Luchau
Boulder, Colorado, USA 2015

Reference

Lisa, PJ 1994 The assault on medical freedom. Norfolk, VA: Hampton Roads Publishing Company.

Love what you do, do what you love

This book is for you, the dedicated hands-on practitioner who recognises the power of touch in affecting chronic pain. It is designed to be many things to many people and many things to the same person. It is at once a practical textbook, a tome of bodywork philosophy, and a beautiful picture book. Yet above all, this book is a love story, a love story about the bold and beautiful art of bodywork, a story that proves the adage 'if you love what you do you will never work another day in your life'.

Massage Fusion was written for the millions of therapists worldwide who love massage and bodywork, for those who have found meaning and sense in their lives through the simple yet profound act of touching other human beings with reverence and respect. This book is written for every therapist, everywhere, who helps others with their hands, head and heart. Our own love of massage has brought us a life that has fulfilled all our dreams. It has given us a sense of purpose, a true vocation, a community and some of the most beautiful and transcendental moments of our lives. We hope that this book connects or reconnects you to that journey.

The *Massage Fusion* story

The *Massage Fusion* story began many years ago in the city that unites the dreamers of dreams – New York. We, the authors, met while working at a magical, vibrant new spa offering specialised hot stone massage treatments to bohemian New Yorkers. As we worked, laughed and played with our fellow therapists – a creative, funny and intelligent bunch – we whiled away the hours talking about our hopes and dreams for the future. Rachel's dream was to open a school in her native UK offering the high level of training common in the USA but unavailable in the UK. She had great ambition for not only herself, but for the entire profession of massage therapy. By making education accessible, she could in turn make the profession more professional. Through this process, she would pave the way for the public to be able to rely on educated massage therapists that could offer essential options for those living with chronic pain. Meg's dream was always to help people help themselves. As a counsellor, business coach and massage therapist, she was determined to create spaces for productive communities to form and allow change to happen on the personal and professional level. She strived to combine her love of psychology, law, art and business to empower others to achieve their greatest potential. Together our visions combined and, in 2003, we travelled to the UK and began offering the first courses that became the basis of our school and professional development organisation: Jing Advanced Massage Training.

With nothing more than enthusiasm and great passion, we started teaching small groups of keen therapists, eager to learn how they could improve their results with the chronic pain situations so familiar to complementary therapists everywhere. To our delight the 'Jing thing' spread like wildfire, therapists loved our fusion of techniques that combined art and science, great touch with precise knowledge and the wisdom of East and West. Most importantly people were getting results using the 'Jing method' – a return to ancient notions of understanding the whole person through a combination of targeted biopsychosocial assessment, effective soft tissue modalities and self-care advice. The first few workshops blossomed in number to over 30 and eventually, in 2011, to a degree level course in Advanced Clinical and Sports Massage – the first of its kind in the UK.

This book is what our students have been requesting for years – the summary of our approach and philosophy from both a practical and theoretical perspective. Our aim with this book is to give you a shortcut to getting results in the tricky business of chronic pain and, in addition, to summarise the current evidence behind the techniques and methods used. Our hope is to give you a strong foundation to relieve pain whilst stimulating your curiosity about why this might be happening.

Getting the most out of your *Massage Fusion* journey

Like most good journeys it is always best to start at the beginning and finish at the end. However if you prefer to find your own way, here is a map to help your navigation:

- Chapters 1–4: these chapters outline some of the fundamental principles of good bodywork including equipment, body mechanics, developing touch, working with client emotions and an exploration of our current level of understanding of chronic pain.

- Chapters 5–11: these chapters look at the theory and evidence base for the use and practice of the different modalities in the Jing method, namely targeted assessment, use of hot and cold, fascial technique, trigger point therapy, acupressure and meridian approaches, and stretching and self-care techniques.

- Chapters 12–19: these are step-by-step protocols to treating pain in different areas of the body using the Jing method, and are illustrated by detailed photos of each of the techniques. If you are tempted to go straight to these practical chapters, we recommend you read Chapter 1 first

to give you an understanding of the massage fusion approach of how and why these techniques are combined to give optimal results.

- Self-care resources: the self-care resource website (uk.singingdragon.com/catalogue/book/9781909141230) gives you a wealth of sheets that you can easily print out and share with your clients.

It's all about you

Most of all, this book is for you. Use it, abuse it, stain it with oil and coffee rings, take it on subways and aeroplanes, disagree with it, quote it and cogitate on it. Our favourite massage books are treasured bedside companions and we hope this is where *Massage Fusion* will live. Enjoy the book; enjoy your bodywork journey!

Rachel Fairweather and Meghan S. Mari, 2015

We would like to sincerely thank all of those who have helped us along the way and who have contributed to making this book possible. The list cannot possibly be all-inclusive due to the number of extraordinary individuals who have had an influence on where we are today; however, we would like to give a special mention to the following.

Our own inspiring teachers from the past including Steve Gough, Gerry Pyves, Jordan Weiner and Carol Carpenter of NHI (National Holistic Institute, San Francisco). Carla Ciuffo and Adam Schwartz for bringing us together, giving us invaluable experience and connecting us with the amazing therapists and friends we met at the Stone-Spa, New York. Angela Mahandru for giving us our first exposure in the UK; Zoe Campell and the Diversified team for continued support via the glorious annual camexpo show; all our wonderful Jing teachers over the years including Jem Pickford, Kasia Robertson, Tracey Kiernan, Sue Ingram, Mel Smith, Yvonne Cervetti, Sarah Symonds, Kathryn Jones, Sydel Hodsen, Fiona Searle, Bettina Karsten and Suzy Daw. Thanks also to Tracey Kiernan for her contribution to the 'Temporomandibular Joint Pain Protocol' chapter and Amanda Oswald for her behind the scenes work in helping our degree level course become accredited. Thanks to those who give their time in service to enable Jing courses to achieve an unsurpassed level of quality, the one-to-one teaching team (TOTOs) and course supporters.

We thank all our support staff at Jing, past and present, particularly Nina Frizoni for her tireless enthusiasm, loyalty and sharing the dream, Anne-Marie Williams, Val Walsh and Nigel Jeffrey. Thanks also go to, our dear friend and colleague, Andrew Dineley for his creative genius in all things 'Jing' and his unwavering patience in helping us develop in so many ways.

We are indebted to Handspring Publishing, in particular Sarena Wolfaard, for the wonderful synchronicity of literally springing into existence at the very right time and taking the idea of this book off the 'to do list' and into reality. We thank them for their vision for manual therapy literature and their immense experience in the field that has made this experience a smooth and ultra-professional ride. Special thanks go to Anita Barrat for sharing her exquisite photography that illustrates the beauty of the work we teach. She is also to be thanked for years of support and her contribution to making the whole Jing experience beautiful.

We would like to thank our own friends and families.

From Rachel's heart: grateful thanks to my beloved partner Kate for the many days, nights and weekends of personal together time that have been sacrificed for this book, for her laughter and the wise words that keep me whole; also to my darling parents who taught me the immense value of 'doing my best' and never giving up. I would also like to thank the many wonderful friends of the 'commune' (you know who you are!) who have uncomplainingly listened to endless stories about massage, and the trials and tribulations of self employment, and have never failed to bring me back to earth when I start to take myself too seriously.

From Meg's heart: massive gratitude to my Sara for her light heart and her unique ability to support me in everything I do and all things Jing, and in helping me to always laugh no matter how hard it gets. My inspirational parents, William and Jacqueline Mari, who infused in me from day one that anything and everything is possible if you say I can. My sister Elizabeth Mari and all my friends and family on both sides of the pond, that have always supported me, my wanderlust and my endless inspiration for following dreams, even when it has meant missing being nearby for so many years.

The largest thanks is to the Jing global community made up of extraordinary individuals whose thirst for knowledge and positivity encourages us to 'keep on keeping on'.

To all who have supported and loved us along the way, we hope this book makes you proud. Thank you for being there.

We must also give thanks to whatever universal alignment occurred all those years ago to bring us together on this crazy journey and we recognise it has only just begun.

Self-care resources

As a companion to this book we have also developed a sister website. This website provides you with a host of useful resources for your clients, such as self-help exercises, self trigger point treatment, meditation and mindfulness suggestions, a pain diary and useful worksheets.

The self-care resources can be downloaded (from uk.singingdragon.com/catalogue/ book/9781909141230) and the opening page to the website contains a list of all the sheet titles so you can easily find what you are looking for.

The sheets are 'made for sharing' – for you, the therapist, to share with your clients, other massage therapists and interested professionals. You can print them out and hand them to clients personally at the end of their treatments. You can also choose to share them electronically via email, social media or links on your website.

Feel free to mix and match the sheets in whatever creative way you choose and which best meets the needs of your clients. Here is a list of the contents to whet your appetite:

- Sheet 1: Prompt questions for client consultation
- Sheet 2: Mindfulness
- Sheet 3: Body scan
- Sheet 4: Positions for relaxation and meditation
- Sheet 5: Seated positions for relaxation and meditation
- Sheet 6: Helpful visualisations for pain relief
- Sheet 7: Static stretches for back pain
- Sheet 8: Active isolated stretches (AIS) for low back pain
- Sheet 9: Tips for neck and shoulder pain
- Sheet 10: Tips for headaches and migraines
- Sheet 11: Tips for shoulder girdle pain
- Sheet 12: Tips for forearm, hand and wrist pain
- Sheet 13: Hip pain
- Sheet 14: Leg and knee pain
- Sheet 15: Self trigger point treatment and exercises for temporomandibular joint (TMJ) pain
- Sheet 16: Decatastrophising worksheet
- Sheet 17: Pain diary

All sheets are available at uk.singingdragon.com/ catalogue/book/9781909141230.

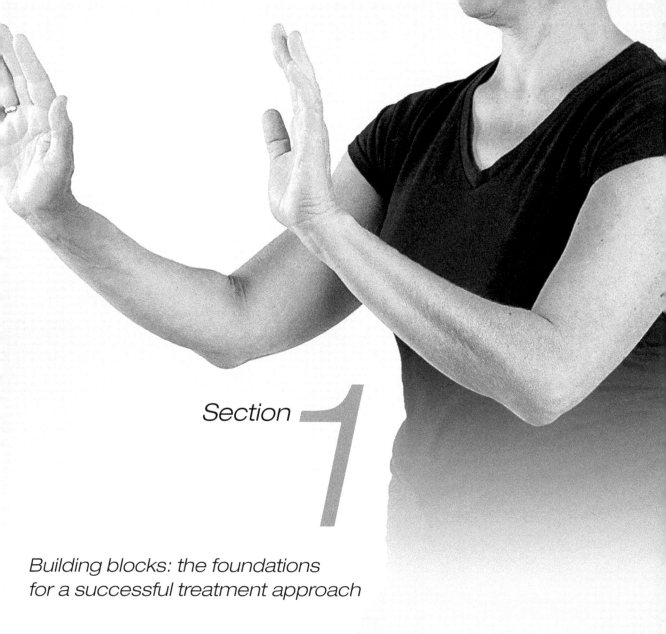

Section *1*

Building blocks: the foundations for a successful treatment approach

Just as houses need firm foundations, the art of massage requires a commitment to getting the basics absolutely right. This section of the book introduces you to some fundamental principles including great body mechanics, the skill of listening touch, working safely with the emotions and the Jing method to reducing pain in 1–6 clinical treatments. In Chapter 4 you will also gain a vital insight into the links between mind and body in the treatment of chronic musculoskeletal pain conditions.

The chapters in this section will give you a solid understanding of the philosophy and practice behind the Jing method, which uses a creative combination of advanced soft tissue techniques to treat common pain conditions.

1

Massage fusion: the art and science of a multi-modal approach to massage therapy

One who works with the hands is a labourer.
One who works with the hands and the head is a craftsman.
One who works with the hands and the head and the heart is
an artist.
ST FRANCIS OF ASSISI

Passion for massage

Excellence is a very close kin to passion.
ANON

The principles expounded in this book are born out of a lifelong passion for massage and a desire to achieve the best possible outcomes for clients in emotional and physical pain. We truly believe that most of us who enter this profession are bodywork 'artists' and we have a profound desire to help other people with our 'hands, heads and hearts'. As an illustration, here is a touching story recounted by an attendee at the memorial service of John Upledger, founder of craniosacral therapy, who died in 2012:

In her simple testimony Lisa Upledger (John's wife) told us that she had more than once during John's last months asked him to state, to define, the overarching intention or mission of his life and his work, as perhaps a message for all of us. Sitting in that room we wondered how would he, this great original thinker, encapsulate for us more than 50 years of groundbreaking course development, teaching, treatment and authorship with its legacy of literally roomfuls of catalogued articles and other research paperwork? What final guidance would he offer? Twice, Lisa told us, he would not be drawn, discouraging her from pursuing the matter. A third time, and when she reckoned would be, during his decline, possibly the last opportunity, she made the same request. Following brief and typically curmudgeonly resistance he at last made his statement: 'Helping people.'
PAGE 2013

Like Dr John, we all just want to 'help people' and yet the million-dollar question for every massage therapist is always: how BEST can we help people? It's a confusing world out there – so many techniques to learn, so many different types of clients. That great success you had with cheery Mrs Smith's back pain after two treatments is just not being replicated with her nervy neighbour, Mr Jones. The literature can be even more confusing: research can be scanty, contradictory, poorly conducted, or just impossible to understand. Some researchers even tell us that massage doesn't do ANYTHING apart from, the slightly bland, 'promote wellbeing'. We desperately want to be able to achieve the best results in the quickest possible time but making sense of the minefield of information can be overwhelming.

The Jing method: the whole is greater than the sum of the parts

Our own personal journey with the evolution of the Jing approach to the treatment of musculoskeletal pain has risen out of such a dilemma. Even if you are only offering relaxation massage, most massage therapists will be familiar with the list of persistent pain conditions that are presented by clients who are desperate for relief. Back pain, neck pain, headaches, repetitive strain syndrome, irritable bowel syndrome, fibromyalgia, jaw pain, tennis elbow, golfers elbow, frozen shoulder – does this list sound familiar? Persistent musculoskeletal pain is complex to treat and baffling to most orthodox medical practitioners, who have little to offer from their 'cut and drug' toolbox. Most of us as novice (or even experienced) massage therapists, are also at sea trying to make a difference in the complex puzzle of persistent pain, not knowing which techniques work best or why. Real results only come through thousands of hours of clinical practice, experimenting with different approaches and client conditions. All of us have longed for a shortcut at some point in our career – I know we certainly have.

The approach outlined in this book aims to give such a shortcut and has come from years of clinical practice, teaching and endless study. Two decades of 'hands on bodies' has informed us of what does and does not work. Between us we have learned dozens of different bodywork techniques in our quest to get the best results for our clients and to give the best teaching to our students. Our pragmatic approach has been literally 'Throw it against the wall and see what sticks.' In other words, try techniques in the clinic on real people in real situations. What worked stayed in the mix; what didn't work has been thrown out.

Slowly but surely, the combination of modalities that has become the Jing approach evolved over the years. Powerful, flowing relaxation massage achieved some results by itself but when combined with trigger point therapy, even greater outcomes were attained. Putting fascial work into the mix helped get results with clients who did not respond to pure trigger point therapy, as did knowledge of acupressure and stretching. More excitingly, each approach used seemed to enhance the effect of the others, e.g. using heat and fascial techniques at the beginning of the treatment reduced the amount of trigger points that needed to be treated. So it was perfectly feasible to work with slowness, focus and precision and combine a number of techniques within a normal clinical hour of 50 minutes. Using a creative combination of techniques seems to mean we work less not more!

This approach parallels the philosophy of Gestalt psychology that is famous for the phrase: 'The whole is greater than the sum of its parts.' A logical approach to multi-modal treatment suggests that the combined effect of a number of skills is magically greater than would be gained through the individual sum of these techniques alone. Each technique enhances and reinforces the effects of the others.

The 'treatment sandwich': psychology is just as important as physiology

Significantly, the multi-modal approach outlined in this book puts an emphasis not just on the hands-on techniques used but also the quality and content of the practitioner–client interaction. A big part of the massage therapist's job is to connect with the client, enable them to feel heard, and also educate and empower them to take control over their own healing. This is a significant part of the session and should not be glossed over. Evidence shows that these aspects in themselves can do as much to promote recovery as our hands-on work. The massage therapist has two significant opportunities to interact and connect verbally with the client: the first is during the client consultation at the beginning of the treatment; the second is at the end where feedback and self-care suggestions can be given. We call this the 'treatment sandwich' as manual techniques are slotted in between the beginnings and endings of slices of verbal client–therapist interaction.

The importance of these verbal components in enhancing client recovery from pain conditions cannot be over-emphasised. Pain is a complex phenomenon and for many of the clients we work with the 'issues are not just in the tissues'. Research shows that all pain is a perception of the brain rather than what is actually happening at the tissue level; in the case of chronic pain even more so. Thus, the sensation of pain can be mediated by a variety of factors including emotional state, previous experience, expectations and sense of control over the pain.

Hence the consultation aspect of the treatment enables the practitioner to connect with the client about both physical and emotional aspects to their pain, provide support and reassurance, reduce fear, and educate about outdated beliefs or attitudes to their condition.

Similarly, the self-care suggestions form an important part of the healing process as they aim to empower the client to take control of their health. Simple principles drawn from meditation, mindfulness, cognitive behavioural therapy and exercise can have powerful effects. The massage therapist can act as cheerleader or coach, setting simple self-care goals and encouraging and supporting progress.

A massage therapist's manifesto for the 21st century

This book and our teachings aim to empower massage therapists to reclaim a sense of confidence in our profession. More than any other occupation, we are best placed to help people with our hands, heads and hearts.

Over the past few decades there has been a shift away from traditional bodywork teachings that emphasised spirituality, connection and the skill of the practitioner. Instead there has been a move towards reliance on 'technique', the reductionism of evidence-based research and structural models borrowed from osteopathy, chiropractic or physical therapy. The psychological and emotional concerns of our clients started to take more of a back seat. The term 'holistic' became watered down and unfashionable for the serious practitioner interested in treating pain. We wanted to prove ourselves, to be 'remedial', 'clinical' and 'sports therapy' orientated. In doing so, we threw the metaphorical baby out with the bathwater. Mind and body can never be separated. Research is increasingly showing us that we can only seriously address pain by taking into account emotional and psychological factors; that the structurally based models of errant tipped pelvises and leg length differentials have no relationship to pain and that our connection and empathy for our clients can help them get better to the same degree as our hands-on work. Researchers are busy re-inventing the wheel with the 'biopsychosocial' model being the new buzzword in health care, the re-branding of 'holistic' for the 21st century. Our call to arms is for massage therapists to rise up and embrace an approach that is rightfully ours. After all we have been doing this stuff for centuries, so we must be pretty good at it!

Massage as art and science

The passionate bodyworker for the 21st century needs to reclaim the historical roots of bodywork whilst embracing new ideas and research. Research is important but over reliance on the findings of randomised controlled trials (RCTs) means that we overlook the need to develop our skills as practitioners. RCTs by their very nature are reductionist, aiming to find the one factor that makes a difference. At the end of the day, people, not techniques, help other people. The bodyworker in pursuit of excellence should be continually working on their own personal development. Ultimately becoming a better massage therapist means becoming a better person. That means keeping up to date with the latest research, being prepared to continually question what you are doing, examining your own motives, beliefs and reactions, and constantly learning.

This book aims to straddle the bridge between art and science, and show the research evidence for a combined creative approach that many massage therapists have been doing naturally for years. At the same time we aim to embrace and reclaim the true art of massage. Exquisite body mechanics, touch and connection are as much part of our teachings as anatomy and technique.

Our methods do not claim to be anything new, simply a careful curation of the best techniques and approaches developed over centuries of bodywork. We feel we are standing on the shoulders of giants in the approach we use, which is informed by amazing pioneers, such as Janet Travell and Ida Rolf, the humansim of Carl Rogers and a rich Eastern tradition. Yet we hope that by stepping back and taking a big picture approach we can see how different methods reinforce and enhance one another. A few quotes from therapists who have trained with us exemplify this East meets West, art meets science view:

> *The Jing way doesn't just treat the body but also the person in it.*
>
> Jing puts together people that care, with techniques that make a difference.
>
> *Jing has allowed me to work scientifically with my heart.*
> THERAPISTS TRAINED IN THE JING METHOD

East meets West: a unifying thread

> *The Jing approach is a fusion of East and West resulting in an effective treatment specific to the person. Jing somehow manages to teach you the power of an informed touch, with the support of an informed toolbox of techniques, you follow your intuition and find the cause of the pain.*
> JING THERAPIST

One of the hallmarks of the Jing approach has always been 'East meets West'. We take the best of both worlds: from the East, the knowledge of meridians, acupressure points and Thai stretching, and an emphasis on self care, holism and the graceful body mechanics of t'ai chi; from the West, the insights of Janet Travell into trigger points, the deep fascial work of Ida Rolf, the flowing moves of Pehr Henrik Ling of Swedish massage, insights from osteopathy and person-centred counselling.

East and West are not natural bedfellows in bodywork as they are mired in different traditions and different languages. Yet stepping back and taking a big picture approach has led us to conclude that the techniques from both worlds offer similar effects but with different explanations. New research explored in this book suggests that fascia is the basis of the meridian system. It seems likely that trigger point work, acupressure points, meridian work and stretching all mediate their positive effects on the body via the fascial system. Moreover, that the fascial system is communicating in a complex way with the brain, not just about motor movements but also, more importantly, about emotional and cognitive factors in our perception of pain. It may well be that the fascia is indeed the physical representation of the mind–body interface that has fascinated bodyworkers for centuries.

Summary of the massage fusion multi-modal approach: HFMAST

So what exactly is the Jing approach? In addition to a targeted consultation, the techniques that form the cornerstone of the Jing method can be summarised by the mnemonic HFMAST. They are:

- **H** The use of **H**eat or cold.

- **F** The use of **F**ascial techniques: both direct and indirect methods.

- **M** Treating **M**uscles with precise trigger point therapy: specifically treating ALL the muscles around an affected joint to release trigger points.

- **A** Treating relevant **A**cupressure points.

- **S** **S**tretching: using techniques such as static, proprioceptive neuromuscular facilitation (PNF) or active isolated stretching.

- **T** **T**eaching the client self-help strategies that lie within the massage therapist's scope of practice. This would include, for example, self trigger point treatment, simple breathing techniques, stretching or mobilisation exercises.

Signifcantly, we recommend that all these techniques are integrated within a 50-minute treatment and the protocol chapters (see Chapters 12–19) outline a step-by-step approach for doing this for different areas of the body. In essence we are giving you a massage 'recipe book' – the protocol chapters outline a great recipe that works for most clients, most of the time, for specific areas of the body. In doing so we are not aiming to stifle creativity – quite the opposite. The protocols allow you to learn a tried and tested approach, enabling you to get results and build confidence. As you grow as a bodyworker we encourage you to play around with the basic recipe, adding or taking away techniques or simply putting your hands on the body and seeing what happens. The approach is intended to act as a 'bodywork blueprint', a safe place from which to be creative. Feel free to experiment, come up with your own ideas and add your own favourite treatment approaches to the mix.

The golden secret: the magic of six

> *If you only knew the magnificence of the 3, 6 and 9, then you would have a key to the universe.*
> TESLA

Not sure about the nine, but three and six certainly play a major part in the Jing method. For some reason many massage therapists feel they have to completely reduce people's pain in one session or they have failed. Conversely, other practitioners see clients week in and week out, for months without anything changing.

A golden secret is the 'power of six'. If you are presented with a client in pain, you will need to recommend that they come to see you once a week for up to 6 weeks to achieve a reduction in their pain. Once you see a consistent reduction in pain that lasts between treatments (usually around the dawn of the other magical number: week 3) you will increase the time between treatments (maybe now seeing them once every 2 weeks). Eventually, if they remain pain free between the lengthened duration between treatments, move them onto maintenance treatments of once a month or whatever suits. In our experience, clients who have had one musculoskeletal pain problem will end up with another, so maintenance treatments are a great part of everyone's health care routine.

This lets your client know exactly how much time and money they need to spend before expecting to see a result. For most musculoskeletal pain problems you will see a reduction in pain by at least week 3. If at this point you are seeing no improvement you will need to change something about what you are doing or refer the client onto someone else you think may be better placed to help.

The 6-week approach is a ballpark figure that works for most musculoskeletal problems. If the problem is longstanding or central sensitisation is a big component (see Chapter 4) then the time period to recovery will be lengthened. On the other hand, some problems can be easily resolved after a couple of treatments.

How to use this book

In summary, the purpose of this book and the proposed model for integrating multiple modalities therefore exists in the spirit of fulfilling the dictum 'the teacher's job is to shorten the journey'. The model outlines a logical step-by-step procedure for integrating different approaches in a way that is complementary and seeks to maintain both the art and science of good massage therapy. The following chapters examine the available clinical and scientific evidence that endorses these approaches and provide step-by-step protocols for their combination.

The book is divided into sections as follows:

- **Chapters 1–4**: Foundations: these chapters outline some of the fundamental principles of good bodywork, including equipment, body mechanics, developing touch and working with client emotions. Chapter 4 also examines the modulation of pain states by the brain that is essential to our understanding of how body and mind work together in the pain experience.

- **Chapters 5–11**: these chapters look at the evidence base for the use and practice of the different modalities in the Jing HFMAST approach, namely targeted assessment, use of hot

and cold, fascial techniques, trigger point therapy, acupressure and meridian approaches, stretching and self-care techniques.

- **Chapters 12–19**: these are step-by-step protocols for treating pain in different areas of the body using the HFMAST approach.

- **Self-Care Resources**: self-help sheets you can use with your clients (available at uk.singingdragon.com/catalogue/book/9781909141230).

In a nutshell

The most important thing is to work with your 'hands, head and heart' and go forth and perfect your own unique art of massage – as Seth Godin, famous inspirational blogger and speaker puts it in his book 'Are you indispensable?'

> Art isn't only a painting. Art is anything that's creative, passionate, and personal. And great art resonates with the viewer, not only with the creator.
> Art is a personal gift that changes the recipient. The medium doesn't matter. The intent does.
> Art is a personal act of courage, something one human does that creates change in another.
> GODIN AND HAGY 2010

Go forth, brave bodyworkers, and make a difference with our beloved art of massage. As President Obama famously said 'We are the people that we've been waiting for.'

References

Godin S, Hagy J 2010 Linchpin: Are you indispensable?, 1st edn. York: Portfolio.

Page J 2013 Dr John's Memorial Service, from John Page. Somerset, UK: Upledger Institute. Available at: http://www.upledger.co.uk/blog/dr-johns-memorial-service-from-john-page.html [accessed 20 August 2014].

Back to basics: the art of advanced massage

Introduction

Just as solid houses need firm foundations, the art of massage requires a commitment to getting the basics absolutely right. With these fundamentals firmly in place you will be assured of giving a treatment that feels amazing and keeps you and your client injury free. This chapter covers the founding principles that we find have often been ignored or glossed over in initial training, such as:

- Choosing the right equipment.
- Stance and graceful body mechanics.
- The art of listening touch.
- Developing critical thinking around contraindications.

Elegant equipment

Our top table tips
Choosing the right massage table

Many moons ago when I was a novice massage therapist, finding a good table was not easy, particularly if you lived outside the massage mecca of the United States. My first purchase was an old fixed height medical couch that my doctor produced from an outside storage shed (complete with dust and cobwebs) for the princely sum of a £25 donation! When Meg and I started Jing it was impossible to find good tables in the UK and we would instead buy them while in New York and bring them back as luggage (possible only with a winning smile at the check-in desk). Fortunately times have moved on and these days it is easy to find a great massage table for a good price, thanks to the marvels of the World Wide Web.

When choosing a massage table, consider the following features:

- **Ease of adjustment**: you need to be able to lower your table to the correct height for your size, so fixed height tables are pretty much a no-no.

We are not a fan of the tables with metal legs and the pop out buttons that seem to have a short shelf life. The wooden screw type tables are much more hardwearing. **See Figure 2.1**

- **Face cradle**: go for a lovely padded, fully adjustable face cradle. Some massage tables only have a hole that can leave the client's neck at an uncomfortable angle. **See Figure 2.2**

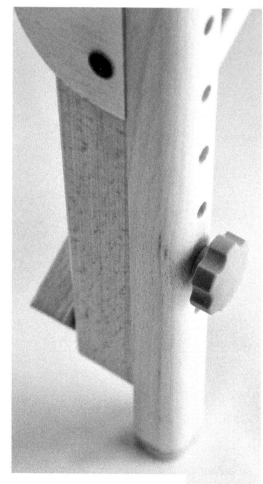

Figure 2.1

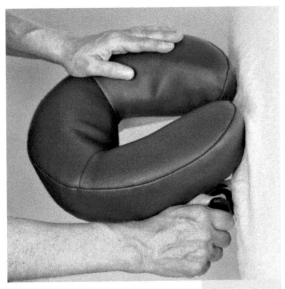

Figure 2.2

- **Width**: choose a table that is wide enough to allow room on either side. The work that we advocate in Jing is creative and fuses a number of different massage styles including adaptations of shiatsu and Thai massage. These involve kneeling on the table in order for the therapist to be able to work deeper without working harder. To do this effectively you will need a table that is at least 28 inches (70 cm) wide.

- **Beauty**: last but not least, make sure your table pleases you aesthetically. Let's face it, there aren't really any major expenses involved in setting up a massage business and buying a table will probably be your biggest outlay. So why not get a table that you REALLY love! Take time choosing something that totally appeals to you in colour, comfort and looks. I spent hours poring over catalogues

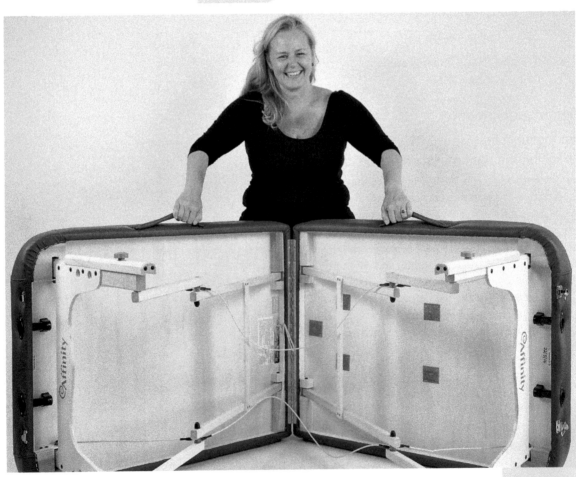

Figure 2.3

when I bought my first proper massage table, deciding on the finer virtues of 'Reiki end plates' (whatever they were), depth of padding and type of vinyl. I was devastated when my first massage table was finally retired after decades of hard use as it had become a treasured and beloved companion. Meg's first table is still in use on Jing courses 20 years on!

Setting up the table

Here are a couple of our top tips for setting up your table quickly and easily:

- Standing behind your folded table with the padded side towards your body, unlock the catch and grab both handles to unfold with ease. Make sure the cables aren't caught around the legs – which is a common mistake that will give your massage table a short lifespan. **See Figure 2.3**

- Putting up a massage table by yourself can be a clumsy and cumbersome business but not if you know this golden secret. Stand in front of the table, put one foot on the table leg and pull the table up using leverage. I know, I know – just that one tip is worth the book price alone. **See Figure 2.4**

- **Table height**: adjust your table so that it is fist height or below – this is essential for doing effective and specific massage work without injuring yourself. Make sure all the legs are screwed in securely and they are all at the same height.

- **Face cradle**: adjust your face cradle so that it is on a slight downwards angle. Make sure the lock is screwed securely – as there is nothing more disconcerting for a client than having the face cradle give way (usually with a loud dramatic crack) in the middle of a relaxing treatment.

Ingredients for a perfect massage

Just as with choosing the right table, take time to invest in other equipment that will give your client the most professional and satisfying experience possible. Aesthetically pleasing linens that thrill both your own and your client's senses contribute as much to building businesses as fancy techniques do.

Our essential ingredients for a top massage are:

- **Two big fluffy towels**.
- **Face cradle cover or pillowcase**.

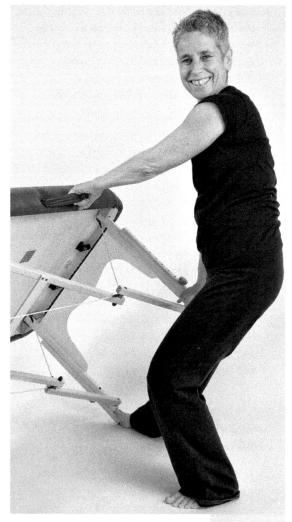

Figure 2.4

- **Couch cover that fits properly**. Therapists often use a flat sheet as a couch cover but these can slide around and be irritating to the client.

- **Two bolsters, cushions or pillows plus a few smaller bolsters**. Pillows and cushions tend to be more adaptable than the harder specialised massage bolsters as they can be squashed and folded as needed. Make a habit of collecting the small pillows given out on aeroplane flights as these are ideal for a range of situations including bolstering under the belly, using as padding when kneeling on the floor or supporting the arms when doing specific forearm work.

- **Stones**: even if you don't offer full specialised stone treatments, a small stone kit is great for applying hot or cold to the body when you are doing specific work. The use of hot and cold is an important part of the work that we teach and stones are just about the best way we have found for applying this.

- **Massage wax**: although technically any medium (oil or lotion) can be used for doing massage, we love using massage wax. It is less messy than oil and better for doing the deep specific work that we teach. We both had a habit of losing and abusing our oil bottles, constantly kicking them over, and being unable to find where we had put them in the dimmed light of a massage treatment. (A compelling reason to gain expertise in fascial work that requires no lubrication.) Wax suits us much better as only a small amount is needed to provide the slight glide that is essential for good soft tissue work. Wax also helps reduce the habit of slathering too much oil on the body – as Tom Myers, author of *Anatomy Trains*, says 'Easy on the oil – they're a client not a salad.' **See Figure 2.5**

The massage therapist's forgotten art: draping and bolstering

Draping your client so they feel safe psychologically and physically is a very important part of professional massage therapy and should not be overlooked. Good draping not only helps your client feel appropriately protected but is also a mindful and meditative act on the part of the practitioner – and the equivalent of massage feng shui. Here are a number of top tips to help you drape without fumbling and fussing.

Prone draping

- **Diamond draping for the gluteals**: to expose the gluteal muscles safely, while the client is in a prone position, we recommend placing a stone on the sacrum and folding the large towel over the top. The stone is not compulsory but adds a bit of extra weight to the drape to keep it in place.

- Take the edge of the drape and, with a diagonal fold, tuck it securely under the thigh to expose the client's muscles fully whilst still protecting their gluteal cleft. **See Figure 2.6A,B**

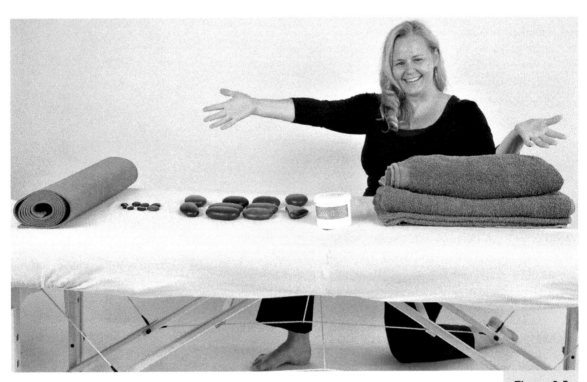

Figure 2.5

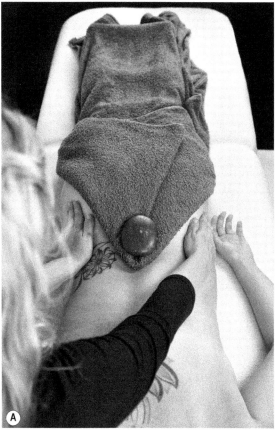
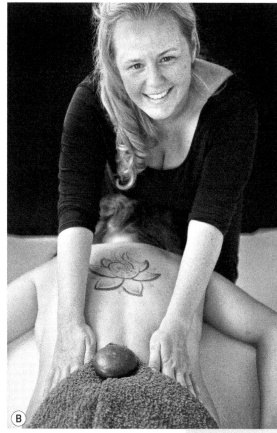

Figure 2.6A,B

- **Draping the legs**: take the bottom corner of the drape and use a long diagonal fold from the client's hip, tucking firmly above their same-side knee. Avoid tucking underneath their opposite leg as this creates a bit of a wind tunnel–which is not so comfortable for your client. **See Figure 2.7, p. 14**

Side-lying draping

- **T draping**: have one towel lengthways along the whole length of the client's body, then place another horizontally on their torso.

- To turn the client from a prone to a side-lying position, hold both towels down on your side and get the client to turn towards you. **See Figure 2.8, p. 14**

- With the client's bottom leg straight and their top leg bent, bolster under the client's head and their top knee to ensure hips and spine are in line. You can also position the client with both knees bent and a bolster between them for comfort.

- Rest the client's upper arm on top of the drape and then fold the top towel over this arm to reveal their back. **See Figure 2.9, p. 14**

Supine draping

- To turn the client from a side-lying to a supine position, stand in front of the client, hold the towel and ask them to turn away from you onto their back.

- **Breast draping**: have one long towel placed from chest to toes on your client. To expose the

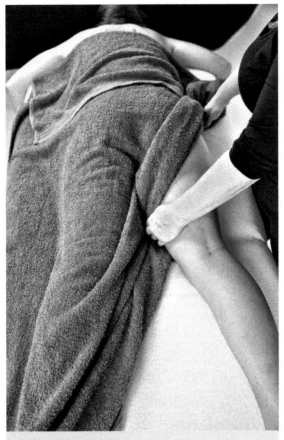

Figure 2.7
Draping the legs

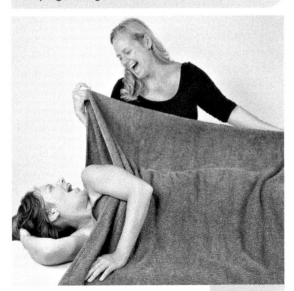

Figure 2.8

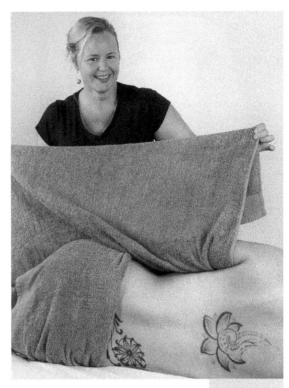

Figure 2.9

abdomen, use another large towel folded in half or thirds lengthwise. Lie this towel in a T shape so that it covers the breasts.

- Hold the top towel with one hand then pull the bottom towel out from underneath to expose the client's belly. Fold the top towel over. **See Figure 2.10**

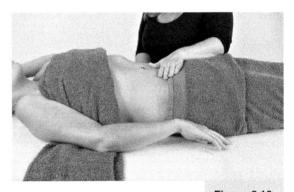

Figure 2.10

T'ai chi for the therapist: beautiful body mechanics

The energy is rooted in the feet, developed in the legs, directed by the waist and expressed through the fingers.
T'AI CHI CLASSICS

Employing good body mechanics while you work not only helps you to avoid injury but also enables you to use a more sensitive and powerful touch. The equivalent of a secret handshake, we like to joke that good body-workers are able to spot each other across a crowded room by the grace, composure and sense of focus of their body mechanics. A good massage therapist moves with ease and fluidity, avoiding techniques that place strain on hands, wrists, neck and back. In this way massage becomes a dance and moving meditation, following the principles of t'ai chi, using breath and energy and from a firm rooted foundation.

Good body mechanics relies on several basic principles:

- **Power of grounding**: as expressed in the quote above, t'ai chi masters understand that power, strength and grace come ultimately from the connection with the earth. Before you start working, take time to establish a strong energetic connection with the ground through your feet, legs and belly (known as the Hara or Tan Tien in the East). In Traditional Chinese medicine the Hara is the 'centre of being' and martial arts emphasise moving from this place to achieve graceful power and strength.

  A good visual to help establish a strong connection with the ground is to imagine roots extending from the soles of your feet and penetrating all the way down into the centre of the earth. On the in breath imagine you are drawing up light, warmth and energy into your belly. On the out breath imagine that energy is shooting up your spine, down your arms and out of your hands. This is a great visualisation to help you work deeper without working harder and encourages you to operate from your legs and belly rather than the upper body and arms. In this way you are able to give a deeper and more sensitive massage without

strain. It does, however, mean that you will develop muscular horse-riding thighs from doing massage rather than buff Madonna arms.

- **Use of the Hara**: a good principle of body mechanics is to ensure that your Hara points in the direction you are working. Imagine your Hara as a strong light attached to your belly which functions to illuminate your workspace. This helps you to avoid twisting your body into uncomfortable positions while massaging.

- **Use your body weight, not muscular strength, to work deeper**. If your table is at the correct height you should be able to lean into the body to achieve depth rather than pressing and straining with the hands and arms. As Ida Rolf, founder of the deep fascial technique known as Structural Integration, said 'Strength that has effort in it is not what you need; you need the strength that is the result of ease' (Rolfresearchfoundation.org 2014).

- **If your client needs deeper work, avoid the temptation to strain and instead bring yourself back to your breath and Hara**. Soften your body, shoulders and arms, breathe out and imagine the breath flowing down your arms as you lean into your client's body to achieve depth. This approach also keeps your body in a sate of receptivity where you can sense changes in the tissues. Tight muscles and locked arms reduce our ability to actually feel.

- **Keep your joints stacked but soft**. Avoid techniques that place your hands or wrists in ulnar or radial deviation or cause the elbows to bend excessively. The wrists should be in line with the elbows and the elbows in line with the shoulders. However, at the same time, ensure your joints are not locked but have a slight softness within them. **See Figure 2.11**

- **Feet, breath, belly**: when we work it is easy to get completely caught up in the task at hand, both psychologically and physically. This can lead to us working harder or faster than we need to and reduces our capacity for listening to the body and using the principle of less is more. Using your own breath as an anchor is a good way to avoid this. Always find the quiet part within yourself by re-connecting with the breath flowing in and out

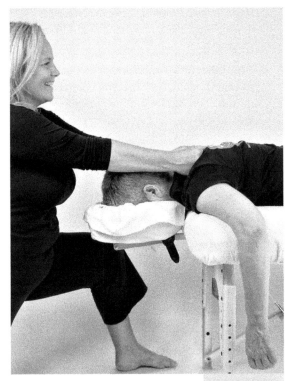

Figure 2.11

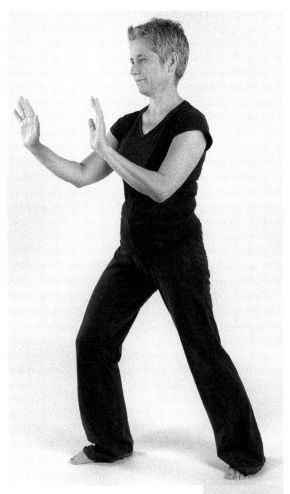

Figure 2.12

of your belly and by noticing the sensation of your feet against the floor. Keep checking back into your own body and noticing how you feel. A good mantra while you work is 'feet, breath, belly'. This really helps you to remain grounded at all times.

- **Keep your chest and heart area open** and avoid the temptation to hunch over or stare at your client's body. The massage therapist's quest for X-ray eyes doesn't help, honest!

- **Use of massage stances:** never bend your back to carry out a move. Use one of the four stances outlined below that will enable you to keep a natural and graceful alignment at all times.

Mighty massage stances

While working, your body should mainly be in one of the four stances below. Remember, massage is a dynamic dance and you may flow seamlessly from one stance to the other depending on what is best for your body at any one time.

- **Forward t'ai chi stance:** stand with your feet hip width apart and slide your right leg forward a step. If you drew an imaginary box on the floor, your right leg would now be on the upper right corner and your left leg on the lower left corner. Make sure there is width to the imaginary box. **See Figure 2.12**

As you exhale, lean forward with the centre of power coming from your hips and belly. Bring your hands into the move as if you are carrying out an effleurage stroke from the head of the table. Breathe in as you bring your pelvis back to centre. In this way you can transfer weight between the front and the back leg to give power. The torso can stay reasonably upright between the forwards and the backwards move, which enables you to give power without hurting or bending your back.

- **Horse stance**: have your feet and legs wider than hip width apart and go down into a slight squat keeping the torso reasonably straight. Make sure your knees roll outwards (laterally) rather than inwards (medially) to prevent strain. Transferring weight in a flowing fashion between your legs enables you to work the full length of the body, e.g. when doing forearm work or when gaining power doing 'pulling up' type strokes. Again the power and direction of movement comes from your pelvis and Hara. **See Figure 2.13**

- **Kneeling t'ai chi stance (proposal stance)**: this can be used to maintain good body mechanics when you need to be at a lower level than standing would allow. The stance looks like you are about to do an old fashioned proposal: one knee is on the floor with the other leg up as if you are about to go into a kneeling lunge. Use a small bolster under the knee if you find this uncomfortable. This is a great stance to avoid bending over, e.g. working on the arms while the client is in a prone position, or the feet or neck while they are in a supine position. **See Figure 2.14**

- **Seated**: a seated position is excellent for some strokes and especially neck, head or detailed work on the feet. Have your legs wide apart (on most tables you can get your legs just either side of the table legs) and both feet firmly connected to the ground. Make sure

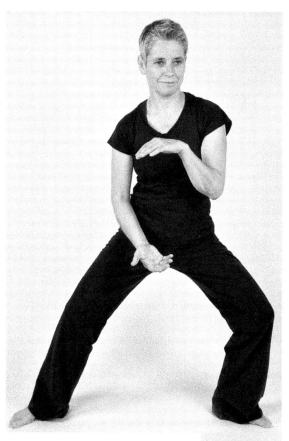

Figure 2.13

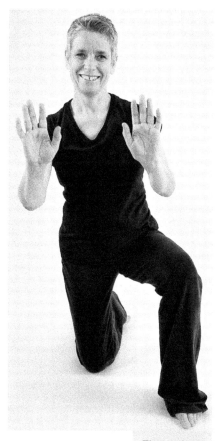

Figure 2.14

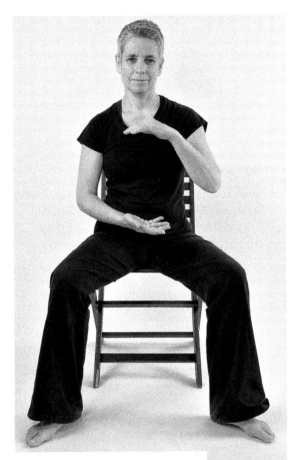

Figure 2.15

We all have two hands, but who among us really knows how to use them? No one argues with the wine taster who, by using their palate, can tell us the characteristics of the wine – its region, its vineyard or even its vintage. The education of touch can go at least as far.
BARRAL AND MERCIER 2005

Presence is more important than technique. Beginners want to learn more and more techniques. When you achieve mastery, one technique will do. It is amazing how much how little will do. Approach touching the client with the utmost respect for her sanctity – that is with reverence. This form of touch allows for transformational change to occur at a level of being that might take years to reach in non-touching therapies.
MILNE 1998

Truth is found in the depths of our listening. Find the stillness that takes you beyond the form. It is from an intrinsic stillness, that is both still and yet dynamic, that this truth is found. The Breath of Life arises from stillness and returns to that stillness. In Taoism, the Tao is neutral and still. Yet within it are images, the blueprint of eternity. From it all motion arises and to it all returns. It is a dynamic process of generation and creation. It is always in present time. Past and future are holographically enfolded within the present. Healing occurs in this eternal present.
SILLS 1997

your own spine is not slumped. The feet stay grounded while the torso can move with the hands and arms flexibly as required so that you can get your whole body into the work.
See Figure 2.15

Transformative touch: the art of listening touch

At Jing we firmly believe that technique alone is not enough to obtain good results with clients. A more important element is the art of touch, the ability to

There are no limits to sensitivity.
J-P BARRAL, OSTEOPATH AND FOUNDER OF VISCERAL MANIPULATION

literally develop 'fingers with brain cells in their tips, fingers capable of feeling, thinking, seeing' (Sutherland 1914). The key to true transformation lies not in learning technique but in our ability to connect with the client, really listen to the tissues and be directed by the body, rather than our intellect. This skill is beyond science, beyond textbooks. This is the quintessential art of bodywork, the sweet place where we are able to let go of our ego, our fear of not knowing, and enter a place where we can just simply be. The place where there is just you, your hands, the body, the breath, the interface. In that state lies the key to genuine change.

When we truly connect with the client's body though focused touch in this way we have the ability to enter a state that the psychologist Mihály Csíkszentmihályi (1990) calls 'flow'. Csíkszentmihályi describes flow as:

> . . . being completely involved in an activity for its own sake. The ego falls away. Time flies. Every action, movement, and thought follows inevitably from the previous one, like playing jazz. Your whole being is involved, and you're using your skills to the utmost.
>
> ARCHIVE.WIRED.COM 2014

It is likely that if you have been doing bodywork for any length of time you will have experienced this state. When you are in flow during a treatment, you come to the end of the session and it feels as if you have been there for 5 minutes or sometimes 5 hours or as if you have been in another dimension entirely. You stopped worrying about what you should do next because you just knew. Your 'monkey brain' shut up for a while. There was only you and the connection with the body.

This is the place where you know deep in your core that you chose the right career. This is the place where you realise bodywork is just about tuning in and listening to the body – it doesn't actually matter which 'technique' your hands are doing. Your hands just know. 'When you achieve mastery, one technique will do.'

This state of flow is the place where small and large miracles happen. There was a 1960s counterculture slogan that proclaimed 'tune in, turn on, drop out' – we could adapt this as a bodywork mantra for mindfulness:

- 'Tune in' to the tissues.
- 'Turn on' your healing powers.
- 'Drop out' of everyday reality.

Tips for developing a listening touch

You should constantly be working on developing your sense of touch. This will enable you to feel not only physical restrictions, such as tight muscles and trigger points, but also more subtle energies, such as the flow of qi in the meridians or the cranial rhythm.

Here are a few tips for developing your listening touch:

- **Good body mechanics**: this lies at the heart of everything we do including developing good listening touch. You need to be fully grounded and comfortable in your body to be able to develop the necessary sensitivity in your hands. Make sure you are always in one of the recommended stances (listed earlier) while working.

- **Keep your hands, arms and shoulders soft**: develop the habit of checking into your body especially your shoulders, arms and hands to make sure you are not holding them in a state of tension. Tense muscles affect your ability to really feel; your body should be relaxed but not floppy.

- **Focus**: you need to develop a relaxed curiosity about the body so that your attention is totally focussed on what is going on in the tissues. If your mind is somewhere else (such as when your next client is arriving, how uncomfortable your body is, what you need to do later that evening or even what technique you should be executing next) you are losing a unique opportunity to truly listen to your client's mind–body. Clear your mind as much as possible; good massage is based on principles of mindfulness, of truly being in the present moment. We know this is a difficult skill to develop, just keep bringing your mind back to the body and your hands when you feel it has wandered.

- **Stay grounded**: really make sure you are connected to the earth through your feet at all times.

- **Slow down!** Most massage therapists are working far too fast. When you go slowly you can feel more and give the client a much more relaxing experience. Relaxation is an extremely important part of the process of reducing chronic pain, so never underestimate the power of slowing down your work. Always think to yourself: 'how slow can I go!'

- **Less is more**: when touching the body, avoid the temptation to push, prod, poke and generally engage in a lot of busy work. Instead carry an inner sense of stillness, even when you are doing strokes that require movement. When palpating have a sense of letting the structures come to you rather than straining to find them. Do fewer techniques with more focus to achieve the best results.

- **Still work**: don't be afraid to be still during treatment. Find places on the body where you can just connect with your hands and simply 'be' rather than 'do'.

- **Practice, practice, practice**: developing this ability to connect and really listen to the story of the tissues doesn't come overnight. As Michelangelo famously said 'If people knew how hard I worked to get my mastery it wouldn't seem so wonderful after all.' Developing your listening touch takes practice. For a massage therapist, practice amounts to time spent with your hands on bodies. The more bodies you tune into with focus, mindfulness and reverence, the better results you will get. There are no shortcuts. There are no tricks. There is no such thing as innate genius. No one is special and no one develops these skills without putting in the time.

Never lose an opportunity to touch with focus and intent. Every time you put your hands on someone (or something) with focus and intent you can develop that skill. Tune into your hands whenever you are touching and practise really sensing everyday objects and different textures. Practise palpating structures on yourself, touch the family pets with focussed intent and always be fully present with your clients. In this way you will gradually develop the sensitivity needed to feel increasingly subtle changes in the tissues.

To treat or not to treat that is the question: massage contraindications explored

The subject of contraindications is a tricky one for most massage therapists. When should we treat? When should we leave well alone? Is it possible to actually seriously harm someone through massage? Although the subject of contraindications is an integral part of massage therapy training, many massage therapists still end up with a lack of clarity and a great deal of fear around the subject of safe treatment. Although it is outside the scope of this text to cover the common contraindications and red flags taught on qualifying courses, it is worth examining the topic to bust some myths and encourage critical thinking.

Contrary contraindications

Most of us want a simple answer to a simple question in this world and certainties make us feel safe. This is the thinking behind giving practitioners lists of conditions with guidelines for how safe, or not, it may be to treat with massage. Simple, right? Massage therapists learn the list of contraindications, educate themselves, and make sure clients are protected by never giving massage for any condition that might be contraindicated. Professional associations and insurance companies feel safe because we have a list. You know how paperwork protects us. Doesn't it? Unfortunately not.

The matter is way more complex than this and here's why:

- Many of the contraindications we learn as massage therapists were developed for Swedish massage only. What about those of us who are skilled in many different massage modalities as advocated in this book? For example, trigger point therapy, myofascial release, stretching or meridian based systems such as Thai massage or Amma. These modalities have very different or, in some cases, no taught contraindications. The long list of contraindications developed for Swedish massage is often generalised for these massage techniques, but with no rationale as these techniques work on very different physiological principles from Swedish massage.

- As teachers of advanced techniques we come into contact with students from many different qualifying courses and schools. Personal experience suggests that students are taught widely varying lists of contraindications and there is no reliable consistency among them.

- A study comparing the relevant available literature on massage contraindications in textbooks and journal articles showed that there was a wide variation in the information given. One physical therapy source listed three contraindications for therapeutic massage whereas another listed as many as 86! (Batavia 2004).

- The same study also showed that there was no research evidence supporting many of the recommendations. The views on what was or was not a contraindication was based more on opinion, conjecture and theory than actual hard data.

- Many commonly taught contraindications have not moved with the times and the research. It is frequently propounded in medical literature that it can take a staggering 17 years for research evidence to filter down to clinical practice and it seems that this is no exception in massage therapy (Morris et al 2011). For example, some recommended contraindications suggest scars should not be massaged for up to 2 years. Even surgeons recognise the importance of massage in producing functional scars and self-massage is routinely recommended to improve the appearance of scars post-surgery. Similarly, I have seen recommendations not to massage tendonitis 'in the inflammatory stage'. Although tendonitis is still a very common diagnosis, research increasingly documents that what is thought to be tendonitis is usually tendinosis (Bass 2012). Tendinosis is the result of breakdown of the collagen fibres and no inflammation is involved. The fundamental assumption about why tendonitis should not be massaged in the early stages is incorrect, yet this information is still being routinely taught. And of course the biggest massage contraindication myth is the blanket recommendation to stay away from treating anyone with cancer. This misconception was based on a crude understanding of how cancer might spread and has no basis in fact (Walton 2011).

- Lists of contraindications also routinely neglect any recommendations around psychological conditions. I have NEVER seen any advice around concerns for the client of massaging someone with a background of known severe trauma, sexual or physical abuse or a diagnosis of severe mental health problems such as schizophrenia. In my experience massage

therapists are routinely likely to encounter such issues, yet are left without any relevant support on how to work safely with such clients.

- Contraindication lists often abdicate responsibility to a medical practitioner for deciding whether a patient should receive massage or not. Although it is vitally important to establish good communication with medical professionals, in my experience it is rare for busy GPs to have the time or interest to keep up with the latest research around manual therapy and what may or may not be useful for the patient. This is simply not their area of expertise as confirmed by several GPs who are my clients. It is up to us to become experts and have mature discussions with medical professionals about what is best for the patient based on the latest informed evidence.

- The blanket contraindication list 'don't touch X' rarely reflects clinical reality. Both massage therapists and clients are unique. Client X with a cancer diagnosis may be perfectly safe to massage whereas, because of various medical complications, client Y is not.

Examples of commonly taught contraindications that may need a makeover
Cancer

Twenty years ago we were all taught that we should never massage someone with cancer. This advice is totally out-dated and there is a great deal of excellent work being done with massage and cancer. Yes, you should educate yourself about the whys and wherefores. Yes, you should liaise with the medical team. But yes, you can treat.

Osteoporosis

Much of the advice around osteoporosis is woefully inadequate and assumes the client may fracture into a million pieces if you so much as look at them. Of course we need to exercise care with pressure when working with clients with known osteoporosis but this will vary from client to client and with the degree of progression of the condition. Educating yourself about the condition and your client's own suscep-tibility to fracture makes more sense than blanket recommendations of not treating. Many clients with osteoporosis are leading normal, energetic, exercise-filled lives and subjecting them to a feather-light massage or refusing to touch them could be denying them a valuable service.

Herniated disc

Massage therapists are often advised not to touch clients with a herniated disc in the acute stage. Again there is no evidence basis for this, especially in the light of research showing there is little relationship between the amount or size of herniation and the pain (this is explored fully in Chapter 4). An appropriately informed and educated massage therapist can provide a client with much needed pain relief in the early stages of a herniated disc. Positioning, client communication and your own education about the condition are key factors but there seems no viable reason to not treat.

Pregnancy

It is still commonly taught that massage should be avoided in the first trimester although pregnancy massage experts agree there is no basis for this (Stillerman 2006). The recommendation sprang from the heightened risk of miscarriage in the first 3 months and the fear that the massage therapist will be held responsible. Many spas still routinely refuse to treat women in their first trimester due to liability issues. Understanding that this 'contraindication' is based on fear of litigation rather than science can help your client make an informed choice about whether massage is for them. Pregnant women should not be refused valuable treatment because of a myth.

Scars

As mentioned above, massage therapists are often advised to avoid scars for months or in some cases years after they have healed. Yet even the medical profession are recommending that patients self-massage scars to improve the appearance and reduce the possibility of adhesions that can lead to ongoing problems. Recent research has shown fascial work to be key in improving the appearance and functionality of scars. Waiting too long before receiving appropriate manual therapy work can lead to even more problems for the client.

Towards a more logical approach: contraindications and critical thinking

So if we can't always rely on our lists of contraindications given in the classroom how on earth do we keep our clients safe and ensure we are 'doing no harm'.

The answer lies in our own education as massage therapists. Most massage therapists are ill-informed about different pathologies, particularly in the UK where the qualifying levels are low. Keeping up with current research and really understanding the physiological basis of common conditions can help us make informed decisions about treatment. Swedish massage is only one tool in the box and there are usually many other massage techniques that can be appropriately used, e.g. Swedish massage is often contraindicated for clients with cardiovascular problems as it aims to boost circulation. However, there is no reason why meridian or certain fascia-based techniques shouldn't be used in these cases.

Deciding whether or how to treat is more a process of informed critical thinking than relying on a blanket list of contraindications. As Tracey Walton (2011) advocates with her eminently sensible decision tree approach to working with complex client conditions, the informed massage therapists should ask themselves two simple questions:

1 What is it about the medical condition that contraindicates massage?

2 What is it about massage that is contraindicated?

Both of these questions must be explored and answering them will enable you to draw up a safe treatment plan for your client. In many cases, several factors, such as pressure, technique, positioning, or avoiding local areas, can be modified to allow you to treat safely, even if someone is on the dreaded contraindication list.

So don't throw away your contraindication list. But make sure you understand why the conditions on it are contraindicated. If they are only contraindicated for Swedish massage or have no basis in current research then you can make informed decisions accordingly. Go on courses, surf the Web and talk to other informed medical providers. This will keep you and your client MUCH safer than the list!

References

Archive.wired.com 2014 Wired 4.09: Go with the flow. Available at: http://archive.wired.com/wired/archive/4.09/czik.html [accessed 17 August 2014].

Barral J, Mercier P 2005 Visceral Manipulation, 1st edn. Seattle: Eastland Press.

Bass E 2012 Tendinopathy: why the difference between tendinitis and tendinosis matters. International Journal of Therapeutic Massage & Bodywork 5(1):14–17.

Batavia M 2004 Contraindications for therapeutic massage: do sources agree? Journal of Bodywork and Movement Therapies 8(1):48–57.

Csíkszentmihályi M 1990 Flow, 1st edn. New York: Harper & Row.

Milne H 1998 The Heart of Listening, 1st edn. Berkeley, CA: North Atlantic Books.

Morris ZS, Wooding S, Grant J 2011 The answer is 17 years, what is the question: understanding time lags in translational research. Journal of the Royal Society of Medicine 104(12):510–520.

Rolfresearchfoundation.org 2014 About Ida P. Rolf PhD. Boulder, CO: Ida P. Rolf Research Foundation. Available at: http://rolfresearchfoundation.org/about [accessed 17 August 2014].

Sills F 1997 The fulcrum. The Journal of the Craniosacral Therapy Association of the UK. Available at: http://www.craniosacral.co.uk/articles/art4.htm [accessed 17 August 2014].

Stillerman E 2006 Prenatal massage during the first trimester. Massage Today. Available at: http://www.massagetoday.com/mpacms/mt/article.php?id=13354 [accessed 17 August 2014].

Sutherland WG 1914 'Let's be up and touching'. The Osteopathic Physician.

Walton T 2011 Medical Conditions and Massage Therapy, 1st edn. Philadelphia: Wolters Kluwer/Lippincott Williams & Wilkins Health.

Working with emotions in bodywork

Emotional pain: Is it your business?

Massage has a long tradition of working not just with the body but the mind and emotions. The two are inseparable and, as we shall see in the next chapter, chronic physical problems often go hand in hand with emotional pain and stress. So every time you touch your client you are making an intervention not only with muscles, fascia and joints, but also with the delicate mind–body balance of the spirit and psyche.

Feeling comfortable with the emotional side of bodywork is important as there is also a strong probability that a significant proportion of your clients have experienced severe trauma during their lifetime – and many of them won't tell you about it. There are a disturbing number of adults who have experienced the horrors of sexual and physical abuse or domestic violence. The statistics speak for themselves:

- Nearly a quarter of young adults have experienced sexual abuse during childhood.

- Many young adults (1 in 9) have experienced severe physical violence during childhood at the hands of an adult (Radford et al 2011).

- Many women (1 in 4) experience domestic violence over their lifetime and between 6% and 10% of women suffer domestic violence in a given year (Council of Europe 2002).

This is only the tip of the iceberg for distressing incidents that can affect physical and emotional health. Add to the litany the ongoing trauma of living with an alcoholic partner, the parent with mental health problems, the chronic illness of relatives, the grief of bereavement, and the nightmare of life threatening accidents. The hard fact is that the anguish of severe trauma is omnipresent. Understanding how this might affect our clients is vitally important to massage therapists everywhere.

Many of the conditions that we treat the in clinic are clearly inextricably linked with the effects of stress and trauma in the body. There is extensive literature documenting how chronic pain is linked to a range of traumatic experiences, including child and adult abuse, abuse-related injury, violence from a partner and post-traumatic stress disorder (PTSD) (Wuest et al 2010). Whether you realise it or not, emotional pain is your business. Literally.

Fight, flight and freeze

Both ancient and modern wisdom unite in the assertion that trauma can affect both physical and mental health. The ancient healing practices have recognised the mind and body as indivisible for centuries, i.e. trauma affects the balance of our energetic life field that in turn affects our physical and mental wellbeing.

Long before Western psychology and the fields of psychoneuroimmunology caught on, most ancient systems of healing were clear about the role of stress and imbalance as a fundamental factor in pain and disease. Traditional Chinese medicine views imbalance as a primary causal factor in disease, identifying a particular emotion with each organ: joy for the heart, anger for the liver, worry for the spleen, sadness for the lung, and fear for the kidney. Excess or insufficiency in emotions can cause imbalance and therefore ill health and pain. Likewise, the shamanic approach sees all sickness to be self generated as an effect of stress. The source of stress is seen as resistance – as our desire for things to be different than they are.

More recently, bodyworkers interested in the somatic understanding of trauma are indebted to the work of Peter Levine and his theory of how extreme distress may become encoded in the body (Levine 1997). Just like animals, our reptilian brain (brain stem) still responds to perceived life threatening situations by producing adrenalin so that our body is in flight or flight mode. However, as humans, often our rational brain prevents us from taking action as we are unable to decide between these two choices. This can lead to a third response – the freeze response – also seen in animals when fight or flight is not possible **(Figure 3.1)**. The animal literally 'plays dead', decreasing metabolic activity and collapsing into immobility. Like having your foot on the accelerator and the brake pedal at the same time, the animal appears lifeless yet there is an inner racing of the nervous system. Do any of the fight, flight or freeze reactions seem familiar? Years ago I was mugged in central London and remember literally feeling rooted to the ground with fear, like everything inside me had frozen. Not quite as brave as a friend of mine who, in a similar situation, chased her attackers down an alleyway and beat them with her handbag! In many cases of trauma, the freeze reaction may be the only viable option. Children who are sexually or physically abused by carers have no choice but to remain in the situation, shutting down their emotions and natural reactions. Fleeing or fighting is impossible.

Creatures who have adopted the freeze response will literally shake off the energy following the freezing period and then go happily about their business with apparently no ill effects. However, for a number of reasons humans have lost the instinctual ability to discharge this residual energy leading to a wide variety of symptoms following trauma, e.g. anxiety and depression. In extreme cases the ensuing psychological responses to trauma can also cause neuropathic, endocrine and immune system changes that lead to an increased risk of chronic pain problems. Studies have shown that individuals with PTSD have excess inflammatory immune activity similar to that associated with chronic pain (Gill et al 2009).

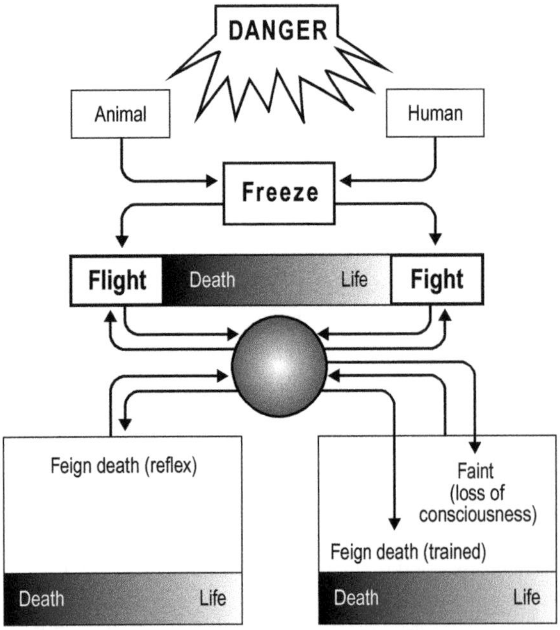

Following trauma, as the system is now stuck in hyper-arousal, any situation that in any way looks or feels like the original trauma will lead to the client re-experiencing symptoms. This is a vital understanding as there is a high possibility that bodywork can recreate the effects of the traumatic situation unless we understand the fundamentals of how to create a safe space for our clients. As you are unlikely to always know which of your clients have experienced sexual or physical abuse, it is vital that this is part of good practice for ALL clients.

Creating a safe space for all clients: 'first do no harm'

Given the strong link between trauma and chronic pain, what do we need to know to help us treat effectively? It is not uncommon for powerful bodywork to evoke emotional release or memories of a previous trauma. This process can either be helpful or harmful depending on your knowledge and confidence in dealing with the situation.

The first rule of good bodywork is to create a psychologically safe space for your clients. This is well known in talk therapies but is often overlooked in bodywork. A safe space involves factors such as:

- **Good communication**: adopt an open listening style when taking a case history; be non-judgemental, maintain good eye contact and ask questions that enable your client to give answers in their own words. As outlined in Chapter 4, be comfortable with asking about stress and emotional factors in addition to physical issues – as this can help to give you an all round picture of the person you are dealing with.

Figure 3.1
The freeze response is seen in both animals and humans when fight or flight is not possible

- **Letting the client know they are in control**: clients who have been physically or sexually abused have had their boundaries completely violated. Their bodies will be hypersensitive to any perceived re-creation of this. They need to know that you are trustworthy and that you will do what you say. Explain exactly what is going to happen in the session, how they should position themselves and how they will be draped. Ensure a safe space emotionally and physically by letting the client know that everything that happens during treatment is confidential. Let them know they are in control and if anything doesn't feel right in any way you will back off and change what you are doing. Remind them that pain does not lead to gain during therapeutic massage and to let you know if you are doing anything that is making them grit their teeth or clench their fists.

- **Explain what will happen at the end of the session**: this prevents your client from feeling anxious about what they should do. For example, say something such as:

At the end of the session, I will leave the room and let you get dressed in your own time. When you are ready, just wait in the chair and I'll come back after a few minutes. It is really great for me to get feedback on how you found the session as that will help us in future sessions to design a treatment plan that is most appropriate for you.

- **Professional draping**: draping is there for a reason. It lets the client know where they will be touched and which areas are private. NEVER work under a drape unless you have a really good reason and have explained to your client why you are doing this and gained their permission. Keep your draping clear and tight and remain mindful of any potential exposure during the session.

- **NO means NO**: always respect your client if they ask you to stop or not to work an area. This may seem obvious but I have seen excellent and well-meaning bodyworkers overrule something a client has said because 'your body needs it'. This is the quickest route to re-traumatising a client

or allegations of misconduct. If you feel an area needs work but your client has asked you not to, you will need to gain trust over several sessions, months or years and work towards this with full permission.

- **As part of the feedback, ask them if anything didn't feel OK** (emotionally or physically) and respect that in the next session.

- **Maintain good boundaries**: you are a massage therapist. Do not slip into the role of counsellor, friend or spiritual guru for any client. Be clear about who you are and what you provide. Be precise about your timing and do not give extra time for sessions unless this has been asked for and paid appropriately. All of this helps your clients to feel safe and that you are trustworthy, i.e. you will do what you say and say what you do.

Dealing with emotional release or re-traumatisation during a session

It is extremely important to be able to recognise the signs of re-traumatisation during a session as this can be damaging and distressing to the client. There is a distinct difference between someone having a healthy and manageable emotional release on the table and the client who is becoming re-traumatised. Red flags to watch out for which mean that you need to intervene are:

- Rapid body movements that are becoming uncontrollable.

- Feeling uneasy in your own body.

- A feeling that the client 'isn't there'.

- Client refusing to engage with you verbally: not answering questions or staring blankly.

- Uncontrollable crying, shaking or laughing.

- Sudden change in breathing pattern.

- Client putting their hands over their eyes or refusing to look at you.

In these cases it is vital that you re-orientate your client back to reality and the here and now as it is very easy to disappear into a literal black hole of trauma where they are unable to think, feel or react to you clearly.

Use the following steps as a guide to deal with the situation:

- Ground yourself: take a deep breath, feel your feet against the ground and breathe out any anxiety or helplessness you are feeling.

- Orientate your client to the here and now by directing them to current sensory experiences. A good start is to ask the client to wiggle their toes and nose. Then ask them to open their eyes and look at something neutral. Ask them to describe the colour of the ceiling tiles or count how many there are or something similar.

- If your client is not doing as you ask you will need to keep asking and be very firm until you get an appropriate response. This point cannot be overemphasised, e.g. if your client is covering their eyes, refusing to answer or staring blankly, they could be in a dissociated state. Keep gently but firmly repeating what you need the client to do in a neutral and safe tone of voice, e.g. 'Everything's fine. You are here with me in the clinic and you are safe. I just need you to wiggle your toes for me so I know you are with me.'

- Do not get involved in conversation about recounting the traumatic event. Your job is to bring the client back to the here and now.

- If your client is crying or upset do not ask them 'what's wrong?' Just maintain a grounded, comforting presence and say something like 'It's fine to feel what you are feeling. Just be aware of the feeling of your body against the couch at the same time.' In this way the trauma does not become overwhelming.

- When your client is clearly back in the here and now you can discuss whether it is appropriate to continue the session or not. If you decide to continue the session, make sure your client stays in a position where they are able to feel in control of any cathartic energy release, e.g. tell them to feel what they feel but to notice the feeling of their body at the same time.

- At the end of the session discuss ways forward together. Unless you have been appropriately trained in bodywork and trauma you may need to suggest additional support, such as talk therapy or another appropriately trained bodyworker.

Energetic boundaries: protecting yourself as a therapist

Without doubt, a true connection with your client is a key component to the therapeutic relationship. In bodywork, our empathy for the client is expressed largely through our sense of touch when we are working on the body. Just as with talk therapy, our touch, focus and positive therapeutic intent can enable our clients to feel heard and accepted.

Working with presence, sensitivity and listening touch while being really tuned into your client can be profoundly healing but can bring it's own challenges for the therapist. Clinical experience and our teaching careers have shown time and time again that it is common for massage therapists to be influenced by their client's conscious or unconscious emotional state while they are working on the body. Therapists will often describe 'picking up' client issues and this can manifest in dizziness, light-headedness, changes in breathing patterns, distress or sensing the physical or emotional pain that the client is experiencing. This phenomenon is also well documented in psychotherapy and dance therapy where it is known as body-centred countertransference: 'the spontaneous arousal of physical feelings in the therapist' (Field 1989). A large percentage of therapists working with people in trauma have reported physical sensations ranging from yawning, sleepiness, nausea, headaches, becoming tearful, raising of a therapist's voice, unexpectedly shifting of the body, genital pain, muscle tension, losing voice, aches in joints, stomach disturbance, and numbness (Booth et al 2010). Why this happens is unclear. Energy-based explanations centre on the role of auras or electromagnetic fields around the body that can be sensed by the practitioner (Brennan 1987) (**Figure 3.2**). Another more scientific rationale could be the potential involvement of mirror neurones: neurones that fire both when you perform an action and when you see another person doing the same action (**Figure 3.3A,B**). These neurones are believed to be the basis of empathy, e.g. if you see someone crying you feel that distress within yourself (Blakeslee 2006).

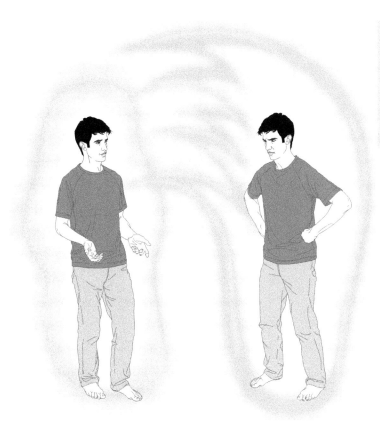

Figure 3.2
Therapists often report 'picking up' emotions and physical sensations from their clients. Energy-based explanations centre on the role of auras or electromagnetic fields around the body that can be sensed by the practitioner

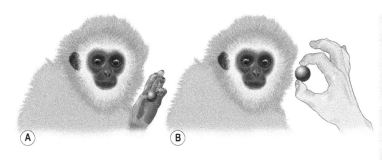

Figure 3.3A,B
A more scientific explanation for transfer of physical and emotional sensations could be the role of mirror neurones. (A) These fire both when you perform an action (i.e. monkey picking up a ball) and (B) when you see another person doing the same action (monkey seeing someone else pick up the ball)

Whatever the mechanism of action, it is important to know how to deal with these feelings when they arise. Some therapists find the sensations overwhelming and treating clients can end up being an emotionally and physically exhausting experience. However, it is important to recognise that these sensations are a way of your client unconsciously communicating with you about their internal state that often cannot be expressed verbally. The following guidelines will help you manage these feelings when you are treating a client:

● Grounding: it is important to be able to distinguish your own energetic field from that of your client and the key to this (as ever) lies in grounding. At the start of a session make sure you are grounded, calm and still. We always recommend starting each session with some still work so that both you and your client can enter a state of mindfulness. If your body feels like a calm still pond then you know that if you start to feel any unusual feelings then these are probably your clients and not your own.

However, if you start the session feeling anxious, irritated, or in a rush then it will be impossible to ascertain which feelings are your own and those which you are picking up from the client.

- If you find yourself experiencing unusual physical sensations (such as anxiety, dizziness and nausea), just visualise breathing the sensations out of your body and back down through your legs to the floor and through your grounding roots to the earth. **See Figure 3.4A,B**

- If you find the sensations overwhelming every time you treat then there are certain visualisations or rituals that can help you feel energetically 'protected', e.g. you can imagine that you are putting on an invisible purple cloak before treatment. Some therapists find that cleansing rituals such as rinsing their hands in cold water or smudging the room with herbs after treatment are helpful.

- Be aware of the energetic interface: the invisible but perceptible boundary where you end and your client begins. You need to be energetically at the point where you are aware of your client but still mindful of your own body. This is a bit like trying to help someone out of a hole in the ground. If you are too close they will pull you in. If you are too far away you won't be able to help them climb out. Bodywork is the same – which is why you should always be aware of your own solid base of support, close enough to connect but not so close you become overwhelmed.

- If you have unresolved issues within yourself it is much more likely that you will feel overwhelmed by similar issues in your clients. Always work on yourself through receiving appropriate therapeutic intervention – this could be through supportive bodywork or talk therapy.

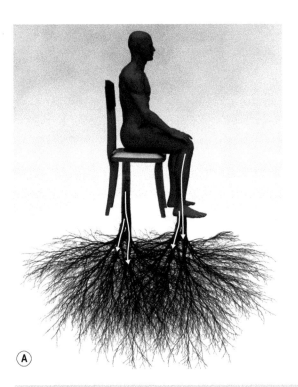

(A)

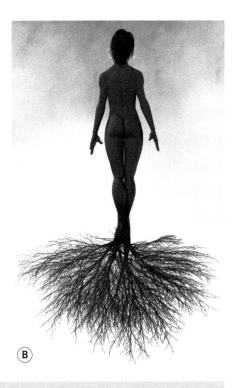

(B)

Figure 3.4A,B
If you experience unusual physical sensations during a treatment visualise breathing the sensations back down through your grounding roots to the floor

References

Blakeslee S 2006 Cells that read minds. New York Times Jan. Available at: http://www.nytimes.com/2006/01/10/science/10mirr.html?pagewanted=all&_r=0 [accessed July 23, 2014].

Booth A, Trimble T, Egan J 2010 Body centred counter-transference in a sample of clinical psychologists. The Irish Psychologist October: 284–289.

Brennan B 1987 Hands of Light. New York City: Bantam Press at Random House.

Council of Europe 2002 Recommendation 2002/5 of the Committee of Ministers to Member States on the Protection of Women Against Violence. Council of Europe, Strasbourg, France.

Field N 1989 Listening with the body: an exploration in the countertransference. British Journal of Psychotherapy 5(4):512–522.

Gill JM et al 2009 PTSD is associated with an excess of inflammatory immune activities. Perspectives in Psychiatric Care 45:262–277.

Levine P 1997 Waking the Tiger, 1st edn. Berkeley, CA: North Atlantic Books.

Radford L et al 2011 Child Abuse and Neglect in the UK Today. London: NSPCC.

Wuest J et al 2010 Pathways of chronic pain in survivors of intimate partner violence. Journal of Women's Health 19(9):1665–1674.

4

Chronic pain: are the issues in the tissues or is the pain in the brain?

One good thing about music, when it hits you, you feel no pain.
Bob Marley

The complex puzzle of pain

Being a massage therapist is not always an easy business. Massage therapists, often more so than any other manual therapy profession, are constantly faced with the issue of chronic pain – that is, pain that persists long beyond the usual healing time for an injury. We are often the last point of call for clients who have run the usual gamut of the medical equivalent of the butcher, the baker and the candlestick maker (GP, MD, physiotherapist, chiropractor and osteopath). These increasingly desperate clients eventually turn to massage, way down the line, often after months or years of dealing with constant daily pain.

Ask any successful massage therapist about the problems that make up their caseload and you are likely to hear the following shopping list of client woes:

- Back pain: including sciatica and ongoing pain from herniated discs.

- Chronic neck and shoulder pain (including whiplash associated disorder (WAD)).

- Repetitive strain injury (RSI) and carpal tunnel syndrome.

- Tennis and golfer's elbow.

- Shoulder girdle problems: frozen shoulder or generalised shoulder pain and restricted range of motion.

- Sporting overuse injuries including Achilles tendinosis and knee complaints.

- Ongoing pain from old injuries that has not resolved after months or years.

- Arthritis: both rheumatoid and osteo.

- Temporomandibular joint (TMJ) or facial pain.

- Headaches and migraines.

- Fibromyalgia, irritable bowel syndrome (IBS) and chronic fatigue syndrome.

- Mysterious pain that is persistent and debilitating but has no diagnosis despite extensive medical tests.

- Mysterious pain that has a diagnosis of an extremely long polysyllabic name that you have to look up on Google (my students love to ask me about their client with blah de blah de blah-itis).

Maybe some lucky massage therapist somewhere has a practice consisting entirely of psychologically stable and physically fit 25 year olds whose back 'hurts a bit after I did a lot of gardening yesterday', but they are certainly not the norm! The hard truth is that if you want to be good at your profession you need to become an expert in treating chronic pain. The public certainly seems to be voting with their feet in that respect and are increasingly seeking our services for pain relief. A survey by the American Massage Therapy Association (AMTA) found that, in 2013, 43% of individuals sought massage for medical reasons with 88% believing that massage can be effective in reducing pain and 24% who had actually used massage for pain relief (Amtamassage.org 2014). Surveys estimate that as much as one-third of the population of the USA are experiencing chronic pain (Johannes et al 2010). Meanwhile over the pond, a staggering 45% of the UK population is suffering from musculoskeletal pain (Carnes et al 2007). That's an awful lot of Brits with bad backs!

So if you haven't yet got a thriving business, being able to provide therapeutic outcomes for chronic pain conditions is one of the most consistent ways of building your practice. As most of us are well aware, clients in chronic pain are rarely able to find long-term relief via more orthodox medical routes, leaving them knocking at the door of alternative health care providers. If you gain a reputation for successful treatment of these conditions you will never again be waiting for the phone to ring wondering where the next client is coming from!

The simple truth is that the orthodox medical profession is rarely equipped with the education, skills, tools and, most importantly, TIME to deal effectively with chronic pain problems. Research over the past few decades, plus more recent developments from brain imaging studies, unequivocally points towards the fact that chronic pain is a complex and multi-factorial phenomenon. As we shall see, traditional medical and structural notions that your back hurts because a disc is herniated or a facet joint is awry are being shown to be severely outdated and only a small piece of the puzzle. This leaves traditional orthopaedic surgical approaches and management by medication without a scientific basis. In its absence, the door lies wide open for … us … super educated massage therapists with our intrinsic holistic approach, healing with our 'hands, head and heart' (ta da!).

Clients who don't get better: the issue is not always in the tissues

Consider these two cases who approached the Jing pain clinic several years ago:

Anna, aged 25, developed pain in her right forearm. Working as a marine biologist she was fit and healthy, her job involved a great deal of physical activity and she had no significant emotional stresses. She presented as cheerful and positive about our ability to help her pain.

Martha, aged 60, developed a similar pain in her right forearm. She was tearful and stressed. Her office job was really getting too much and she felt overwhelmed by the day-to-day demands. She would love to retire but was worried about the financial implications. Her arm had been hurting for a few months when she finally came for treatment, having received no answers from her doctor and some exercises from the physiotherapist that 'made it worse'.

Who do you think got better first? Yes of course you're right. Anna was pain free within a miraculous single treatment (wish all our clients were like that!), whereas Martha (treated with the same techniques) was still in pain several sessions later. She subsequently made the decision to retire at which point the pain started to gradually subside.

Herein lies the dilemma of the working massage therapist: the 'issue is not always in the tissues'. What is going on in the tissues (muscle or ligament damage, inflammation, joint degeneration, trigger points and myofascial adhesions) is only ONE factor that leads to the client's experience of pain.

Research over the past few decades has shown that the subjective experience of pain is not just due to tissue damage but is heavily influenced by both psychological and social factors. This approach has come to be known as the biopsychosocial model (a bit of a mouthful, hence commonly abbreviated to BPS) as first proposed by the psychiatrist George Engel (1977, 1980) (**Figure 4.1**). The biopsychosocial model contrasts strongly with the still prevailing biomedical view that sees pain as a result only of biological factors such as disease, abnormalities of structure or tissue damage.

For many of you the biopsychosocial model may not seem like a new concept – as the 'mind–body' paradigm

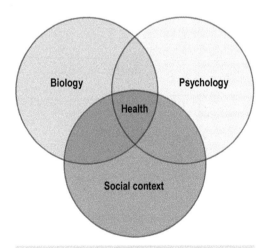

Figure 4.1

The biopsychosocial (BPS) model sees health as a function of biological, psychological and social factors

is firmly part of the belief system of most complementary practitioners. However, recent advances in brain imaging studies have now taken the mind–body model into the realm of science and shown that pain is indeed heavily influenced by our brains. Hence psychosocial factors including beliefs, feelings, emotional state and sense of control over our circumstances have a much larger role than previously believed. The BPS model is now becoming widely accepted in medical and scientific circles as the most relevant model for the treatment of chronic pain (Gatchel et al 2007).

The biopsychosocial model: why feelings really do hurt and why pain is political

Broken down into its component parts the biopsychosocial model postulates that pain is due to the following factors:

- **Biological (the 'bio' bit)**: the biological components of the pain condition include factors such as disease, tissue damage or abnormalities of structure. For example, in musculoskeletal conditions the 'biological' components would be nociceptive inputs such as damaged soft tissues (sprains and strains), degenerative joints (osteoarthritis), disease processes (rheumatoid arthritis) and herniated discs. Our prevailing biomedical model of health usually assigns these components primary importance; however, as we shall see they are only one piece of the jigsaw.

- **Psychological**: psychological and cognitive factors also contribute to the pain experience. These include:

  - **Emotions**: there is a complex and often self-perpetuating relationship between pain and emotion, e.g. depression can lead to episodes of chronic pain and chronic pain can lead to depression (Tunks et al 2008). A systematic review showed that stress, distress and anxiety are significant factors in the development of neck and back pain (Linton 2000), while another study showed a strong correlation between a diagnosis of anxiety and chronic widespread pain (Benjamin et al 2000). It seems that our brains are literally able to turn up or down the volume of our pain

experience depending on how we are feeling. Recent brain imaging studies have shown that when experimental subjects were shown pictures that provoked different emotional states this caused corresponding changes in relevant structures involved in pain processing in the brain (Roy et al 2009).

Have you ever noticed that your more anxious and upset clients are less likely to get better? And that often they have had the same complaint or something similar before? A 12-year survey following low back sufferers found that this is indeed the case. Those likely to be most disabled from low back pain were those in emotional distress with earlier experiences of the problem (Brage et al 2007).

- **Pain related beliefs**: our belief about the pain condition can also have a huge effect. A common belief is known as 'fear avoidance' (**Figure 4.2**). Often individuals in pain become terrified of movement, believing that this will cause more injury and therefore more pain. The reality is, however, that fear avoidance and lack of movement by itself leads to increased pain and disability (Rainville et al 2011). As thoughts themselves are nerve impulses they can be powerful enough to maintain pain states.

- **Catastrophising**: another common psychological feature of chronic pain is 'catastrophising'. This refers to unhelpful thought patterns that basically foresee the worst possible outcome (**Figure 4.3**). You all know this syndrome: 'I've hurt my back … I won't be able to work … I will lose the house … I won't be able to feed the kids and they will all be taken into care … I will end up in a wheelchair like Great Aunt Betty.' A more helpful thought pattern would obviously be 'I've hurt my back; it will get better in a few days; it shouldn't stop me going into work but I'll maybe come home earlier this week and take it easy in the evenings.'

Research has demonstrated a consistent relationship between the tendency to catastrophise and the heightened pain experience. This has been demonstrated to be

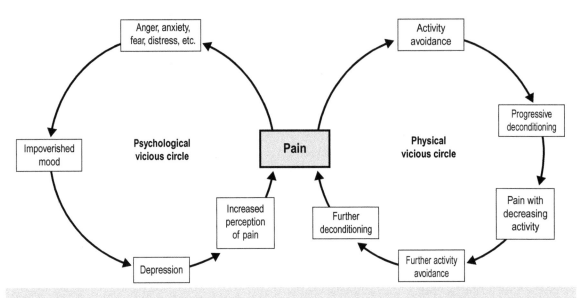

Figure 4.2
The fear avoidance model. Pain leads to fear of movement and decreased activity that in turn leads to more pain

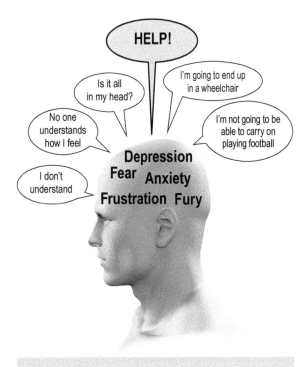

Figure 4.3
A tendency to catastrophise about the pain is correlated with heightened pain experience

the case for many types of common conditions including mixed chronic pain, low back pain, rheumatoid arthritis and whiplash. Furthermore, those with a tendency to high levels of catastrophising thoughts are more likely to become disabled because of their condition, use more health care services, take more medication and stay in hospital longer (Sullivan et al 2001). Talk about thoughts creating reality.

Unfortunately the medical profession sometimes doesn't help with offsetting this tendency to catastrophise. A friend of mine who went to the GP with a simple back pain was referred to the disabled hydrotherapy group! She was convinced she was going to be in pain for the rest of her life whereas in actuality the pain was likely to be a simple soft tissue injury.

- **Social**: sociological factors can also play a part in our experience of pain. Unfairly, pain favours the poor, not to mention other groups who are similarly disadvantaged through social injustice.

The relationship between lower socio-economic status and chronic pain problems is well documented. You are more likely to experience chronic pain if you have lower education, low income and are unemployed (Bonathan et al 2013, King et al 2011, McBeth and Jones 2007). Staggeringly, if you are in the lowest social class you have nearly a three-fold increased risk of chronic widespread pain, such as shoulder, forearm, low back and knee pain (Macfarlane et al 2009). Race can also play a factor as black people experience more chronic pain than white people (Fuentes et al 2007, Green and Hart-Johnson 2012). Women are also more likely to experience chronic pain (Johannes et al 2010). One study of those suffering from long-term whiplash pain discovered that poor recovery was associated with factors such as:

- Being female

- Older age

- Having dependents

- Not having full-time employment (Harder et al 1998, Suissa 2003).

Clearly working with pain conditions is not a straightforward issue. Pain is not just about whether there are injuries or restrictions within the soft tissues and joint structures of the body but is the result of a number of factors including attitudes, beliefs, expectations, context, behaviour, poverty, oppression and social inequity.

It is hard to know where we, as individuals, can be most effective. Should we be working with the tissues, addressing psychological factors or out campaigning against social injustice? Without a doubt, physiology, psychology and politics all intertwine in the individual experience of pain.

Down with Descartes!

The prevailing views about pain, medicine and treatment are still firmly derived from the dualistic thinking of the French philosopher Descartes. Descartes was the first to suggest that the mind and body were distinct and separate entities. He suggested that the body works like a machine while the mind or soul are non-material and do not follow the laws of nature. Our traditional views of pain are heavily influenced by Descartes' theories, e.g. pain is seen as a one-way transmission system from the hurt body part to the brain. **See Figure 4.4**

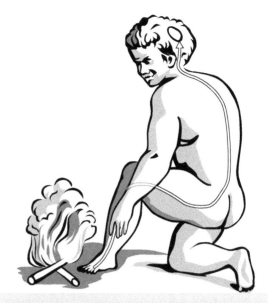

Figure 4.4
French philosopher Descartes saw pain as being primarily 'bottom up' – a one-way transmission system from body to brain

Descartes was clearly a brilliant thinker and his ideas took root at the very heart of Western thinking; this 'Cartesian dualism' eventually gave rise to our practice of different professions with expertise in either body pain or emotional pain. Pain in the heart after bereavement? See a psychologist. Pain in the heart after going for a long run? See a doctor.

This is in sharp contrast to Eastern philosophy and medicine which rejects the idea of dualism and sees mind and body as inseparable. Interestingly as we shall see, modern neuroscience has finally come round to this point of view. Brain imaging research over the past two decades has shown the strong influence of the brain in our experience of pain.

The issues in the tissues versus the pain in the brain

The biggest newsflash in pain biology research over the past decade is this:

The amount of pain you experience does not necessarily relate to the amount of tissue damage sustained. There can be tissue damage without pain and pain without tissue damage.

Yes, that's right. You can be riddled with bulging discs, rotator cuff tears and crumbly joints but be in no pain whatsoever. Conversely, you can have real, excruciating and debilitating pain without a single iota of damage to any of your muscles, ligaments or joints.

Consider these strange but true facts from research studies:

1 Tissue damage without pain seems to be reasonably common. Studies have shown that:

   A Of those with no low back pain, 52% have bulging discs and 27% a disc protrusion (Jensen et al 1994). Another study (Savage et al 1997) found that 32% of asymptomatic subjects had 'abnormal' lumbar spines when examined by magnetic resonance imaging (MRI).

   B Partial or full rotator cuff tears can be found in 34% of people with no pain or other symptoms. An amazing 15% of people with full-thickness tears have no pain (Sher et al 1995).

   C A study that carried out MRIs on 45 pain-free participants with no history of hip pain revealed abnormalities in 73% of hips, with 69% of participants having labral tears (usually considered a major cause of pain and ensuing surgery)(Register et al 2012).

   D In another study, 61% of subjects who had meniscal tears in their knees had no pain, aching or stiffness during the previous month (Englund et al 2008).

2 Findings from MRIs and X-rays are NOT related to the pain experienced in musculoskeletal complaints. This will come as a great relief for those of you who are proudly handed X-rays by your clients with the expectation you will confidently know which way up to hold them (by the way if this does happen, to enhance the belief in you as a therapist, I find it's best to gaze at them at arm's, length against the light and stroke your chin thoughtfully. As the joke goes: amateurs say 'oops!' and professionals say a knowing 'ahhh!').

For example, a study examining MRIs of the shoulder in patients with arthritis found that the thinning cartilage in the shoulder joint or the amount of bone spurs has no correlation with pain or function. Clients could be riddled with bone spurs or severely diminished joint space and have little evidence of any problems (Kircher et al 2010).

Similarly, MRIs of the spine of sciatic patients show no relation between symptoms and degree of disc displacement or nerve root entrapment. Some people have huge disc protrusions and no pain while others have tiny bulges and are in excruciating pain (Karppinen et al 2001). Another study proved that there really is no such thing as normal, at least where spines are concerned. Comparing MRIs of patients in pain with asymptomatic subjects, the research found that many (32%) had crumbly, funny looking, bone spur ravaged 'abnormal' lumbar spines with bulging discs. Which, according to the doctors, should mean they were in terrible pain, except they weren't. On the other hand, 47% of the sample had prize-winning 'normal' lumbar spines. Which obviously meant they were pain free, right? Err, no! They were all back pain sufferers. An epic fail for the orthopaedic approach (Savage et al 1997). Also, in a 12-month follow-up period of the subjects, those who developed low back pain for the first time had no change in the MRI appearance of their lumbar spines. The authors damningly concluded that MRIs were fabulous sci-fi toys to play with but didn't actually serve much purpose:

Although MRI is an excellent technique for evaluating the lumbar spine, this study shows that it does not provide a suitable pre-employment screening technique capable of identifying those at risk of low back pain.
SAVAGE ET AL 1997

Another 7-year follow-up study found that the findings on MRIs were not predictive of the development or duration of low back pain. Individuals with the longest duration of low back pain did not have the greatest degree of anatomical abnormality on their original scans (Borenstein et al 2001).

To be fair, there is some association between MRI findings and pain but this is fairly low and as such not particularly clinically useful (Endean et al 2011).

3 Just as there can be tissue damage without pain, there can also be pain without tissue damage or structural abnormalities. The majority of low back pain (85%) is now classified as 'non-specific', i.e. there is no identifiable structural cause such as herniated discs, spondylitis or irritated facet joints. The horrible and persistent pain of RSI in the wrists and hands has no associated tissue damage, neither does the debilitating pain and hypersensitivity of fibromyalgia or chronic headaches. As we shall see later, this feature of pain without tissue damage is particularly true in chronic or persistent pain conditions and is known as 'central sensitisation'.

4 Taking the pain without tissue damage concept one step further is the finding that there can be real pain coming from a structure that doesn't exist, e.g. 60–80% of amputees suffer pain from their phantom limbs. Although the severity of phantom pain usually decreases with time, severe pain persists in 5–10% of patients (Nikolajsen 2012). The sensation of phantom limb pain is so real that subjects report such sensations as morning stiffness and an increase in pain when stressed.

5 Our experience of pain is also dependent on context. For example, the same minor finger injury will cause more pain in a violinist than a football player (Butler and Moseley 2003). Patients who are given more information about a surgical procedure need less pain medication and stay in hospital for a shorter time (Kol et al 2014). The context and social cues given about pain can be of prime importance in our experience of its intensity. You see this clearly with toddlers who fall and look to their parents for information before deciding whether to howl blue murder or move on to the next game. My own parents, brought up in the 'keep calm and carry on' ethos

of wartime, had a hale and hearty approach to my own childhood aches and pains. Here is a sample conversation:

Me: 'Dad it hurts if I do this.'
Dad, barely looking up from his newspaper: 'Don't do that then.'

I undoubtedly have their non-pandering policy to thank for my marvellously pain-free life and the fact that I visit the doctors so seldom I keep getting struck off.

No brain, no pain!

The brain decides whether something hurts or not – 100 % of the time with no exceptions.
BUTLER AND MOSELEY 2003

So if the pain condition is not always coming from damage to the tissues, what exactly is going on? Research over the past two decades has confirmed that pain is a perception of the brain rather than always being an accurate representation of what is happening at the tissue level. Thus, the sensation of pain can be mediated by a variety of factors including emotional state, previous experience, expectations, sense of control over the pain condition and other social and contextual factors.

Our old model of pain, originating with Descartes, holds that there are sensory receptors in the tissues known as nociceptors. These receptors detect noxious stimuli such as tissue damage or inflammation and send messages via the neurones to the spinal cord and brain. In the old model, nociceptor stimulation is always interpreted by the brain as pain. Pain indicates that the body is in danger and the brain can then choose appropriate actions (remove sharp object from foot; go to hospital; wrap self in blanket and watch re-runs of 'Friends'). In this model, we have a 'bottom up' system where the tissues send an email to the brain saying 'tissue damage', the brain receives the email and duly interprets the sensation as pain.

Famous pain researchers, Melzack and Wall (1965), were the first to suggest that this nociceptive input was not the only factor that led to the perception of pain.

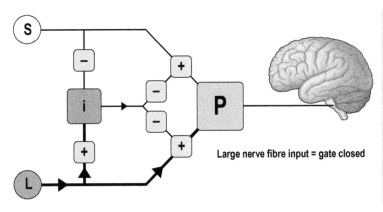

Large nerve fibre input = gate closed

Figure 4.5

The gate control theory: both thin (associated with nociception) and large diameter (associated with touch, pressure and vibration) nerve fibres carry information from the site of injury to two destinations in the dorsal horn (the 'gate') of the spinal cord. If there is more large fibre activity relative to thin fibre activity at the inhibitory cell, this closes the 'gate' to the nociceptive input and less pain is felt

(S) Small nerve fibres   (L) Large nerve fibres   [i] Inhibitory neurone   [P] Projection cells

Their famous 'gate control theory' suggested that both thin (associated with nociception) and large diameter (associated with touch, pressure and vibration) nerve fibres carry information from the site of injury to two destinations in the dorsal horn (the 'gate') of the spinal cord. If there is more large fibre activity relative to thin fibre activity at the inhibitory cell then less pain is felt (**Figure 4.5**). This is the explanation of why massage works for temporary relief of pain, i.e. touch increases the amount of large fibre activity to the brain and thus closes the 'gate' to the nasty nociceptive input. Importantly, the gate control theory also proposed that these pain signals from the body are also modulated by descending influences from the brain, e.g. psychological variables such as past experience, attention, emotional state and other cognitive activities (Melzack 1982).

From the gate to the neuromatrix

Neo: 'I thought it wasn't real.'
Morpheus: 'Your mind makes it real.'
Neo: 'If you're killed in the matrix, you die here?'
Morpheus: 'The body cannot live without the mind.'
THE MATRIX 1999

The year 1999 was a critical time. For a start we all partied like it was indeed 1999. Also, in a strange parallel universe, while the general public drooled over Keanu Reeves in *The Matrix*, the pain geeks got their own version with science hero Melzack publishing 'From the Gate to the Neuromatrix' (Melzack 1999). This seminal paper built on Melzack's theories of pain and emphasised the role of the central nervous system in the sensation of pain. Both *The Matrix* and neuromatrix heroes were united in their belief that 'the mind makes it real'.

Over the past few decades advances in pain research have built on the ideas suggested by Melzack and Wall and have shown that there is in fact no straightforward relationship between nociception and pain. The receptors in the tissues are sensitive to all kinds of stimuli and if these stimuli are perceived to be dangerous to the tissues (nociception literally means danger reception) an alarm signal will be sent to the spinal cord that may be sent on to the brain. But the crucial point is that nociception by itself does not cause pain. The messages sent to the brain only report 'danger' not pain; it is the brain and spinal cord that have to make sense of these inputs and create a meaningful experience based on all the other information available, both past and present. This involves many areas of the brain and not just one 'pain centre' as previously thought. The truth is that pain is created by the brain, not just passively perceived by the brain as a sensation that arrives from the body. This neural network that integrates multiple inputs to produce the output pattern of pain is known as the neuromatrix (Melzack 1999).

The brain is the boss of pain

Nociception is neither sufficient or necessary for pain.
MOSELEY 2007, P. 81

We have travelled a long way from the psychophysical concept that seeks a simple one-to-one relationship between injury and pain.
MELZACK 1999

The new neuromatrix model puts more emphasis on 'top down' inputs from the brain, not just the receiving of 'bottom up' messages from the tissues (**Figure 4.6**).

If you think of how complex the brain is, this model makes much more sense. The brain is more like the top boss receiving multiple emails from the tissues; it then quickly has to sift through all the information it has received and also refer to many other archived sources of information. The brain then makes a decision based on all this evidence as to whether the arriving sensations should be interpreted as pain or not. Remember that pain is a result of the body's belief that you are in

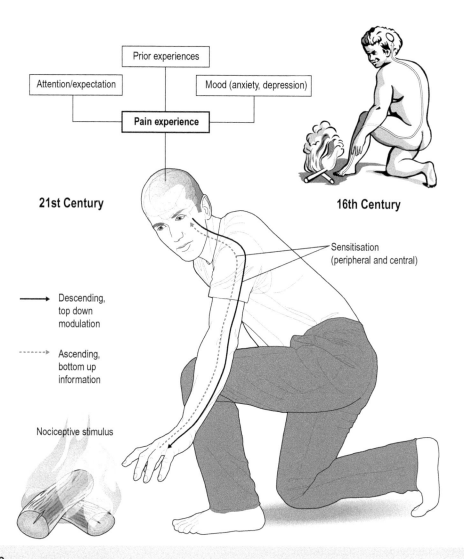

Prior experiences

Attention/expectation

Mood (anxiety, depression)

Pain experience

21st Century

16th Century

Sensitisation (peripheral and central)

Descending, top down modulation

Ascending, bottom up information

Nociceptive stimulus

Figure 4.6
The new neuromatrix model of pain puts more emphasis on 'top down' inputs from the brain, not just the receiving of 'bottom up' messages from the tissues

danger and need to do something to ensure your survival. So the 'brain as boss' may or may not decide to take notice of the emails from the tissues with subject heading and three exclamation marks: 'Danger, danger, high voltage!!!' Just like your real boss does.

A good example is a memory of when I was a child and was racing home on my bike (probably too late for the time my Mum had stipulated) and careered into some bramble bushes. I picked myself out and, as it was dark and I couldn't see myself, I carried on home happily with no ill effects. When I arrived back, and into the light, I suddenly saw that my arms were terribly scratched and bleeding and I suddenly realised I was in terrible pain, immediately bursting into tears. In this case, at the time of the accident, my brain had received the nociceptive input (damaged tissue) but chose not to interpret this as pain. Presumably the message was not backed up by the visual stimuli that would report I 'should' be in pain. Later on, seeing my scratched and damaged arms immediately caused my brain to amend its earlier report to 'danger and pain'.

As Moseley puts it 'Nociception is neither sufficient or necessary for pain.' For example, thoughts can activate alarm signals in the brain without there being any nociception anywhere in the body. Equally, if the nociceptive input is not perceived by the brain as a danger then there will be no pain. This could be one reason why, in the MRI studies of asymptomatic individuals reported earlier, many people have bulging discs or arthritic joints but no pain. If this damage has happened gradually over a period of time the brain may have concluded that this was no threat to survival; therefore, no need to feel pain.

The hill of pain story

The following is a great example of how a real sensation of pain can be the result of inputs other than nociception, as reported by blogger Todd Hargrove from attendance at a conference with pain specialist Lorrimer Moseley:

Lorimer told a great story that illustrated the power that cognitive inputs can have over the output of pain. He once worked with an elite biker who had back pain with riding. After a great deal of progress,

she could ride the flats but was still experiencing pain while climbing hills. Most therapists would assume that the problem with hills was related to some mechanical factor that comes into play when the relationship to gravity is changed.
But Moseley was curious whether hill climbing was problematic for visual or cognitive reasons. So he set up some cameras on a bike treadmill in a way that created an illusion of hill climbing for the rider, even as she rode over flat ground. She immediately reported back pain, based solely on the new visual input. After it was explained to her that this was an illusion, she regained the ability to climb without pain. Apparently the recognition that her pain was not caused by a mechanical factor modified her cognitive inputs in a way that convinced the brain that hill climbing was not dangerous.
BETTERMOVEMENT.ORG 2012

Persistent pain and sensitisation

So what happens in cases of chronic persistent pain? Most injuries will heal within 3–6 weeks (even fractures only take 6 weeks), yet, as we know, in clinics we are often presented with cases of extreme pain that have persisted for months or years. In these cases it is unlikely that there is any real tissue damage remaining, yet there is definitely real pain.

This phenomenon is known as sensitisation. As the nociceptive signals travel to the brain via the neurones and the spinal cord, their input can be modulated (turned up or turned down) at several places along the way. In sensitisation the nociceptive signals are facilitated or magnified in some way that can serve to enhance the sensation of pain (**Figure 4.7**). Sensitisation can be both peripheral (the tissues and peripheral nerves) and central (brain and spinal cord).

- **Peripheral sensitisation**: this is where there is facilitation of primary nociception at the tissue level, e.g. inflammation will increase sensitisation. Under normal circumstances, such as after injury, sensitisation is a good thing, causing the injured area to feel hypersensitive to touch or movement and thus protecting the tissues from further damage. Usually this pain and sensitisation will diminish as the person

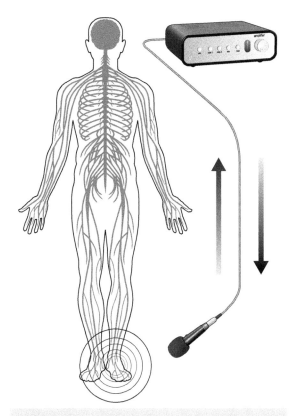

Figure 4.7
In sensitisation, the nociceptive signals are magnified by the nervous system which can enhance the sensation of pain

heals and the pain response will return to normal levels.

- **Central sensitisation**: this is where the central nervous system can 'change, distort or amplify the experience of pain in a manner that no longer reflects the noxious stimuli from the periphery' (Lederman 2013, p. 127). In other words the spinal cord and brain can act like a faulty amplifier that turns up the volume of the pain: the client is in (real) pain even though there is no longer any injury or damage. This persistent pain sensitisation has been shown to be a feature in many of the client conditions that are staples of the massage therapist's clinic. This includes fibromyalgia, osteoarthritis, musculoskeletal disorders with generalised pain hypersensitivity, headache, TMJ disorders, dental pain, neuropathic pain, visceral pain hypersensitivity

disorders and post-surgical pain (Woolf 2011), carpal tunnel syndrome (De-la-Llave-Rincón et al 2012), whiplash (Curatolo et al 2001), chronic low back pain (Roussel et al 2013), and tendinopathies including tennis elbow (Jespersen et al 2013), overuse sports injuries (Van Wilgen and Keizer 2011) and patellar tendinopathies (Van Wilgen et al 2013).

Central sensitisation is somewhat like the oversensitive car alarm that keeps getting triggered even though there is no danger or damage to the car. In cases of central sensitisation we need to make sure, as bodywork therapists, that we are addressing the faulty and over-sensitised alarm system and not just focussing on the tissues.

'Uncle Homunculus': the little man inside your brain

Being in pain not only affects your physical body but also makes visible changes to a virtual map of your body, located in your brain. Yes, as you always suspected, there really is a person living in your head and he goes by the name of 'homunculus' (**Figure 4.8**). The homunculus is a thin strip of brain above the ear that contains a sensory body map – so we all have a virtual body inside our heads that represents our real bodies. The homunculus looks rather grotesque as it is usually drawn with bigger body parts for those areas with more sensory receptors, i.e. the lips, hands, feet and sex organs have more sensory neurons than other parts of the body, so the homunculus has correspondingly large lips, hands, feet and genitals. In fact, if he really was living inside your head you would probably want to issue him with an eviction notice for frightening the neighbours.

Brain imaging studies have shown us that there are marked changes in the virtual map in our head with chronic pain. For example, if there is a persistently injured limb, that part may show 'smudging' in the brain map, i.e. the edges become altered or distorted. The map also changes with usage; as a massage therapist and therefore using your hands a lot, you are likely to have a homunculus with even bigger hands than the average person.

This has implications for treatment as it is likely that manual therapy and movement can affect this inner map.

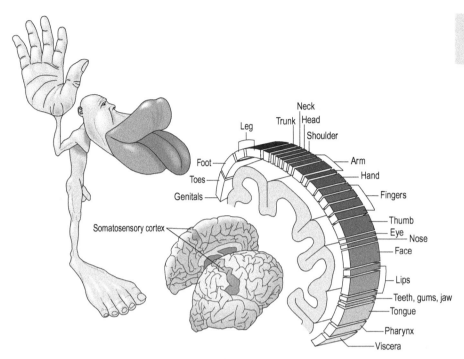

Figure 4.8
The sensory homunculus

Smudging is reversible and it is interesting to postulate how bodywork and movement therapy may have a positive effect on the poor old homunculus.

The vicious cycle of pain

Jordan, 55, came to me in extreme chronic pain. He needed a stick to walk, had recurring low back pain and persistent violent headaches. He had been unable to work for about 10 years. There was no medical diagnosis despite repeated testing.

Whilst taking a case history I found that Jordan used to be a promising athlete and spent much of his younger years running at an elite level. Back in the day, knowledge of training and recovery was less advanced and he reported training day in, day out, with no rest periods. He started getting injuries (a calf pull here, a hamstring strain there), yet usually had no time for treatment or rest and was just advised by his coach to 'push through it'. The pains and injuries started taking longer to recover and Jordan then developed persistent low back pain. He was advised to have surgery. The pain persisted so a second surgery was attempted. The pain was now constant and debilitating so Jordan had to stop running; the back pain continued and Jordan was now

so exhausted he spent a lot of his day in bed. Then he started getting chronic headaches. Eventually he gave up work and resigned himself to a life of disability and constant unrelenting pain.

You may well have clients like Jordan where their original pain has not resolved satisfactorily, leading to more and more pain. Some fancy terms for this are:

- Hyperalgesia (things that used to hurt and now hurt more).

- Allodynia (things that didn't hurt and now hurt).

For some clients in chronic pain this sensation can be extremely severe. In his informative TED (Technology, Entertainment, Design) talk on chronic pain, Elliot Krane likens the sensation of allodynia to feeling as if you are being attacked with a blowtorch, when in fact you are being stroked by a feather (Krane 2011). This feature of persistent and chronic pain is a consequence of a neural process called long-term potentiation; in other words, the more times the brain uses a certain neural pathway, the easier it becomes to activate that pathway again. It is the same as always walking the same route to work or an oft-trodden path through the woods or a well-worn ski-groove in the snow: the neural pathways become ingrained and automatic. Moseley likens the brain to an orchestra with the different players representing the different parts of the brain that may be involved in the output of the pain response. In chronic pain the orchestra is so accustomed to playing the 'pain tune' it has forgotten how to play anything else and the tune has become automatic (Butler and Moseley 2003). The poor body in pain is pretty much stuck at a bad wedding where the DJ brain only plays the Macarena. Ouch!

Why does acute pain become chronic?

It is not yet clear what factors contribute towards a pain experience turning into a chronic problem. Research shows some strong evidence for the influence of certain psychological factors, such as:

- **Psychological distress, depression and somatisation** (the tendency to experience psychological symptoms as somatic and to seek medical help for them) (Pincus et al 2002).

- **Poor expectation of recovery**: Henry Ford allegedly said 'Whether you think you can, or you think you can't – you're right.' This is certainly true for pain where research has shown that those who think they can get better do get better. This has been shown in WAD where those who expected to get better soon recovered over three times as quickly as those who expected that they would never get better (Carroll et al 2009). For low back pain, expectation of recovery has been shown to have a strong correlation with a return to work (Iles et al 2008).

- **Pain intensity at outset**: it seems that in addition to patients' perceptions about whether their back pain will persist, the amount of pain they experienced at onset was also a significant predictor of poor outcome at 6 months and at 5 years (Campbell et al 2013). Studies with patients suffering from whiplash have also indicated that high levels of initial neck pain post-collision are correlated with low levels of expectation around return to work (Ozegovic 2010).

Without a doubt, early intervention and education is key to helping your client's problems heal normally without turning into chronic pain. Pain research shows that the relationship between pain and the state of the tissues becomes less predictable as pain persists. The longer your client has been in pain the less likely it is to be due to perpetuating tissue damage and the more likely it is to be due to sensitisation factors.

Should I tell my clients that the pain is 'all in their head'?

No! Understanding the role of the central nervous system in persistent pain sensitisation is very different from dismissing pain as being 'in the head' or 'psychosomatic'. These kinds of beliefs are unhelpful to the client and will not solve the problem. The pain is very real, not imaginary, as anyone in long-term pain can testify. However, thoughts, feelings and expectations that are ruled by the brain have a much larger influence in the sensation of pain than commonly believed. Unfortunately, the core belief that bodily pain = damage is highly culturally ingrained due to the dominant belief that mind and body are separate. This means that you need to have excellent communication skills to explain these concepts to your clients in a helpful way.

Good education in itself can go a long way to reducing your client's pain. It can be incredibly liberating for clients to realise that their bad back is not 'damaged'. Changing this core belief in itself can help them to initiate positive healing behaviours such as returning to activities they enjoy, moving and exercising more and reducing negative thought patterns.

The good news: everything is temporary anyway

Everything is changeable, everything appears and disappears.
THE BUDDHA

The good news is that it is possible to change the sensitivity of the nervous system. The life of a sensor is short and your sensitivity is constantly changing, so you always have an opportunity to take control and affect what is going on. The Buddha was right: everything is always changeable.

What is your pain telling you?

*Criticism may not be agreeable, but it is necessary.
It fulfils the same function as pain in the human
body. It calls attention to an unhealthy state of things.*
WINSTON CHURCHILL

Remember the important fact that pain is telling us something, i.e. if you are in pain, the brain believes at some level that your very survival is at threat. Your brain is telling you to take action, as Winston Churchill put it, against 'an unhealthy state of things'. Often our view of what actions we can take has become extremely limited (go to doctor, take pills, stop doing the things you enjoy). An educated massage therapist can play a valuable role in helping people reflect on the story that our pain is trying to tell us and this can be an extremely important part of healing. Consider these real client stories:

Sally came to me with RSI: extreme pain in her arms and hands that was extremely sensitive to the touch. Trigger point and fascial techniques just seemed to make the pain worse. In discussion, Sally revealed she was feeling extremely stressed and overwhelmed trying to combine a college degree with full-time work. I reflected back to her that this probably had a component in her pain condition. She took control, transferred to part-time college status and the pain gradually subsided, assisted by regular massage sessions. I also taught her some self-care techniques that enabled her to practise relaxation and mindfulness between sessions.

John came to me with extreme knee pain. His knee was sore and swollen and it was difficult for him to walk. He was working extremely hard and long hours at the time, commuting to London to support his young family. He had been to a chiropractor who 'thought he might have meniscal damage'. He was terrified as he had looked the problem up on the Web and saw a lot of information about needing surgery. He was worried he would be unable to continue working and would fall into financial difficulties. I talked to him about the biology of pain and that most pain problems resolve naturally within a few weeks. As he was young and healthy there was no reason for this not to be the case. I pointed out that it was unlikely the chiropractor could accurately diagnose the meniscal problem without an MRI scan and talked to him about the studies that show there is little correlation between structural damage and pain. We discussed him working fewer hours for a couple of days as his job required standing all day long, which he found excruciating. The next week John returned much improved and was pain free by session three.

Several years ago (after years of priding myself on my body mechanics and not overusing my hands in treatment) I developed a condition called De Quervain's tenosynovitis. This coincided with a time when I was building up my teaching and clinical business. Every day felt packed to the hilt but, as I am good at 'keeping on, keeping on', I carried on pushing through, despite waking up every day feeling overwhelmed. After several sessions of bodywork from the best colleague in town and a stint of acupuncture the problem remained. Everyday activities such as picking up a cup of tea were extremely painful. I resigned myself to the fact that it would probably go away eventually, yet the issue remained stubborn. At some point I borrowed a time management book from my friend, which I really enjoyed, and this helpful information gave me the sense that I could get back in control of my time and business. The very next day the pain in my thumb started to disappear.

What these stories all share in common is the theme that regaining control of our pain through understanding or changing circumstances removed the perceived threat to the brain. Our pain is unique to us and we all hold the key to unravelling its message. A skilled massage therapist can assist the healing and desensitisation process greatly through education around pain, self-care suggestions and not letting the client fall into processes of catastrophisation.

Placebo and nocebo effect

The new knowledge of neuroscience and pain also explains the intriguing effects of placebos. The placebo effect (literal meaning in Latin is 'I shall please') describes observable and real changes in health measures following a sham procedure or inert drug treatment. For decades the placebo effect has been used mainly as a comparison in randomised clinical trials (RCTs) so that the 'real' effects of drugs can be studied. For example, in the RCTs, beloved by researchers, two groups of patients are compared; one group takes an active drug while the other group (matched for variables like age, sex, health status, etc.) takes a dummy drug that looks exactly the same but has no active ingredient. In a single-blinded study the subjects are unaware of whether they are taking the real or dummy pill; in a double-blinded study neither researcher nor patient is aware of who is receiving what. A drug is only considered effective if it has effects above and beyond the placebo group (known as 'statistically significant' in academic speak). What is striking in many RCTs is that the placebo group also show marked improvements even though the drugs are clear fakes. Ted Kaptchuk, a leading acupuncturist turned placebo researcher, has remarked 'We were struggling to increase drug effects while no one was trying to increase the placebo effect' (Feinberg 2013). After being dismissed for years as somewhat of a nuisance, evidence is now accumulating to suggest that placebos can be highly effective in certain circumstances – particularly in treating pain (Finniss et al 2010). Research is now focussing on how the placebo effect can be ethically manipulated to increase healing outcomes.

Although the placebo effect is often an accusation tossed at complementary practitioners as an explanation for any observed benefits of their treatments, it is worth noting that orthodox medicine is not immune from these mechanisms. A societal belief in the power of doctors, surgery and pills greatly enhances healing outcomes. Some of the most shocking findings have been found with the use of sham surgery. These studies involve comparing real surgical procedures against a hilarious doctors and nurses' charade where surgery is simulated using real situations, sights and sounds but no actual treatment; sort of like 'Grey's Anatomy' but without the love affairs.

Amazingly, patients who had fake surgery for a broken back had as much pain relief and improvement in function as those receiving the real surgery (Buchbinder et al 2009, Kallmes et al 2009). Similarly, patients with osteoarthritis of the knee who underwent placebo arthroscopic surgery were just as likely to report pain relief as those who received the real procedure (Moseley et al 2002). A recent well-reviewed Finnish study found that one of the world's most common orthopaedic operations – arthroscopic partial meniscectomy of the knee – is also no more effective than sham surgery (Sihvonen et al 2013). Staggeringly in this study, a year after the procedure both groups of participants were equally delighted with the results of their 'operation'. Of the patients who underwent the real operation, 93% would choose the same treatment, while 96% of those in the placebo group would do so. These findings have massive implications for health care spending and priorities; particularly as it is estimated that the number of these operations in the USA is close to a million. Maybe hospital TV shows should team up with real hospitals to provide patients as extras – they could both save each other a fortune!

Much of the effect of drug therapy may also be attributable to the placebo effect. Meta-analysis of antidepressant medications has reported only modest benefits over placebo treatment (Kirsch et al 2008) and it is estimated that 50% of the pain relief obtained from taking migraine medication is due to the belief that the medication is effective, i.e. placebo effect (Kam-Hansen et al 2014).

Above all, the placebo effect demonstrates the powerful effect of the unconscious processes of our mind in affecting health outcomes. Yet what implications can this have for the ethical massage therapist? Placebo studies often rely on deception to achieve results, which is clearly undesirable. The most important factor is realising that anything you can do to honestly and ethically increase the client's belief or confidence in you and your treatment is likely to enhance the outcome. Often alternative therapists employ these tactics unwittingly. For example, I remember many years ago starting to have joint pains in my elbows; I was young and not long into my massage career and started an immediate process of catastrophisation about arthritis, disability and having to give up my newly found passion. I mentioned the issue to a herbalist friend who said cheerfully 'Oh I should be able to sort that out for you, no problem.' I felt instantly relieved and comforted with her confidence. Of course the herbal medicine did the trick, but why? Was there an active ingredient, a placebo or both? Frankly who cares – I got better which was the main thing. On a similar note, I have also been to bodyworkers who have made statements like 'The treatment will carry on working for several days.' Although I'm not sure there is any physiological basis for this, planting the notion in my mind that this was going to happen undoubtedly meant that it did! Client expectation of outcome is correlated with functional improvement – which has been shown for example in acute low back pain (Myers et al 2008).

Note that we are not recommending lying or deceiving your client or claiming to cure them, all of which would be totally unethical. Yet be aware of how your words and behaviour can either promote confidence and the expectation to heal or have the reverse effect. For example, it's fine to say to clients who have pain issues 'That sounds like something I should be able to sort out' or 'I've had good results with problems like that before' or 'Research shows massage gets good results in helping reduce low back pain.' These are all true statements that will help the positive mindset of the client whilst avoiding the trap of 'claiming to cure'. Clients are also likely to feel reassured by social cues that suggest you know what you are doing: this might include your qualifications, experience, positive recommendations by friends, knowledge of research studies, the look or feel of your treatment room or your own sense of confidence and gravitas.

Conversely using language such as 'herniated discs take ages to heal', 'you have a scoliosis', 'sounds like arthritis' will set up a different set of expectations in your client's head. This effect is the lesser-known cousin of placebo: the nocebo. Our expectations of negative effects will also often lead to those very events happening. In an interview, Ted Kaptchuk talked about a study where he compared the effects of placebo acupuncture versus placebo pills for forearm pain. Patients in both groups were warned about different possible side effects, e.g. drowsiness for the sugar pill takers, redness and swelling from the needles for the sham acupuncture group. Lo and behold, a large percentage of patients in both groups reported exactly those side effects even though the treatments they received were completely inert (Feinberg 2013).

In short, having an awareness of the power of the placebo effect in treatment can help to enhance our outcomes. The placebo effect demonstrates what ancient healers and holistic practitioners have known for decades; namely, that the mind can have an extremely powerful influence on our recovery from illness and pain.

Implications for treatment

The big question, as always, is: how does our new knowledge of pain inform our treatment approach? The good news is that the massage therapist can play a pivotal role in treating chronic pain and it is likely that, if you have been in business for a while, you have already become an unwitting expert in the mix of psychological and physical approaches needed to help your client resolve their problems.

Firstly, being able to recognise the potential role of central sensitisation in client pain should be a key part of the assessment process. Do not be afraid to gently draw your client out about psychosocial factors including stress, emotional state, family support and their attitude to the pain condition. This can help you recognise key factors that may point the finger at central sensitisation processes rather than tissue damage or structural abnormalities. Too scared (or British) to ask your client how they feel? Then stay tuned for more on this in the following chapter, which explores the assessment process in greater detail.

Secondly, it is important to see the treatment session as a stage for client education, pain management approaches and self-care suggestions. There are simple common sense approaches that fall well within the massage therapist's role that can be incredibly useful to the client. Of course in some situations emotional or cognitive components involved in the client's pain may warrant referral to another professional (such as a cognitive behavioural therapist or another talk therapist) but in many cases a common sense approach to the problem can be invaluable. Massage therapists are in a prime position to carry out this task as they often have an intrinsic understanding of the joint role played by mind and body. This expands the potential role of massage therapist to one of health care educator and facilitator of the client taking control of their healing process. Want to know more? Then head straight for the Self-Care Resources (available at uk.singingdragon.com/catalogue/book/9781909141230).

But what about the massage itself? Does this new understanding of pain mean that we should not be addressing the tissues at all but just talking to our clients about pain science and sending them to therapy to address their anxiety? Not at all, clinical experience over many decades suggests that the bodywork techniques advocated in this book may well be effective because they help to reduce peripheral and central sensitisation. Research has suggested that trigger points and fascial adhesions may well play an important role in perpetuating both peripheral and central sensitisation. (For more on this see the respective chapters. Yes indeedy, hold on to your seats)

Moreover, the interplay of emotions and chronic pain is interesting for massage therapists who have long main-tained the link between body and emotions. Massage is now well documented as having a positive role on emo-tions, including depression and anxiety, with 'a course of treatment providing benefits similar in magnitude to those of psychotherapy' (Moyer et al 2004). Although previously thought to be mediated via a lowering of cortisol, recent research suggests that massage has less effect than previously thought on cortisol levels and that the positive effects of massage must be explained by a different mechanism of action (Moyer et al 2011). What-ever the physiological basis, reducing emotional pain is likely to have a corresponding effect on somatic pain. Mind and body are interlinked and cannot be treated separately.

In summary, a massage treatment is an ideal stage for the BPS approach. This is entirely because we have been doing it for decades. Alone and unsung in our treatment rooms, massage therapists across the world have been dealing with tears and trauma in our quest to 'help people'. We have combined the roles of counsellor, bodyworker and personal coach to do the very best for our clients. It's simply what we do best.

Reinventing the wheel?

We shall not cease from exploration, and the end of all our exploring will be to arrive where we started and know the place for the first time.
TS ELIOT 1943

Although the new research around pain biology is exciting, in a sense it tells us nothing new. Ancient forms of medicine have always emphasised the unity of body and mind and the influence of both on pain and disease. Psychotherapists have been asking their patients for years 'What is the pain telling you about your life?' I myself went into massage as I thought dealing with physical pain would be more straightforward than the complex challenge of being a mental health social worker – only to find that most of my patients with back pain, fibromyalgia, RSI and headaches were suffering from anxiety, depression, a history of sexual abuse or other unresolved emotional issues. As they say, you can take the girl out of social work but you can't take social work out of the girl. The concept of holistic medicine, the BPS model and the psychosomatic medicine of the 1970s all share the common view that mind, body and social factors are interlinked.

So now the research has caught up, maybe once and for all we can finally change the dominant medical view that mind and body are separate. Mind, body, spirit and social context are indivisible and cannot be separated if we are to successfully treat pain and disease.

Move over Descartes, your time is up!

References

Amtamassage.org 2014 Consumer Survey Fact Sheet – American Massage Therapy Association. Available at: http://www.amtamassage.org/research/Consumer-Survey-Fact-Sheets.html [accessed 17 August 2014].

Benjamin S et al 2000 The association between chronic widespread pain and mental disorder: a population-based study. Arthritis and Rheumatism 43:561–567.

Bettermovement.org 2012 Review of Conference with Moseley and Hodges on Pain and Motor Control. Better Movement. Available at: http://www.bettermovement.org/2012/review-of-conference-with-moseley-and-hodges-on-pain-and-motor-control/ [accessed 17 August 2014].

Bonathan C, Hearn L, Williams AC de C 2013 Socioeconomic status and the course and consequences of chronic pain. Pain Management 3(3):159–162.

Borenstein DG et al 2001 The value of magnetic resonance imaging of the lumbar spine to predict low-back pain in asymptomatic subjects: a seven-year follow-up study. The Journal of Bone and Joint Surgery Am 83–A(9):1306–1311.

Brage S, Sandanger I, Nygård JF 2007 Emotional distress as a predictor for low back disability: a prospective 12-year population-based study. Spine 32:269–274.

Buchbinder R et al 2009 A randomized trial of vertebroplasty for painful osteoporotic vertebral fractures. The New England Journal of Medicine 361(6):557–568.

Butler D, Moseley G 2003 Explain Pain, 1st edn. Adelaide: Noigroup Publications.

Campbell P et al 2013 Prognostic indicators of low back pain in primary care: five-year prospective study. The Journal of Pain : Official Journal of the American Pain Society 14(8):873–883.

Carnes D et al 2007 Chronic musculoskeletal pain rarely presents in a single body site: results from a UK population study. Rheumatology (Oxford, England) 46:1168–1170.

Carroll LJ, Holm LW, Ferrari R et al 2009 Recovery in whiplash-associated disorders: do you get what you expect? The Journal of Rheumatology 36(5):1063–1070.

Curatolo M et al 2001 Central hypersensitivity in chronic pain after whiplash injury. Clinical Journal of Pain 17:306–315.

De-la-Llave-Rincón AI, Puentedura EJ, Fernández-de-las-Peñas C 2012 New advances in the mechanisms and etiology of carpal tunnel syndrome. Discovery Medicine 13(72):343–348.

Eliot TS 1943 Four quartets. New York: Harcourt, Brace and Co.

Endean A, Palmer KT, Coggon D 2011 Potential of magnetic resonance imaging findings to refine case definition for mechanical low back pain in epidemiological studies: a systematic review. Spine 36(2):160–169.

Engel GL 1977 The need for a new medical model: a challenge for biomedicine. Science (New York, NY) 196(4286):129–136.

Engel GL 1980 The clinical application of the biopsychosocial model. The American Journal of Psychiatry 137(5):535–544.

Englund M, Guermazi A, Gale D et al 2008 Incidental meniscal findings on knee MRI in middle-aged and elderly persons. New England Journal of Medicine 359:1108–1115.

Feinberg C 2013 Ted Kaptchuk of Harvard Medical School studies placebos. Harvard Magazine Jan–Feb 2013. Available at: http://harvardmagazine.com/2013/01/the-placebo-phenomenon [accessed 17 August 2014].

Finniss DG et al 2010 Biological, clinical, and ethical advances of placebo effects. Lancet 375(9715):686–695.

Fuentes M, Hart-Johnson T, Green CR 2007 The association among neighborhood socioeconomic status, race and chronic pain in black and white older adults. Journal of the National Medical Association 99(10):1160–1169.

Gatchel RJ et al 2007 The biopsychosocial approach to chronic pain: scientific advances and future directions. Psychological Bulletin 133(4):581–624.

Green CR, Hart-Johnson T 2012 The association between race and neighborhood socioeconomic status in younger Black and White adults with chronic pain. The Journal of Pain: Official Journal of the American Pain Society 13(2):176–186.

Harder S, Veilleux M, Suissa S 1998 The effect of socio-demographic and crash-related factors on the prognosis of whiplash. Journal of Clinical Epidemiology 51(5):377–384.

Iles RA, Davidson M, Taylor NF 2008 Psychosocial predictors of failure to return to work in non-chronic non-specific low back pain: a systematic review. Occupational and Environmental Medicine 65(8):507–517.

Jensen MC et al 1994 Magnetic resonance imaging of the lumbar spine in people without back pain. The New England Journal of Medicine 331:69–73.

Jespersen A et al 2013 Assessment of pressure-pain thresholds and central sensitization of pain in lateral epicondylalgia. Pain Medicine (Malden, Mass) 14(2):297–304. Available at: http://www.ncbi.nlm.nih.gov/pubmed/23279601 [accessed 3 April 2014].

Johannes CB et al 2010 The prevalence of chronic pain in United States adults: results of an Internet-based survey. The Journal of Pain: Official Journal of the American Pain Society 11(11):1230–1239.

Kallmes DF et al 2009 A randomized trial of vertebroplasty for osteoporotic spinal fractures. The New England Journal of Medicine 361(6):569–579.

Kam-Hansen S et al 2014 Altered placebo and drug labeling changes the outcome of episodic migraine attacks. Science Translational Medicine 6(218):218ra5.

Karppinen J et al 2001 Severity of symptoms and signs in relation to magnetic resonance imaging findings among sciatic patients. Spine 26(7):E149–154.

King S et al 2011 The epidemiology of chronic pain in children and adolescents revisited: a systematic review. Pain 152(12):2729–2738.

Kircher J et al 2010 How much are radiological parameters related to clinical symptoms and function in osteoarthritis of the shoulder? International Orthopaedics 34(5):677–681.

Kirsch I et al 2008 Initial severity and antidepressant benefits: a meta-analysis of data submitted to the Food and Drug Administration. PLoS Medicine 5(2):e45.

Kol E, Alpar SE, Erdoğan A 2014 Preoperative education and use of analgesic before onset of pain routinely for post-thoracotomy pain control can reduce pain effect and total amount of analgesics administered postoperatively. Pain Management Nursing: Official Journal of the American Society of Pain Management Nurses 15(1):331–339.

Krane E 2011 The mystery of chronic pain. Technology, Entertainment, Design (https://www.ted.com). Available at: http://www.ted.com/talks/elliot_krane_the_mystery_of_chronic_pain [accessed 17 August 2014].

Lederman E 2013 Therapeutic Stretching: Towards a Functional Approach. Churchill Livingstone Elsevier.

Linton SJ 2000 A review of psychological risk factors in back and neck pain. Spine 25:1148–1156.

McBeth J, Jones K 2007 Epidemiology of chronic musculoskeletal pain. Best Practice & Research Clinical Rheumatology 21(3):403–425.

Macfarlane GJ et al 2009 The influence of socioeconomic status on the reporting of regional and widespread musculoskeletal pain: results from the 1958 British Birth Cohort Study. Annals of the Rheumatic Diseases 68:1591–1595.

Melzack R 1982 Recent concepts of pain. Journal of Medicine 13(3):147–160.

Melzack R 1999 From the gate to the neuromatrix. Pain (supplement 6):S121–126.

Melzack R, Wall PD 1965 Pain mechanisms: a new theory. Science (New York, NY) 150(3699):971–979.

Moseley G 2007 Painful yarns, 1st edn. Canberra, Australia: Dancing Giraffe Press.

Moseley JB et al 2002 A controlled trial of arthroscopic surgery for osteoarthritis of the knee. The New England Journal of Medicine 347(2):81–88.

Moyer CA, Rounds J, Hannum JW 2004 A meta-analysis of massage therapy research. Psychological Bulletin 130(1):3–18.

Moyer CA et al 2011 Does massage therapy reduce cortisol? A comprehensive quantitative review. Journal of Bodywork and Movement Therapies 15(1):3–14.

Myers SS et al 2008 Patient expectations as predictors of outcome in patients with acute low back pain. Journal of General Internal Medicine 23:148–153.

Nikolajsen L 2012 Postamputation pain: studies on mechanisms. Danish Medical Journal 59(10):B4527

Ozegovic D, Carroll LJ, Cassidy JD 2010 What influences positive return to work expectation? Examining associated factors in a population-based cohort of whiplash-associated disorders. Spine 35(15):E708–13.

Pincus T et al 2002 A systematic review of psychological factors as predictors of chronicity/disability in prospective cohorts of low back pain. Spine 27:E109–E120.

Rainville J et al 2011 Fear-avoidance beliefs and pain avoidance in low back pain – translating research into clinical practice. The Spine Journal: Official Journal of the North American Spine Society 11(9):895–903.

Register B et al 2012 Prevalence of abnormal hip findings in asymptomatic participants: a prospective, blinded study. The American Journal of Sports Medicine 40(12):2720–2724.

Roussel NA et al 2013 Central sensitization and altered central pain processing in chronic low back pain: fact or myth? The Clinical Journal of Pain 29:625–638.

Roy M et al 2009 Cerebral and spinal modulation of pain by emotions. Proceedings of the National Academy of Sciences of the United States of America 106(49):20900–20905.

Savage RA, Whitehouse GH, Roberts N 1997 The relationship between the magnetic resonance imaging appearance of the lumbar spine and low back pain, age and occupation in males. European Spine Journal: official publication of the European Spine Society, the European Spinal Deformity Society, and the European Section of the Cervical Spine Research Society 6:106–114.

Sher JS et al 1995 Abnormal findings on magnetic resonance images of asymptomatic shoulders. The Journal of Bone and Joint Surgery (American) 77:10–15.

Sihvonen R et al 2013 Arthroscopic partial meniscectomy versus sham surgery for a degenerative meniscal tear. The New England Journal of Medicine 369(26):2515–2524.

Suissa S 2003 Risk factors of poor prognosis after whiplash injury. Pain Research & Management: The Journal of the Canadian Pain Society = Journal de la Société Canadienne pour le Traitement de la Douleur 8(2):69–75.

Sullivan MJ et al 2001 Theoretical perspectives on the relation between catastrophizing and pain. The Clinical Journal of Pain 17:52–64.

The Matrix 1999 [film] Dir. Andy Wachowski and Larry Wachowski.

Tunks ER, Crook J, Weir R 2008 Epidemiology of chronic pain with psychological comorbidity: prevalence, risk, course, and prognosis. Canadian Journal of Psychiatry. Revue Canadienne de Psychiatrie 53:224–234.

Van Wilgen CP, Keizer D 2011 Neuropathic pain mechanisms in patients with chronic sports injuries: a diagnostic model useful in sports medicine? Pain Medicine (Malden, MA) 12(1):110–117.

Van Wilgen CP et al 2013 Do patients with chronic patellar tendinopathy have an altered somatosensory profile? A Quantitative Sensory Testing (QST) study. Scandinavian Journal of Medicine & Science in Sports 23(2):149–155.

Woolf CJ 2011 Central sensitization: implications for the diagnosisand treatment of pain. Pain 152 (supplement 3):S2–15.

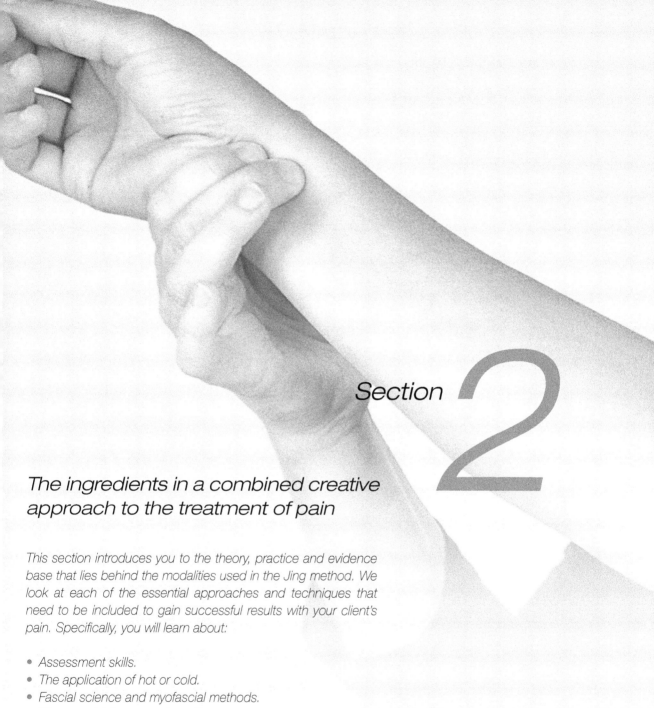

Section 2

The ingredients in a combined creative approach to the treatment of pain

This section introduces you to the theory, practice and evidence base that lies behind the modalities used in the Jing method. We look at each of the essential approaches and techniques that need to be included to gain successful results with your client's pain. Specifically, you will learn about:

- *Assessment skills.*
- *The application of hot or cold.*
- *Fascial science and myofascial methods.*
- *Trigger point theory and practice.*
- *The links between acupressure-based approaches and new fascial research.*
- *The evidence for using stretching in treatment and the different methods, including static, PNF, MET, active isolated and fascial stretching.*
- *Teaching self-care approaches to your client.*

5
Clinical assessment

Good clinical assessment is a crucial skill for massage therapists, yet unfortunately one that is often poorly taught, overlooked or misunderstood. It is common for massage therapists to carry out minimal assessment, especially if working in spa settings, or when doing relaxation massage. Due to lack of knowledge of adequate assessment procedures, many therapists end up terrified of treating pain related conditions as they are unclear about the potential sources and causes of pain. Is the tingling down our client's hand and arm a result of a nerve compressed by soft tissue (well within our scope of treatment) or something more serious? Is our client's bad back a muscular problem or should they be referred back to their doctor? How much should we ask about stress and emotional factors – after all we are not trained counsellors?

Precise and targeted clinical assessment should be a vital tool in any therapist's toolbox and will not only help give you better outcomes but will increase your professional standing with other professionals and clients. As we shall see, a thorough assessment that takes into account the wide range of physical, emotional and social factors involved in your client's pain experience is the cornerstone to achieving optimal results.

What is the difference? Assessment vs diagnosis

Assessment: A judgement about something based on an understanding of the situation.
Encarta World English Dictionary
Soukhanov 1999

An assessment is an educated evaluation of a client's condition and physical basis for his/her symptoms in order to determine a course of treatment.
Rattray et al 2000

A mantra drummed into most massage therapists is that we are 'not trained to diagnose' and this makes many of us feel twitchy and unconfident about assessment in general. Yet assessment is not the same as diagnosis and it is important to understand the difference with respect to your role and scope of practice. As exemplified by the Rattray et al quote above, massage therapists usually use the word assessment when evaluating which soft tissue structures may be involved in a client's musculoskeletal pain condition, e.g. is the problem primarily to do with the muscle, ligament or joint? Although this is a useful definition of the massage therapist's role in assessment it is also not the whole picture. Consideration must be given to the effects of stress, emotions and central sensitisation in any pain condition. As we have seen from Chapter 4, psychological and social factors can play a huge part in the experience of pain and it is important to also evaluate these factors.

Assessment is very different from diagnosis which is a term used by the medical profession who have a different category of possible causes to consider. Doctors will also consider medical causes outside of the domain of massage therapists, e.g. is the pain due to a cancerous growth or problems with the central nervous system. By way of illustration, chronic low back pain could be the result of a tumour pressing on the spine or spinal infection, both of which are clearly medical issues. However, if other causes of pain have been ruled out by the GP, your consultation and assessment can focus on whether the condition is being caused by soft tissue issues such as trigger points and fascial adhesions, or the exacerbating effects of emotional stress, the complications of central sensitisation and/or any of the other factors that lie within your scope of practice.

Why do an assessment?

Four things belong to a judge, to hear courteously, to answer wisely, to consider soberly and to decide impartially.
Socrates

Quite simply, a good assessment enables us to plan effective treatments that achieve the goals or outcomes that the client desires. Assessment enables us to narrow down the factors that may be contributing to a pain condition and to rule out others. Doing an assessment enables you to be the equivalent of a massage Sherlock Holmes, picking up clues from your client in various different ways to help you figure out what is going on and how you can best help. A good assessment enables you to see whether your treatment is working and gives you measurable benchmarks so both you and your client are able to assess progress.

Assessment is important as it helps us to have a better idea of how long a condition may take to respond to treatment. For example, is your client's painful shoulder due to a problem with the tendon (e.g. supraspinatus tendonitis), trigger points in the subscapularis, the joint (e.g. adhesive capsulitis otherwise known as frozen shoulder) or a chronic pain issue where there is no longer any tissue damage but a continued heightened central nervous system response? All of these issues may present with similar symptoms but assessment can help us drill down and really figure out which one is most likely. Although all may be treated in a similar way through the Jing combination of advanced techniques, a true frozen shoulder or long lasting chronic pain problem will typically take longer to show full improvement. However, trigger points in the subscapularis may be resolved in a couple of weekly sessions. Of course, as we know, pain is multi-faceted and in most clinical situations we are not faced with a single cause but a complex combination of causative and perpetuating factors. This can make our job tricky, but never boring!

Being there: the importance of the therapeutic relationship

> *Too often we underestimate the power of a touch, a smile, a kind word, a listening ear, an honest compliment, or the smallest act of caring, all of which have the potential to turn a life around.*
> LEO BUSCAGLIA

Reflect on the last time you had a successful healing or a personal growth interaction – perhaps with your doctor, an alternative health care provider, teacher or talk therapist. Chances are you really liked that person, felt they were on your side and you get a bit of a warm fuzzy glow when you think about them. From the other side of the therapeutic relationship, you may also notice an unusual feeling of fondness when you think about some of your clients; an empathy and concern for their welfare that goes beyond the superficial.

Whether you are a medical doctor, massage therapist, talk therapist or acupuncturist, a key component of facilitating wellness in your client is this therapeutic relationship or alliance. This refers to the sense of 'collaboration, warmth, and support between the client and therapist' (Ferreira et al 2013). Research shows that if you have a good relationship with your doctor then this means you are likely to have an improved health care outcome regardless of what treatment you receive (Kelley et al 2014, Kaplan et al 1989). As one reviewer put it 'Successful interactions between patients and their practitioners lie at the heart of medicine' (Griffin et al 2004). This is just as true for our work with musculoskeletal pain. Studies have shown that positive therapeutic alliance ratings between physical therapists and patients are associated with improvements in outcomes for low back pain and increased treatment satisfaction for clients with musculoskeletal problems (Ferreira et al 2013, Hall et al 2010). Really? Can our client's bad back be improving just because they like us? Is being smiley more important than soft tissue release? Research suggests that the interpersonal dynamic is certainly a factor and points to the importance of the practitioner–client bond as part of a competent and truly holistic healing process.

Taking time with your clients in the assessment process will pay off handsomely in terms of results. Kaptchuk et al (2008) found that the quality and length of the initial interaction with a practitioner was strongly correlated with improvement measures. Clients receiving placebo acupuncture for irritable bowel syndrome (IBS) were randomly divided into three groups: 'waiting list condition', 'limited interaction' or 'augmented interaction'. In the waiting list group the patients had no interaction with the practitioner. In the limited interaction group the acupuncturist introduced himself and said that 'he knew what to do', after which the conversation ceased and the treatment began. In the augmented interaction group the patient and the practitioner had a 45-minute conversation, before the treatment began, where the practitioner expressed empathy, asked the patient about symptoms, and told the patient that he had very positive experiences with treating these symptoms.

The results showed how powerful the interaction with the therapist is, independent of what happens in the actual treatment. Patients in the extended consultation group had a significantly greater improvement and more pain relief when compared with the group exposed to the limited interaction of the confident but somewhat abrupt practitioner. The latter, in turn, had significantly more improvement than the waiting list group who had no human interaction other than the sham acupuncture treatment.

Moreover, if any of you out there are worried about litigation, investing in the therapeutic alliance is probably your best insurance policy (I feel an infomercial coming on). In landmark research by Dr Wendy Levinson, where she studied hundreds of conversations between patients and physicians (half of whom had been sued at least twice and the other half had never been sued), she found that the difference was entirely due to how the doctors talked to their patients. Those who had never been sued spent longer with their clients, were more active listeners and were funnier! However, they gave exactly the same quality of information as the poor old, socially unskilled doctors with bad jokes who were spending their days immersed in litigation suits (Levinson 1997).

Power to the people! Individual qualities of successful practitioners

At the end of the day, techniques don't get results, people do. We all know that some therapists seem to consistently get good outcomes whereas others who are using the same techniques do not. What are the characteristics of these successful healers – these enviable practitioners who enjoy word of mouth fame and are usually talked about in hushed and reverential tones? Psychologist Bruce Wampold has outlined a number of attributes of talk therapists that are correlated with successful outcomes. In my experience, the list could equally apply to those bodyworkers who consistently get results:

1　**Excellent interpersonal skills.** Effective therapists have sophisticated interpersonal skills, including warmth, acceptance, empathy and a focus on others, not themselves.

2　**Ability to help you feel you can trust the therapist.** According to Wampold, people determine whether or not they can trust someone within the first few minutes of the interaction. Effective therapists create the conditions of warmth, acceptance and expertise both verbally and non-verbally within seconds of that first crucial interaction.

3　**Willingness to establish an alliance with you.** As we saw above, the ability of the therapist to build on those initial feelings of trust and establish a strong therapeutic alliance is critical to achieving a successful outcome. Good therapists are able to do this with a wide range of individuals and not just those who they like or are most similar to them.

4　**Ability to provide an acceptable explanation of your symptoms.** Successful therapists are able to provide an explanation for the experience of pain and distress that crucially makes sense to the client. This may mean that explanations for symptoms are presented in a different way depending on the client's beliefs and worldview. Some will need a scientific rationale, others will respond more to simple 'big picture' explanations.

5　**Commitment to developing a treatment plan that is consistent with the explanation.** Successful therapists involve clients in understanding the treatment plan and lay out a route for progression that is consistent with the client's conception of why they are in pain.

6　**Communication of confidence about the course of therapy.** In Wampold's words, an effective therapist is 'influential, persuasive and convincing'. They provide the client with a believable explanation for their symptoms and communicate strongly their belief that the therapy will be worthwhile.

7　**Monitoring progress.** Good therapists are continually monitoring how their clients are responding to treatment and show their clients that they care about their progress. Checking in at every treatment or providing more full progress reviews after a few sessions are ways that the massage therapist can achieve this.

8   **Flexibility**. Good therapists are able to pick up on client unresponsiveness to treatment and to change approaches. In the words of the great Albert Einstein 'The measure of intelligence is the ability to change.'

9   **Inspiration of hope and optimism**. A good therapist is able to balance hope for desired recovery with realistic goals. Many clients struggling with chronic pain feel overwhelmed and despairing, leading to a negative cycle of increasing disability and distress. Being able to communicate that things can change with time and the right approach is crucial to the healing process.

10 **Sensitivity towards social and cultural backgrounds.** Good therapists understand that context is important to a full understanding of why a client is in pain. Family, religion, gender, class and other factors can have a huge impact on our experience and potential recovery from pain.

11 **Possession of self-insight**. An effective therapist is self-aware and is able to separate their own issues from those of clients. This is very important in bodywork where it can be easy for us to energetically 'pick up stuff from our clients'. Knowing where our clients end and we begin is vital to being a grounded and competent bodyworker.

12 **Reliance on the best research evidence.** With the Internet it has never been easier to keep up with the latest research evidence. There are so many exciting developments in bodywork with the rise of investigation into fascia, chronic pain and many other areas. There is no excuse not to stay abreast of the latest cutting edge advances in manual therapy, not just in massage but complementary fields such as osteopathy, chiropractic and movement therapy.

13 **Involvement in continued training and education.** Excellent bodyworkers are always passionate about new learning, leaving no stone unturned to discover the best techniques and approaches for their clients.

Obviously the result of treatment depends on many factors, but evidence shows that these 13 qualities in a therapist play a key role in increasing the odds of a successful outcome, regardless of whether the primary focus is improvement of mental or physical health. Many successful bodyworkers will realise that they unconsciously and naturally integrate the attributes above into their assessment and treatment process. As always, it is useful to ascertain which aspects of your approach are helpful. Improvement in your work relies on the simple process of doing more of what works and less of what doesn't.

The assessment process: initial client enquiry

Remember your assessment starts as soon as your client makes contact with you: from the initial phone call or conversation with a colleague about a pain problem. Never lose any opportunity to gain information about your client's physical, spiritual and emotional make-up. Even if you have an online booking system, it is worthwhile also calling the client beforehand to glean some basic information. Making a connection in this way will also reduce the possibility of a no-show and enable you to screen out those who are not suitable for what you offer (including those seeking sexual services, regrettably still a hazard in the industry).

In the initial phone call, find out what the client wants out of the treatment. Reasons for seeking massage tend to fall into four categories:

1   **Medical**: I want to be out of pain and/or improve mobility.

2   **Emotional/nurturing**: I want to relax/take time out/be looked after/feel safe in my body.

3   **Personal growth**: I want to understand my body better; access emotional hurts that may be locked away.

4   **Exploratory**: I want to know what a hot stone massage feels like.

The first two reasons tend to be the most common. According to an American Massage Therapy Association (AMTA) survey in the USA, 75% of individuals surveyed claim their primary reason for receiving a massage in the previous 12 months was medical (43%) and stress (32%) related (Amtamassage.org 2014).

The following points are worth remembering during that initial phone call. If you don't get a chance to cover these areas before the visit, then they will form part of the assessment process during the first appointment:

- **Be positive, cheerful and professional.** Remember your potential client will be forming a strong opinion of whether you can help them or not within those first few minutes of speaking.

- **Listen to what the issues are in a general sense (without getting into taking a detailed case history).** Use open questions to draw the client out and jot down notes if needed for future reference.

- **Find out how the client heard about you.** This is helpful for your marketing and also to screen out anyone about whom you feel suspicious. I remember giving one poor male caller a grilling about his (genuine) groin strain until I found out he was the husband of an extremely trustworthy colleague.

- **Explain about your approach, relevant training and background; describe what they can expect in terms of your approach to working with pain conditions.**

- **Talk about your scope of practice and why this may be different from that of the surgeon/ physiotherapist/osteopath/chiropractor/other massage therapist.** This is important if the client has had previous treatment that they found ineffective and will also inform you about what existing approaches didn't work. If the client is having current treatment explain how massage can work well in conjunction with another therapy (if it does!).

- **Give some idea of treatment duration.** Working within the approach outlined in this book, this would generally be 1–6 weekly treatments initially to see a decrease in pain.

- **Explain practicalities.** This would include how to get to the venue and an exploration of any special needs (i.e. if they are unable to negotiate stairs). Also let your client know how long the treatment will take (then stick to it as this is the essence of good boundaries!).

- **Don't forget to tell them how much you charge and how you take payment.**

- **Let them know you are looking forward to seeing them and working together.** This is the start of forging a therapeutic alliance that is crucial to the healing process.

The what, why and how of effective assessment

Like any skill, good assessment relies on fully understanding the what, why and how of the process:

- What information do I need to elicit?

- Why is it useful?

- How can I best obtain that information from the client? Do I need to ask them, look at them or touch them to get the information. An effective assessment usually includes all of these aspects.

There are many different models for assessment in bodywork and our own approach is a creative combination of numerous skills and perspectives culled from various disciplines we have been exposed to over the years.

An outcome based approach to bodywork

A key factor in effective assessment is being very precise about the exact desired outcome for the client. If you are not clear about your goal, how will you or the client know if you have achieved this? Many massage therapists confuse outcomes (the end result desired such as pain reduction) with the methods used to get there (the best bodywork techniques needed to achieve the outcome). For example, I often get potential clients asking for a 'deep tissue massage'. I will then ask why they want this type of tissue massage: is it for relaxation or for a pain problem? If pain is the issue I will explain that this is my area of expertise and my goal will be to reduce their pain in the shortest possible time (using the once a week for up to 6 weeks formula). To get them out of pain I will use a variety of soft tissue techniques, some of which might be similar to deep tissue massage and some of which will be very different, like fascial release or cranial work. This is an important distinction – it is your job to provide the desired outcome for the client and not for them to tell you what tools you should use to achieve this. This is similar to any other skilled profession. If I take my car to the mechanic I tell them what's wrong (the engine is rattling) NOT how to fix it (I want you to use an 8 mm spanner to dismantle the carburettor …).

If you are successful in attaining the desired outcome, your client will be happy whatever the means used to get to that point. This is exemplified by the great quote from one of my clients for whom I obtained complete relief of her chronic migraine problem of 30 years by mainly using cranial work. She said 'For what I don't feel you doing the results are amazing!'

When working with pain conditions your outcomes will generally be concerned with:

- Decrease in pain.
- Increase in range of motion (ROM).
- Ability to carry out functional activities of daily living that were previously difficult. This will vary from person to person in terms of what is important in their life. Make sure your outcomes are centred on what is important for the client NOT what you think should be important. For example, if their intended outcome is to relax due to personal stresses at work, they will not thank you if you spend the entire session doing painful fascial work on their caesarean scar.

Your outcome should aim to be **SMART**:

- **S**pecific
- **M**easurable
- **A**chievable
- **R**ealistic
- **T**ime line: how long before they can expect to see a difference; this may be different depending on the condition, severity, length of time experienced and your experience of treating similar conditions.

The question 'How would you like to feel after the session that is different from how you feel now?' can be very helpful, especially if your client is having trouble formulating their needs. This is also a great question to ask in relaxation massage to get a clearer outcome.

Assessment: the HOPRS approach

The HOPRS acronym is a fantastic way to remember the key components of an effective consultation (Lowe 2006).

- **H**ealth history questions (usually known as your case history or medical intake).
- **O**bservations (i.e. of posture).
- **P**alpation (of soft tissues including muscles and fascia).
- **R**OM tests. These help us to establish the nature of the soft tissue problem and specifically whether there is tissue damage to joints, ligaments or muscles. ROM tests are subdivided into active, passive and resisted.
- **S**pecial orthopaedic tests that help us to identify problems more precisely.

Your skill set may also mean that you carry out other forms of assessment to help determine the nature of the problem, e.g. the local or general 'listening' techniques used in visceral manipulation, arcing used in cranial work, scanning the chakras for imbalances or taking the pulse if you are trained in traditional Chinese medicine. Depending on your skill, knowledge and scope of practice you may focus more on some areas of the above assessment process than others. However, whether you are doing relaxation massage, sports massage, energy work or pregnancy massage, some form of assessment is vital. You always need to know why your client has come to you, what they are expecting from the treatment and a baseline for any changes you make.

A good assessment process has a dual purpose: it is both holistic and reductionist. You are trying to build a broad picture of your client and their life while looking for specific clues that will help you address the problem they are presenting. Schedule at least half an hour extra on your first appointment with someone to allow adequate time for this. It can also be useful to schedule a longer time on the fourth treatment to review progress and do a more thorough re-assessment.

Health history

A good listener is not only popular everywhere, but after a while he knows something.
WILSON MIZNER

> *When I have been listened to and when I have been heard, I am able to re-perceive my world in a new way and to go on. It is astonishing how elements that seem insoluble become soluble when someone listens, how confusions that seem irremediable turn into relatively clear flowing streams when one is heard. I have deeply appreciated the times that I have experienced this sensitive, empathic, concentrated listening.*
> CARL ROGERS

Taking a case history is often the first real contact you have with your client. This is the point where you can really start to hear your client's story, make a connection with them as a human being and start your detective journey gathering clues as to their physical, emotional and spiritual make-up. It is also the point where your client will start to make judgements about you, your level of skills and professionalism, and ultimately whether they will come back for further treatment. Taking time to do a thorough case history is an investment not only in your client's welfare but your business. Your job at this point is to draw out the information that you require to make an assessment of your client's needs and, most importantly, what outcome they would like to see from this treatment or series of treatments. It is your task as a professional to figure out how you can achieve this outcome and realistically how many sessions this may take.

You can start your assessment the minute your client walks through your door. Getting a sense of how your clients move and present themselves can help you to build up an overall picture of how to make a connection and give the best treatment. Think of both structural and emotional considerations:

- **Structural**: are they able to walk, sit, etc. easily. Do they struggle taking their coat off or getting up the stairs?

- **Emotional**: what are your first impressions? Is your client confident, nervous or frightened. Are they taking ownership of their mind–body or are they looking for someone to fix them?

- Make these observations while keeping an 'open mindset' and be prepared to be proved wrong about your initial assumptions once you have found out more about your client. Don't make judgements about what your client needs or the

source of their issues – the burly bodybuilder doesn't necessarily need a sporty massage with loads of stretching while the medical doctor might love some energy work.

Listening skills in assessment: the principles of metta and unconditional positive regard

Most people in pain need to feel heard. This is your big opportunity to make a lasting connection with your client; a meaningful relationship is the real reason why someone comes back to you. Remember to keep an open mind and look for 'the face behind the face' – clients may have an outward show of defensiveness or cheerfulness but what lies behind that? What is it in this person that helps you to understand and accept them fully? One of the principles of our own practice is the belief in the power of 'unconditional positive regard'; a term coined by humanistic psychologist Carl Rogers to denote the basic acceptance and support of a person regardless of what the person says or does. This fantastic quote illustrates Roger's approach beautifully:

> *Years ago, I was invited to a seminar given by Carl Rogers. I had never read his work, but I knew that the seminar, attended by a group of therapists, was about 'unconditional positive regard'. At the time I was highly sceptical about this idea, but I attended the seminar anyway. I left it transformed. Roger's theories arose out of his practice, and his practice was intuitive and natural to him. In the seminar, he tried to analyse what he was doing for us as he did it. He wanted to give a demonstration of unconditional positive regard in a therapeutic session. One of the therapists volunteered to serve as the subject. As Rogers turned to the volunteer and was about to start the session, he suddenly pulled himself up, turned back to us, and said, 'I realise there's something I do before I start a session. I let myself know that I am enough. Not perfect. Perfect wouldn't be enough. But I am human, and that is enough. There is nothing this man can say or do that I can't feel in myself. I can be with him. I am enough.' I was stunned by this. It felt as if some old wound in me, some fear of not being good enough, had come to an end. I knew, inside myself, that what he had said was absolutely true: I am not perfect, but I am enough.*
> REMEN 1989

Unconditional positive regard is similar to the Buddhist principle of metta (loving kindness), i.e. benevolence towards all beings, without discrimination, that is free of selfish attachment. It is a strong, sincere wish for the happiness of all beings. It is worth remembering that loving kindness lies at the very basis of massage practices. Traditional Eastern massage bodywork, such as Thai massage, is essentially spiritual in nature and considered to be a meditative application of metta.

Key points of effective listening skills

Effective listening skills rely on both good verbal and non-verbal communication and several key elements are involved (Mindtools.com (n.d.)):

1 **Pay attention**: this may seem obvious but you need to give the client your undivided attention, and let them know they are being fully heard. Give warm and accepting eye contact and have an open body posture. Don't sit behind a desk or fold your arms as this instantly creates a non-verbal barrier to opening up. Develop the ability of forming a connection with your client while jotting down relevant information; you may wish to use key words that you can flesh out after the session. Your client's perception of you will be greatly influenced by your body language during the intake; you are likely to gain more information if you are not glued to your note taking during this process.

2 **Show that you're listening**: use your own body language and gestures to convey your attention. Nods, smiles and small encouraging verbal comments like 'yes' and 'uh huh' help the speaker to open up and give you the full story as they feel that you are genuinely interested. **See Figure 5.1**

3 **Reflecting back, mirroring and paraphrasing**: the skills of mirroring and paraphrasing are useful communication skills to help fully draw out your client's story. Mirroring involves repeating back

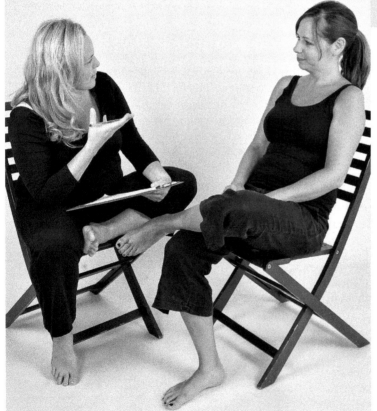

Figure 5.1

keywords or phrases to show you have understood and to encourage them to continue. For example:

Client: My back has been hurting for such a long time I can't even remember when it started.
Massage therapist (nodding sympathetically): It's been a long time, hasn't it?

Mirroring can feel a little awkward at first but is an effective tool; it should be short and simple, repeating back the last few words or keywords that the client has said. Be careful not to over mirror which can be extremely irritating. Anyone who has been on an introductory counselling course will be familiar with the hilarious parody of students bobbing their heads, uh-huh(ing) and mirroring simple requests such as 'Shall I close the window?' (Response: I hear you saying you want to close the window.) As with all good skills, moderation is key!

Paraphrasing involves reflecting back what the speaker has said using different words, showing that you are really trying to understand the meaning of what is said. Sometimes this involves taking in a large amount of information and summarising the meaning. For example, a client has been talking for 15 minutes about the history of their back pain, the times when it has been really bad, the medics and therapists she has seen, etc.

Massage therapist: so it seems like this has been an issue for a really long time and the pain tends to get worse at stressful times of your life when you are feeling overwhelmed and unsupported. And that the lack of a clear diagnosis of why it hurts so much has been really frustrating for you.
Client: Yes that's right actually. I never really thought about the fact that it gets worse when I'm stressed.

4 **Asking questions**: in general you should be listening more than talking; don't interrupt, correct the speaker or start talking about your own experiences. Use questions wisely to get the information you need. There are two main types of question that are useful in the assessment process:

A **Open questions**: these are ones that require more than one word answers. They are great for drawing people out and getting them to expand on what they were saying. Examples of open questions are:

a What does the pain feel like when your back hurts?

b Is there a pattern to when you get the headaches?

c Was there anything else going on for you when you first started to get the IBS symptoms?

d Tell me exactly what happened in the accident when you hurt your knee.

B **Closed questions**: these require only a yes or no answer. These are useful if you want to bring the assessment to a close, narrow down on specific information or make sense out of a rambling client story! Examples are:

a So the pain started last June?

b The pain is worse at night, is that right?

c So although you said you didn't do much exercise you do cycle to work every day?

Red flags, yellow flags

Apart from being a good tongue twister (try saying red flags, yellow flags 10 times quickly), the concept of red flags and yellow flags in assessment is important in understanding the nature of a client's pain condition.

Red flags are warning signs to the practitioner that factors other than musculoskeletal issues may be at work. For example, these would include signs such as the pain being unrelenting even at night, accompanying systemic ill health, unexplained weight loss or a recent accident. The presence of one or more red flags in musculoskeletal pain conditions may be indicative of a more serious pathology and in these cases the client should be referred back to a medical practitioner to have this checked out. Massage therapy may still be appropriate but the primary cause of the complaint should be identified first (Chaitow 2006).

Yellow flags are indicators of psychosocial factors that may be involved in perpetuating the pain issue. In acute situations, unaddressed yellow flags may mean that the pain is more likely to become chronic. In existing chronic pain conditions these elements can be a barrier to recovery. Identifying yellow flags can help focus treatment by emphasising self care and education measures in addition to the hands on work. As we have seen from the chapter on chronic pain, in cases where there are many psychosocial factors at work, the issues are not just 'in the tissues'.

A great mnemonic for remembering the major yellow flags is the 'ABCDEF and W' sound bite (Gifford 2002, Sheffieldbackpain.com (n.d.)). Gentle and open questions around the areas below will help you to tease out the role that psychosocial factors may be playing in perpetuating your client's pain condition:

- **Attitudes:** what is the client's attitude towards the current problem? Is the client optimistic that they will get better with appropriate help and are they expecting to return to normal activities? Or is the client fearful and catastrophising about the future?

- **Beliefs:** unhelpful beliefs about the pain can be absorbed from friends, the media or misinformed professionals. The most common misguided client belief is that they have something serious causing their problem, such as cancer or arthritis. Others include the fear that the condition will lead to permanent disability and that they should rest or not work.

- **Compensation:** is the patient awaiting payment for an accident or work related injury? This in itself can lead to subconscious or non-deliberate perpetuation of the pain condition. Enquiring into the stress of dealing with legal issues can be very revealing.

- **Diagnosis:** there is an emerging body of evidence that what clinicians say to clients may help to create chronic pain situations. For example, complicated diagnoses, terrifying visuals of crumbling spines or 'popped' discs are likely to make the client feel hopeless, out of control and reliant on an expert. Ask the client what they have been told and what it means to them. Try and steer the client towards more accurate and empowering information that emphasises their own role in returning to health.

- **Emotions:** clients with high levels of stress or other emotional difficulties, such as ongoing depression and/or anxiety states, are more likely to have chronic pain issues. It is important that these are not overlooked in the quest to find the soft tissue issues or structural causes of the pain.

- **Family:** it is interesting to ask about the role of the immediate family as both under-supportive and over-protective attitudes can play a role in perpetuating the pain.

- **Work:** understanding your client's work situation can be very helpful. On the one hand, lack of a meaningful occupation can exacerbate pain states. This led Gifford (2002) to state that 'getting people back to work or keeping them in work if at all possible should be a major goal of physiotherapy'. On the other hand many clients can end up trapped in jobs where they feel unsupported, bored or bullied which also leads to persistence of pain conditions. The self-employed are not exempt and are often the worse culprits for driving themselves into the ground and then experiencing bad backs, chronic headaches or repetitive strain injury (RSI). Ring any bells anyone? In these situations, encouraging the client to take a holiday or proactive measures to reduce their workload can be very helpful.

Areas to cover in your case history

- A consultation form is useful to help you remember what areas to cover in the assessment. There are many different types of consultation form; we generally recommend you design your own as this will suit your needs best. Remember a form is only as good as the way it is used. We are not fans of using tick-box forms for clients to fill in themselves (unless you are going to explore this in detail later). People do not fit into tick-box forms and want to know that you have heard them. Leave plenty of room for comments on your paperwork. Examples of helpful questions to ask or include on your consultation form can be found in the Self-Care Resources (available online at uk.singingdragon.com/catalogue/book/9781909141230)

- Talk to your client, using the form as a guide rather than firing questions at them. Much like your massage, the assessment should feel like a flowing dance of true communication. If your client has a tendency to talk a lot about irrelevant matters, try and gently draw them back to the relevant topics without being abrupt. Open questions can help to draw out more minimalist clients whereas closed questions can help to narrow things down with those who tend to ramble.

When taking a case history there are several main areas you should aim to cover:

1. The current pain condition itself

If your client is presenting with some kind of pain problem you will need to be focussed with your questioning to obtain the information you need to treat them effectively. Use the mnemonic OPQRS to help:

- **Origin of the pain.** When did the pain begin? Was there a precipitating factor, e.g. accident, fall or emotional trauma? Has it been going on for weeks, months or years? If clients describe a physical cause (e.g. falling off a horse) it is also helpful to ask 'Was anything else going on for you at that time?' This will help you to evaluate whether stress or emotional factors were also involved. Time after time, I find that the horse fall coincided with parental divorce, bereavement or childhood abuse. Remember it is far easier for clients to point to physical rather than emotional factors as being causative in their pain.

- **Provocation:** does anything make the pain worse, e.g. cold, movement or getting stressed? Conversely does anything make the pain better, e.g. warm bath, moving around, etc.

- **Quality of the pain.** This can help you identify the source of the problem. Nerve pain tends to be tingling or electric. Chronic soft tissue pain can be dull and achy whereas more recent acute muscle pain can be sharp and stabbing. Pain of a muscular origin is often aggravated or relieved by movement. Beware of pain that is deep and unrelenting, even in sleep, and make sure that other causes have been ruled out. This type of pain can often be a sign of a more serious medical issue.

- **Radiate:** does the pain stay in one place or does it radiate to different parts of the body? Referred pain can indicate either the presence of trigger points or nerve pain if it is more electrical in nature.

- **Site:** where is the pain exactly? Get your client to point to the body area to avoid misunderstanding. You would be amazed at client's perceptions of where their 'hip' or 'back' is! It can also be helpful to have a picture of a body on your case history form where the client can draw in the areas of pain.

Find out if the client has been given a diagnosis for their pain state and by whom, and if they understand what it means. People can be notorious for self-diagnosing, e.g. 'It's arthritis, my mother had it'. Unfortunately medics and other practitioners can also be prone to handing out unhelpful or confusing diagnoses that often have no basis or relevance to what might be going on.

2. Past or concurrent pain conditions or medical factors

Make sure you also ask about other pain conditions that may be current or have occurred in the past. This can help you assess the impact of central sensitisation or other factors that may be relevant. Clients often also forget to mention other conditions you may be able to help them with, such as digestive problems or headaches. A good checklist includes asking about:

- Headaches.

- Menstrual pain.

- Digestive issues: any constipation/diarrhoea or IBS type symptoms.

- Any other episodes of the current pain or other pain problems. Find out how it was treated and how long it took to resolve.

- Any accidents or operations: make sure you enquire about any scar tissue as this can also be contributing to the pain issue.

3. The role of stress, emotions and other psychosocial factors

Manual therapists often minimise the effects of psychological and social factors in pain conditions, seeing them as secondary to structural or soft tissue factors. Yet as we have seen 'psychosocial factors are stronger predictors of outcome than any individual biomedical measures' (Gifford 2002). Although we are not counsellors, massage therapists need to develop the ability to ask sensitively about these areas to assess their likely influence in the presentation of pain. A good question to ask is 'Where would you put your stress levels at the moment on a scale of 1–10.' Then use this as a springboard for some open questions about the role of stress or emotions in the client's life. Helpful follow-up questions for example could include:

- Is it home or work factors that are most stressful for you at the moment?

- Sounds like you have a lot going on at work? Do you feel like you are getting any support around those issues?

- Do you have any strategies for helping manage your stress levels?

- Sounds like you have been feeling pretty anxious since your road accident? Have you had a chance to talk that through with anyone like a supportive friend or counsellor?

Ask questions using the areas outlined with the ABC-DEFW mnemonic, outlined earlier in this chapter, in order to gather information about psychosocial factors that might be affecting the pain state.

4. Functional limitations

Find out how the pain is affecting the client's daily life – in other words, what is the client not able to do that they would like to. This might be sporting activities (running and cycling) or less immediately obvious things such as being able to pick up their child without pain or reach the top shelf of the kitchen cupboard without wincing.

5. Physical activity

Assessing how much your client moves during the day and in what way can be very revealing. Inactivity is one of the biggest causes of chronic pain conditions. Does your client exercise? What type and how often? Do they enjoy it or does it feel like a chore? How does exercise make them feel afterwards? How do they get around during the day: walk, cycle or drive? Even moderate levels of physical activity can impact positively on pain. Rather than asking 'How often do you exercise?', which can lead to an immediate feeling of inadequacy for the non-sporty, you may find questions such as 'How do you spend your day' are more helpful and have a greater likelihood of eliciting an honest answer!

Observation

> *Seeing is touch at a distance.*
> IDA ROLF

This part of the assessment process begins the minute you see your client. How do they walk, negotiate the stairs or take off their coat? Are they easy in their body or are there areas of apparent restriction? How do they seem emotionally: do they have a good vital energy or do they seem tired and low? The more you use your powers of observation, the more you are able to develop this faculty to your advantage. Ida Rolf, the founder of Rolfing, was reputedly able to assess the exact location of a lumbar herniation in an unknown client walking through the door in a heavy overcoat.

It is also useful to carry out a more structured process of body reading and the exact way you do this often depends on your training or particular bodywork discipline. Physiotherapists, osteopaths and other structurally orientated bodyworkers are usually trained to observe the body in a systematic fashion, noting for example, relative heights of the shoulders, tilts to the pelvis, rotations of the legs, etc. This can give clues as to what areas of soft tissue may be tight or restricted. For example, a laterally rotated leg could indicate a tight piriformis muscle that may be the cause of a client's sciatica by entrapping the sciatic nerve.

A quick way of assessing visually is simply to look at your client while they are standing and notice any gross, observable differences between the two sides of their body (left to right and front to back). Which areas seem tight or drawn together? These may well be areas you need to work to free up muscular or fascial adhesions.

Observation is a useful skill but remember it is only one part of the assessment process. Recent research indicates that structural considerations may not be as important in our client's pain problem as previously believed (Lederman 2010). So your client's unequal leg length, scoliotic spine or anteriorly tipped pelvis may be one piece of the jigsaw puzzle but certainly not the whole picture. Overall these factors are likely to carry less weight than the psychosocial factors identified in the case history. **See Figure 5.2**

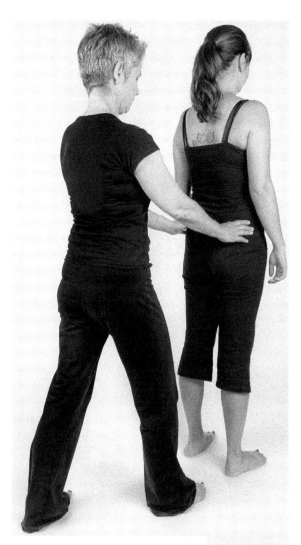

Figure 5.2

Our palpation skills need not be limited to muscle and fascia. A skilled therapist will learn to appreciate delicate movements, such as the cranial or visceral rhythm, or subtle energies, such as the chakras and the meridians. This is what makes massage so magical.

Assessment through palpation should take place during the whole of the treatment not just during intake. At Jing we say 'All assessment is treatment and all treatment assessment.' Every time you touch soft tissue you should be assessing whether it is healthy or riddled with trigger points or fascial adhesions. As you become more skilled at palpation you will find that assessment blends naturally into treatment and re-assessment. For example, while treating a muscle you compress it slowly while feeling for trigger points, and then apply compression and feel the release as the tissue changes. **See Figure 5.3**

Range of motion (ROM) tests

ROM tests assist in the systematic analysis of individual movements that may be involved in the pain condition.

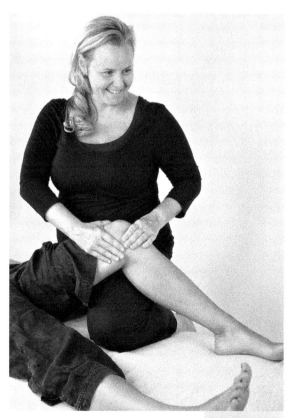

Figure 5.3

Palpation

Palpation cannot be learned by reading or listening; it can only be learned by palpation.
Frymann 1963

Palpation is truly one of the most wonderful tools in our repertoire and is a skill that we develop constantly in our work. There are no limits to palpation as an assessment tool. As we develop our sensitivity as body-workers, we find that we are able to feel more subtle differences in tissues and energy fields.

They can help to delineate which soft tissue structures may be involved in the issue, e.g. whether the problem is primarily due to damage of the ligaments, muscles, tendons or joints. ROM tests also provide a benchmark for re-assessing after treatment.

ROM tests are usually carried out on the major problem joint and the ones that are located proximally and distally. So for an elbow issue, also assess the glenohumeral joint and wrist. For back problems assess the cervical spine and coxal (hip) joint.

ROM tests can be subdivided into:

- **Active ROM tests**: the therapist instructs the client to actively perform each possible movement for a problematic joint. For example, to assess the neck, the client would be instructed to perform flexion, extension, lateral flexion and rotation. The therapist will be observing factors such as ROM and pain for each of the movements. **See Figure 5.4**

- **Passive ROM tests**: for these, the client is completely passive with the therapist moving the body part into the various ranges of movement. For example, to passively assess the shoulder, the client is supine and the therapist takes the weight of the arm and moves it into flexion, extension, abduction, adduction, lateral and medial rotation. Again the therapist is noting ROM and any pain

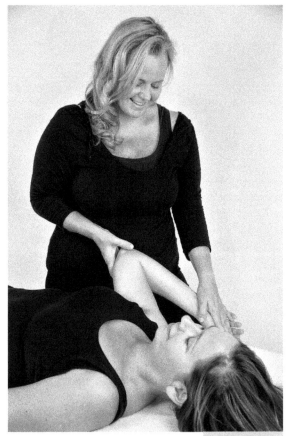

Figure 5.5

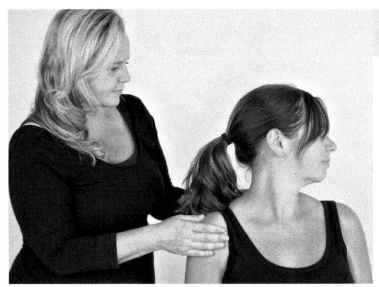

Figure 5.4

on each movement. Passive ROM helps to assess non-contractile structures such as a joints or ligaments. **See Figure 5.5**

- **Resistive tests**: with these tests, the client is instructed to actively engage the muscles in order to take their joint into a certain movement but the therapist resists the actual motion. This causes an isometric contraction of contractile tissues such as muscles or tendons. In this case the therapist is looking for signs of pain or weakness. Resistive tests help to ascertain whether there is a problem with the muscles or tendons.

Special orthopaedic tests

Special orthopaedic tests help to drill down further as to the nature of the problem and can also help to isolate a specific condition. For example, Adson's and Wright's manoeuvres can establish the likelihood of thoracic outlet syndrome. **See Figure 5.6**

Introducing orthopaedic testing to your assessment process

It is beyond the scope of this text to go into detail about ROM and special orthopaedic testing but we would highly recommend Whitney Lowe's excellent text for massage therapists on this subject (Lowe 2006).

For a good introductory step we would suggest using active ROM testing in all your treatments as this will give you an accurate benchmark for measuring which movements are painful and restricted. These movements can be re-tested after the session to show yourself and the client any subsequent differences.

Some tips for active ROM testing:

- Make sure you remember to include all the ranges of movement at a joint (include these on your consultation form so you are sure not to forget).

- Show the client the movement clearly and cleanly and correct them if they do it differently than you have demonstrated. For example, when assessing neck ROM it is very common for a client to take their trunk into the movement in an attempt to get further.

- When testing the arms you can assess both sides at once. This enables you to easily make a comparison and is more time efficient.

- Remember to test the joint above and below. Many upper limb problems come from the shoulder or neck.

- Remember to re-test at the end of the treatment to see if you have made a difference.

Benchmarking

During your assessment and treatment, use measurable benchmarks to determine whether your treatment is effective. These can include pain scales and measures of ROM. You should obtain benchmarks before and after treatment to see if you have made a difference:

- **Pain scales**: use a subjective pain scale of 1–10. Ask your client where the pain is now and also how high it goes or when it changes. Clients

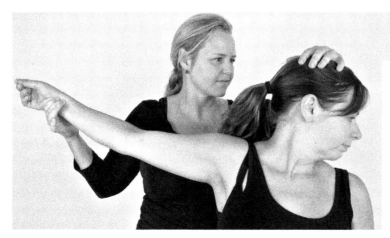

Figure 5.6

forget what it felt like to be in pain, and therefore neglect to give you the credit for getting them out of it! Clients with long-term chronic health conditions, such as fibromyalgia, also find it difficult to see any difference; reminding them of progress over months or in some cases years can be extremely helpful.

- **ROM**: use active ROM testing to determine lack of ROM or pain for specific movements.

- **Activities of daily living**: another good benchmark is to find out from your client what they are unable to do easily in their everyday life, e.g. putting on their seatbelt or picking up their small child. On subsequent treatments you can ask them if this has improved. Your client's ability to carry out functional activities will be far more important to them than whether they have clinically achieved a few more degrees of movement.

Bringing it all together

When you have gathered all of your information from the various aspects of your assessment process you are in a position to make an informed judgement about a treatment plan. Make sure you have really listened to your client, not just with your ears but your informed touch and that your assessment is not based on snap judgements. Be prepared to modify your treatment plan as you go along depending on what you find with further exploration of the tissues and how your client responds.

From your assessment you should have a clear idea of what soft tissue structures might be involved in the pain condition and also the potential role of central sensitisation and psychosocial factors, such as stress or anxiety. It can be helpful to distinguish urgent issues from underlying important issues. For example, with low back pain the urgent issue is 'My back hurts; I need to be out of pain as soon as possible' and the underlying issue may be 'I am chronically stressed and overworked and feel out of control with my life.' A good treatment plan will aim to treat and help resolve the urgent issue while informing and educating about the underlying issues.

When you have finished your assessment take some time to discuss your approach and treatment plan with your client. Explain what you are going to do in the session, how you will address the urgent issue and explain how the 'urgent' issue fits with the 'underlying important issues'. Explain exactly what is going to happen in the treatment, the position the client should take on the table and how they will be draped. Ensure a safe space emotionally and physically by following the guidelines outlined in Chapter 3.

Treatment planning using the HFMAST approach

As this chapter outlines, the assessment process is as much part of your treatment as your hands-on work. Research has shown that using empathy, developing a therapeutic alliance with your client and utilising good listening skills will enhance your ability to decrease your client's pain.

The assessment process is also a good opportunity to start educating your client about their body, the neuroscience of pain, and to explain how they can feel more in control of their situation.

Of course, a thorough assessment should also allow you to gather all the information necessary to devise an appropriate treatment plan. Your treatment plan should emphasise not only the hands-on work but also selfcare, education and empowerment strategies.

The approach outlined in this book simplifies the treatment planning element by providing a suggested series of techniques to use in common musculoskeletal conditions. The combination of modalities used in the HFMAST protocols aims to reduce any peripheral input (such as trigger points and fascial adhesions) that may be contributing to perpetuation of central sensitisation. We know that massage in itself can help to decrease emotional components of anxiety or depression that can be key in maintaining pain states. The emphasis on self care also enables the therapist to educate and inform around strategies such as pacing, countering unhelpful beliefs or exercise.

Think of the HFMAST approach like a really good recipe which outlines the ingredients needed to get a result. The skill of treatment planning lies in the mix of the various ingredients. Clients where central sensitisation is a strong component of the pain state will need more emphasis on pacing, self care and changing unhelpful thought patterns. Other clients may need more fascial work and less trigger point work.

A general blueprint for treatment planning is as follows:

- Once a pain area is identified, treat all the muscles around the joint as outlined in the chapter protocols using the HFMAST formula as a guide.

- Treat the client once a week for up to 6 weeks. In most pain conditions you should see a decrease in pain by week 3.

- Once you have seen a decrease in pain, lengthen the time between treatments.

- When a reduction in pain has been fully achieved, recommend that your client moves onto a maintenance schedule of once a month, or whatever suits. In our experience, people rarely have one musculoskeletal problem in their lifetime. It is much easier to keep someone out of pain than to treat an already established problem. Regular massage should be an essential part of everyone's health care routine.

- If you have not seen any change by week 3 you will need to alter your approach. This may involve changing the mix of the ingredients of the HFMAST approach (more fascial work or more emphasis on self care). If you feel the problem is really beyond your scope of practice then refer to another appropriate professional.

References

Amtamassage.org 2014 Consumer Survey Fact Sheet – American Massage Therapy Association. Available at: http://www.amtamassage.org/research/Consumer-Survey-Fact-Sheets.html [accessed 17 August 2014].

Chaitow L 2006 Making sense of back pain, I. Massage Bodywork Magazine. Available at: http://www.massagetherapy.com/articles/index.php/article_id/1186/Making-Sense-of-Back-Pain-I [accessed 19 May 2014].

Ferreira PH et al 2013 The therapeutic alliance between clinicians and patients predicts outcome in chronic low back pain. Physical Therapy 93(4):470–478.

Frymann V 1963 Palpation – Its study in the workshop. In: Academy of Applied Osteopathy Yearbook. Newark,

Ohio: Academy of Applied Osteopathy, pp. 16–30. Quoted in Chaitow L 2008 The essence of palpation: how do you feel? Massagetoday.com. Available at: http://www.massagetoday.com/mpacms/mt/article.php?id=13822 [accessed 18 August 2014].

Gifford L 2002 Perspectives on the biopsychosocial model, part 2: the shopping basket approach. In Touch, The Journal of the Organisation of Chartered Physiotherapists in Private Practice 99(Spring Issue):11–22.

Griffin SJ et al 2004 Effect on health-related outcomes of interventions to alter the interaction between patients and practitioners: a systematic review of trials. Annals of Family Medicine 2(6):595–608.

Hall AM et al 2010 The influence of the therapist–patient relationship on treatment outcome in physical rehabilitation: a systematic review. Physical Therapy 90(8):1099–1110. Available at: http://ptjournal.apta.org/content/90/8/1099.abstract [accessed 12 May 2014].

Kaplan SH et al 1989 Assessing the effects of physician–patient interactions on the outcomes of chronic disease. Medical Care 27(supplement 3):S110–127.

Kaptchuk TJ et al 2008 Components of placebo effect: randomised controlled trial in patients with irritable bowel syndrome. BMJ (Clinical Research Edn) 336:999–1003.

Kelley JM et al 2014 The influence of the patient–clinician relationship on healthcare outcomes: a systematic review and meta-analysis of randomized controlled trials. PloS ONE 9(4):e94207.

Lederman E 2010 The fall of the structural model. Available at: http://www.cpdo.net/Lederman_The_fall_of_the_postural-structural-biomechanical_model.pdf [accessed 30 March 2014].

Levinson W 1997 Physician–patient communication: the relationship with malpractice claims among primary care physicians and surgeons. JAMA: The Journal of the American Medical Association 277(7):553.

Lowe W 2006 Orthopedic Assessment in Massage Therapy. Sisters, OR: Daviau Scott.

Mindtools.com (n.d.) Active listening: hear what people are really saying. Available at: http://www.mindtools.com/CommSkll/ActiveListening.htm [accessed 18 August 2014].

Rattray F et al 2000 Clinical Massage Therapy, 1st edn. Toronto: Talus Inc.

Remen RN 1989 The search for healing. In: Carlson R, Shield B (eds) Healers on Healing, 1st edn. Los Angeles: JP Tarcher, p. 93.

Sheffieldbackpain.com (n.d.) Yellow flags in back pain. Sheffield Back Pain. Available at: http://www.sheffieldbackpain.com/professional-resources/learning/in-detail/yellow-flags-in-back-pain [accessed 18 August 2014].

Soukhanov A 1999 Encarta world English dictionary. New York: St Martin's Press.

Wampold B Qualities and actions of effective therapists. American Psychological Association. Available at: https://www.apa.org/education/ce/effective-therapists.pdf [accessed 24 November 2014].

6

The warm-up act: the power of hot and cold in advanced clinical massage

After you have completed a precise and targeted assessment, the first step in the Jing HFMAST approach for the treatment of pain is the application of hot or cold. This is literally your warm-up act for the great techniques to follow.

The use of hot and cold as a therapeutic modality has been around for centuries. Physiotherapists, naturopaths and osteopaths are well aware of the efficacy of thermal modalities in bodywork, as was your mother who gave you a hot water bottle to soothe your sore belly when you were a child. Hot and cold were used by our ancestors to treat everything from strains and sprains to fevers and alcoholism. Many early proponents claimed miraculous cures from the use of hot and cold, such as the hardy Sebastian Kneipp who, during the early 1800s in Germany, cured himself of tuberculosis by immersing himself in the freezing cold Danube River (Kneipp (n.d.)). Kneipp subsequently became an enthusiastic proponent of the use of hydrotherapy (administration of hot and cold via water to cure illness) and, in an attempt to prove that indeed there was a method in his madness, refined his treatments to include cold rinses, hot and cold contrast baths, hot and cold wet packs and compresses. These are all still routinely used today.

For the clinical massage therapist, those of you who use hot stones will already be aware of how the deeply relaxing effect of heat can enable you to work deeper but not harder, not only improving your outcomes but saving your own hands and body. Likewise, having a handy cold pack in your clinic can soothe a painful and sore injury within minutes and teach your client the value of this easy and inexpensive self-help technique. Clients and therapists alike enthuse about the power of hot and cold, particularly when applied dynamically using stones and blended with other clinical massage techniques such as fascial work, trigger point work, acupressure and stretching. See the boxes on the right for a few comments from Jing therapists.

Despite the popularity of hot and cold, there still are many misunderstandings about when and how each

One of my clients had been in chronic pain with his neck after whiplash in two consecutive car crashes EIGHT years ago. He had never felt safe or comfortable enough to have anyone touch his neck. He came to me and we worked gently on the area with the heat of the stones. He was so relaxed by the use of the stones but tensed up as soon as I put my (loving!) hands on his neck. We worked very deeply into trigger points and stretching with the stones and the results were incredible. After only two sessions he was pain free.

I have had massages with a therapist who did the stone course with you. I suffer from back pain that ranges from dull to piercing. Normally I would go for a purely therapeutic massage, but wanted to try the stones. Not only was the treatment amazing, but I had more pain relief from the use of placement stones and heated stones used to strip the muscles than I have had from any massage in a long time. While I adore just about every type of massage, the therapeutic qualities of hot stone fusion massage outstrip them all. I got a relaxation massage and a pain relief massage all in the same 85-minute session!

As a writer, I spend long periods sitting at my PC and have experienced a succession of different types of pain in my back and shoulders. After just one session of hot stone fusion massage, my back has improved and my shoulders haven't felt so good in years. Fantastic!

modality should be used. In addition, recent research has shown some traditional beliefs to be without substantiation and it is worthwhile taking a tour through the science and evidence of thermotherapy (use of heat), cryotherapy (use of cold or ice) and contrast bathing (alternation of hot and cold).

Thermotherapy: the helping hand of heat in the chronic pain conundrum

Heat can be used very effectively in cases of chronic pain. The best definition of chronic pain is pain that has persisted beyond the usual healing time for an injury and is characterised by being dull, achy or long standing. In our experience this is a common phenomenon in the massage therapist's clinic and we are much more often confronted with the conundrum of chronic pain than dealing with recent acute issues. If you have a busy clinic you are probably well acquainted with obstinate back pain, neck pain, repetitive strain injury (RSI), plantar fasciitis and other conditions that have persisted beyond an expected healing time.

It is fair to say that chronic pain is much more complex to treat than acute pain and usually requires a multi-faceted approach, as outlined in this book. Adding heat into the mix right at the beginning of your treatment can enhance your outcomes significantly.

The positive effects for heat in chronic pain cases can be summarised as follows:

- **Psychological effects**: heat makes us feel nurtured, relaxed, cared for and positive, which are attributes we want our clients to associate with our treatments. If our clients feel safe under our hands, their bodies relax and let us in to do vital therapeutic work without resistance. We instinctively feel that heat has a 'feel good' factor. My best friend said to me once that if she ever feels out of sorts she just has a bath and it always makes her feel better! Following her advice has stood me in good stead and, likewise, applying heat in a clinical situation invariably has a positive effect. Research has shown that some of the positive effects of heat are indeed modulated via the brain, which suggests that heat works more from a 'top down' process rather than from its local effect on the tissues (Davis et al 1998, Yasui et al 2010).

- **Decreased muscle tightness and trigger point activity**: heat seems to have a direct effect on reducing tight muscles, which is often the primary cause of common pain conditions. Tight muscles also harbour pain referring trigger points – the bad boys of musculoskeletal pain. It seems that heat applications may reduce the firing rate of muscle spindle cells, hence reducing muscle tightness and pain (Therapeutic Modalities (n.d.)).

- **Increased circulation and reduction of rehabilitation time**: the local increase in circulation caused by heat application is thought to be beneficial in healing soft tissue injuries. Bringing fresh blood and nutrients to the areas helps maintain the optimum health of the tissues for injury repair. A 1% increase in temperature results in a 10–15% increase in local tissue metabolism (Nadler et al 2004).

- **Increased pliability of fascia**: heat applications help to improve the viscoelasticity of fascia; therefore, myofascial and therapeutic stretching procedures are much more effective if heat is applied beforehand (Klinger 2012). Heat may also have a key role in helping to restore the sliding and gliding function of fascia which if compromised can lead to myofascial pain and dysfunction. A key player in maintaining the free movement of fascial layers on each other is a lubricating substance called hyaluronic acid (HA). In pain syndromes, chains of HA molecules literally get entangled leading to increased viscoelasticity, tissue stiffness and decreased range of motion (ROM) (Matteini et al 2009). The HA chains can be disentangled by heat of over 40 degrees, which also confirms the role of moist heat as preparation for fascial work (Hammer 2014). This is exactly what is advocated by the Jing HFMAST approach.

- **Decrease in perception of pain**: we naturally turn to the healing properties of heat when in pain. Hot water bottles, baths, jacuzzis and hot compresses are common self-care measures for everything from sore backs to period pains. Heat can help to decrease the individual perception of pain and enable us to feel in control of our pain responses.

Ice for injury: the use of cold

Cold has always traditionally been recommended for acute injuries, i.e. those where the injury is recent (usually less than 72 hours) and characterised by inflammation, swelling, lack of mobility and pain. A recently sprained ankle is the classic textbook example of an acute injury. Most of us are familiar with the RICE protocol of applying rest, ice, compression and elevation for bruising, swelling and pain, and in our own households the freezer cabinet has been raided many times over the years for bags of frozen peas. (Even though we have both been massage therapists for a quarter of a century, neither of us ever actually seems to have an ice pack in the house.)

Massage therapists often get confused about which injuries are acute and as a result sometimes use ice or cold inappropriately. A good example is sudden onset low back pain where therapists are often terrified of mysterious 'inflammation' that is not obvious but they are convinced must be there. Approximately 85% of low back pain is actually known as 'non-specific' – in other words we have no idea what the cause is. There is no injury and therefore no inflammation!

Clinical experience suggests that trigger points and myofascial restrictions are key components of this type of pain, and such soft tissue restrictions actually respond much better to heat. In these cases ice may not be useful as it can trigger the spasm of already overly tight muscles and cause those trigger points to flare up.

The use of cold packs and ice has been used in physiotherapy and sports injury relief for decades. We are all familiar with the image of an athletic trainer rushing onto the sports pitch with an ice pack to revive a fallen comrade writhing in pain. There are several physiological effects that are commonly trotted out by textbooks and teachers to support the use of ice in treating acute injury (Nadler 2004):

- **Pain reduction**: this is the main reason to apply ice to an injury. Numerous scientific papers and your own common sense back this up. Cooling the body down to 10–15 degrees results in a local anaesthetic effect.

- **Reduction in blood flow**: cold causes vasoconstriction and therefore reduces tissue metabolism.

- **Reduction in muscle soreness**: cold is believed to be of benefit in reducing certain types of muscle soreness, especially that associated with increased levels of unaccustomed exercise (known as delayed onset muscle soreness (DOMS)).

Table 6.1
Proposed physiological effects of hot and cold

	Cold	Heat
Pain	↓	↓
Spasm	↓	↓
Metabolism	↓	↑
Blood flow	↓	↑
Inflammation	↓	↑
Oedema	↓	↑
Extensibility	↓	↑

- **Cold slows down the cellular metabolic activity**. In acute injuries, the increase in cellular metabolic activity is one factor that prolongs the healing process. Using cold immediately after injury shortens the recovery period.

- **Decreased swelling (oedema)**: swelling is one of the primary causative factors in the perpetuation of acute pain. Cold is very effective in reducing oedema.

As we shall see later, not all of these proposed benefits of ice stand up to scientific scrutiny. **See Table 6.1**

Best of both worlds: hot and cold contrast applications

To get the beneficial aspects of hot and cold, the technique of 'contrast bathing' is also popular in the clinic. The use of hot and cold is alternated to a particular area. This is believed to cause a flushing of the tissue fluids and improve many of the neurological responses that will create the best environment for healing.

Although invigorating to receive, studies show that contrast bathing may be less effective than suspected. This is mainly due to the fact that the short applications of hot and cold used in contrast bathing have been shown to have little effect on deep muscle temperature. As the scientific rationale for contrast bathing depends on the supposed physiological effects of the substantial fluctuations in tissue temperature, this casts doubt on the therapeutic effectiveness of contrast therapy

(Myrer et al 1994, 1997). It seems there are no additional benefits to using contrast therapy as opposed to using hot or cold alone.

Despite this lack of evidence base for using contrast bathing, the technique remains a popular choice in rehabilitation clinics and has traditionally been employed both in treatment and self care for issues ranging from recovery of sporting injuries to hand pain. A review by Stanton et al (2003) suggested that, for hand pain, empirical evidence indicates contrast baths have a positive effect on the patient, whatever particular protocols are used. A systematic review by Breger Stanton (2009) concluded that the contrast bath procedure might increase superficial blood flow and skin temperature, though the evidence on the impact on swelling is conflicting. No relationship between these physiological effects and functional outcomes has been established. A case of 'so it improves superficial blood flow; so what?'

Hot and cold water immersion treatment is also gaining popularity as a tool for enhancing athlete recovery. Cochrane (2004) stated 'there is overwhelming anecdotal evidence for it's inclusion as a method for post exercise recovery'.

One of the theories for using contrast bathing is that it reduces swelling and removes waste products associated with the inflammatory process. However, Cochrane (2004) argues that this is 'unproven and contentious'. Quoting Myrer et al (1997), he states that a decrease in swelling is caused by the lymphatic system (not the circulatory system) taking away fluid and debris, which in turn is caused by muscle contraction or gravity. Therefore, during contrast bathing, any vasoconstriction or vasodilation in the superficial tissues that may affect the blood flow will not affect the lymphatic system.

All in all, a poor result for contrast bathing in the evidence-based research stakes. However, it is still clearly a popular choice with therapists and athletes and there is strong anecdotal evidence that the technique is useful in some situations.

What does research tell us about the use of hot and cold?

Experimentally, many studies have supported the use of hot and cold for different conditions found in the clinic.

Evidence base for the use of heat
Low back pain

Some research trials have been overwhelmingly positive in their support of the use of heat for pain reduction. In common with experiences in the clinic where effects on pain reduction can in some cases be instantaneous, one trial of 90 participants with acute low back pain found that a heated blanket significantly decreased pain immediately after application. Other trials showed the benefit of daily heat application where participants with a mix of acute and subacute low back pain had significantly reduced pain after 5 days compared with an oral placebo (French et al 2006). Heat (in the form of a continuous low level heat wrap) works even better than painkillers and anti-inflammatories for treating acute non-specific low back pain (Nadler et al 2002).

Combining heat with other known effective treatments can give even better results; this supports the Jing approach outlined in this book. One trial of 100 participants with a mix of acute and subacute low back pain found that using low level heat wrap therapy in conjunction with exercise significantly increased pain relief compared to heat alone, exercise alone or a self-help booklet. The results were quite striking with 72% of the subjects in the heat and exercise group demonstrating a return to pre-injury function compared with 20%, 20% and 19% for heat wrap, exercise and booklet, respectively (Mayer et al 2005). This is an important finding and confirms our belief in the value of self-care suggestions for clients as an important part of the client–therapist interaction. Both local heat application and encouraging exercise and movement are easy and safe suggestions for the client in pain.

In conclusion, evidence is limited but encouraging for to the use of heat in the treatment of low back pain. The gold standard of health-based evidence research, a Cochrane review on the subject (French 2006), concludes:

> *There is moderate evidence in a small number of trials that heat wrap therapy provides a small short-term reduction in pain and disability in a population with a mix of acute and sub acute low back pain, and that the addition of exercise further reduces pain and improves function. There is insufficient evidence to evaluate the effects of cold for low back pain and conflicting evidence for any differences between heat and cold for low back pain.*

Arthritis

Both rheumatoid and osteoarthritis respond favourably to hot and cold thermal application. Traditionally the view has been that cold applications should be used for the treatment of active arthritis (in an inflammatory stage) and heat treatment for less active arthritis and non-inflammatory rheumatic disorders (Berliner 1999). In general the research seems to support the use of cold as being more effective. A systematic review by Brosseau (2003) found that ice massage improved ROM, function and knee strength in subjects with knee osteoarthritis. Cold packs were less effective than ice massage overall as they decreased swelling but had no significant effect on pain. However, there may also be a role for heat in some cases as Kitay et al (2009) found that combining heat with other techniques of continuous passive motion, vibration and local heating significantly decreased pain, improved ROM and the quality of life in patients with osteoarthritis of the knee.

With regards to rheumatoid arthritis, it seems that although thermal therapy is unlikely to tackle the causes of the disease, both hot and cold can be effective for short-term pain relief. Both superficial moist heat and cryotherapy can be used as an effective pain reliever and paraffin wax baths combined with exercises also have beneficial short-term effects for clients with arthritic hands (Robinson et al 2002).

Neck pain

Yasui et al (2010) showed that application of local heat increased subjective feelings of mental relaxation and reduced neck stiffness and fatigue, also demonstrating that the process occurred not just through the direct peripheral effects of the heat on vasodilation but also through the central nervous system involved in controlling stress responses. Nadler (2004) has recommended the use of heat as a way of helping pain relief without drugs, e.g. a wearable heat wrap has been shown to be effective for patients with acute pain and may also be beneficial in patients with chronic pain. Cramer et al (2012) found that self-treatment with a mud heat pack once a day for 20 minutes was effective in relieving pain and improving sensory functioning in patients with chronic neck pain.

Cold also has its place in reducing neck spasm. Chaudhary et al (2013) showed that application of a cold pack along with exercises was a more effective intervention in upper trapezius muscle spasm than exercise alone (although not as effective as myofascial release (MFR) plus exercise).

Wrist pain

Continuous low-level heat wrap therapy has been shown to be helpful for a range of common wrist conditions, including strains and sprains, tendinosis, osteoarthritis and carpal tunnel syndrome (Michlovitz et al 2004). The wrap not only decreased pain but also increased grip strength for sprains and strains, tendinosis and osteoarthritis.

Fibromyalgia

The mysterious debilitating pain of fibromyalgia syndrome (FMS) is hugely helped in the clinic through heat treatment and these clients are often big fans of hot stone massage, especially when combined with fascial work. This is confirmed by research where a comprehensive Internet survey of over 2500 people with fibromyalgia found that heat was rated amongst one of the most effective self-help strategies along with rest, pain medications, antidepressants and hypnotics (Bennett et al 2007). Another researcher (Kurzeja 2003) was less interested in his subjects' preferences and had the bright idea of seeing whether whole body cryotherapy would be a more useful treatment than heat for FMS sufferers. Unsurprisingly, subjects with FMS did not respond too well to being subjected to temperatures of minus 110 degrees Celsius and half the subjects dropped out with panic attacks. (One does wonder how this one got past the ethics committee.) The hardy ones that did make it, however, did show some improvement in symptoms compared to those treated with heat and this led the researcher to muse dispassionately 'Thus, although only 47% of the patients tolerated the whole-body cryotherapy, the results suggest patients with fibromyalgia should test the cryotherapy in the cryo cabin, if possible.' However, as the more appealing options of mud bath or hot air used in the study also showed the same decrease in pain intensity, I think it is safe to conclude that fibromyalgia clients should stick with heat as a preferred treatment option.

Trigger point activity

Both hot and cold are commonly used in clinical situations to decrease trigger point activity and myofascial pain (Majlesi and Unalan 2010, Hong 2002). The mother of trigger point therapy, Janet Travell, was an advocate of cold and found the use of vapocoolant spray combined with stretch (known as the 'spray-and-stretch' technique) to be most effective in treating acute trigger points. She also found the same beneficial effect could be achieved by stroking with ice (Travell et al 1999). Travell and Simons also believed, from their extensive work, that central trigger points (those found in the endplate zone where muscle fibres meet nerves) respond better to heat, whereas trigger points at the distal attachments (tendon, aponeurosis and bone) may become less irritable with the application of cold (Travell et al 1999, p. 145).

From our own clinical experience, we would generally recommend heat as the best supplemental method for treating myofascial pain from trigger points, alongside the additional techniques described in the HFMAST protocol.

Fascial restrictions

As outlined above, the application of heat may enhance fascial work through increasing viscoelasticity and disentangling the HA chains implicated in myofascial pain syndromes.

Stretching and improving ROM

A combination of heat and stretching is definitely more effective than stretching alone and enables greater ROM to be achieved (Cosgray et al 2004, Funk et al 2001, Nakano et al 2012). Although there are studies that also report the effectiveness of ice in increasing ROM (Larsen et al 2013), a systematic review of both modalities by Bleakley and Costello (2013) concluded that 'Heat is an effective adjunct to developmental and therapeutic stretching techniques and should be the treatment of choice for enhancing ROM in a clinical or sporting setting.'

Thus in the clinic, heat can be an excellent complement to stretching for conditions that have resulted in severe loss of ROM such as frozen shoulder. The pain and severe limitations in ROM seen with this condition can be significantly improved with a combination of deep heat and stretching exercises. This combination works better than just stretching by itself or superficial heat and stretching (Leung and Cheing 2008).

Temporomandibular joint (TMJ) disorder

A survey of effective pain measures used with patients with TMJ disorder found both hot and cold packs (along with massage (hoorah!)) provided the greatest relief from pain (Riley et al 2007).

Menstrual pain

Unsurprisingly to most women who spend a few days a month glued to a hot water bottle, continuous low-level topical heat therapy was as effective as ibuprofen for the treatment of dysmenorrhoea (Akin et al 2001).

Evidence base for the use of cold: is this the end of an ice age?

Despite being one of the most commonly used therapeutic modalities for the treatment of acute injuries, the effectiveness of ice has been heavily questioned in recent years. The biggest blow for ice has come from one of its hitherto strongest proponents, namely the man who came up with RICE (Rest, Ice, Compression and Elevation) for the treatment of athletic injuries. Dr Gabe Mirkin coined this term in the 1970s in his best selling book *Sports Medicine* (Mirkin and Hoffman 1978) and coaches, physiotherapists and massage therapists have used the guidelines for years. However, in a recent blog post Dr Mirkin rained on his own parade by citing evidence that ice did not hasten recovery from muscle damage or add any extra benefits over the use of compression alone (Mirkin 2014).

In a U-turn from his previous stance, Mirkin suggested that ice might actually do the opposite and delay healing. The inflammatory response is crucial to healing, he argues, and should not be supressed by icing. He recommended that ice only be used immediately after injury for short 10-minute periods with 20 minutes of rest and should be discontinued after 6 hours.

Naturally this blog post sent Twitter twittering and Facebook into a frenzy with other experts jumping to disagree, opining that ice is still useful in reducing excessive swelling that can delay healing. Many athletics trainers are still firmly convinced of the benefits of ice and argue that inflammation is good but excessive swelling harmful.

RICE, MICE, PRICE and POLICE

For the clinician, the jury seems to be out about exactly how helpful ice is in treating acute injury, not to mention the other components of the RICE protocol. The traditional RICE guidelines have been revised to PRICE (Protect, Rest, Ice, Compression and Elevation) and then to MICE (Movement, Ice, Compression and Elevation) and now to POLICE (Protection, Optimal loading, Ice, Compression and Elevation). Clinicians seem unable to totally throw away a reliance on ice but opinion seems to be leaning towards the early introduction of movement in addition to compression and elevation. Ice definitely still reduces pain so there will always be a role there.

Lack of an evidence base in guidelines for the use of ice

Sports medicine textbooks abound with enthusiasm about the use of ice for acute soft tissue injury yet are lacking in consistent advice about how it should be applied. There is considerable variation in the literature regarding the recommended duration and frequency of advised treatments (MacAuley 2001). A systematic review by Bleakley et al (2004) also found an absence of evidence-based guidelines for the use of ice and studies showed wide variations in the clinical use of cryotherapy. There was also no evidence of an optimal mode or duration of treatment when using ice for soft tissue injury.

Use of cold for different clinical conditions
Acute soft tissue injury

Although widely used in clinical practice, the evidence for the effectiveness of ice in acute soft tissue injury is somewhat underwhelming. With the knack of some evidence-based research for stating the obvious, ice has definitely been proven to reduce pain for different types of soft tissue injury (Hubbard and Denegar 2004). However, the same review concluded that the use of ice to improve other clinical outcomes (improve ROM and decrease swelling) remains inconclusive and ice does not necessarily add any extra effectiveness to other treatments, such as compression or general rehab. Even the traditional wisdom of ice teamed with compression is questionable as Block (2010) concludes that 'While the effects of cold and static compression are clearly

better than no treatment, they do not appear to be directly additive.' In other words, 2 + 2 does definitely not equal a metaphorical 4 in the ice plus compression equation.

A review by Collins (2008) found insufficient evidence to suggest that cryotherapy improves clinical outcome in the management of soft tissue injuries. However, some studies showed a positive result for a cooling gel and that modest cooling reduced oedema (although prolonged cooling could cause tissue damage).

In general, ice is still a commonly used treatment strategy for acute soft tissue injury and pain. Although lacking a strong evidence base, ice is a better option than heat for acute injury where swelling and inflammation is involved and will help to control pain.

Delayed onset muscle soreness (DOMS)

In the Holy Grail quest to find something (anything!) that alleviates muscle soreness after exercise, athletes have recently taken to plunging themselves into freezing waters of less than 15 degrees Celsius. A Cochrane review showed there was some evidence that this strategy is actually effective compared with passive interventions involving rest or no intervention (Bleakley et al 2012). So if your braver sporty clients want to try this as a self-help technique to deal with DOMS they can go right ahead. Personally I prefer the smug soreness of a worked-out muscle to a freezing cold bath, but each to their own. An even more masochistic fringe of the athletic community takes the practice to further extremes with the sci-fi world of whole body cryotherapy, which involves short exposures to air temperatures of less than minus 100 degrees Celsius (brrr!). This allegedly enhances recovery and rehabilitation from injury although a review of the evidence suggests that 'less expensive modes of cryotherapy, such as local ice pack application or cold-water immersion, offer comparable physiological and clinical effects to whole body cryotherapy' (Bleakley et al 2014). However, this probably doesn't give you as much street cred as locking yourself in a freezing chamber. No one ever dined out on the story of how they applied an ice pack to their leg.

Also it is worth noting that, in a counterintuitive study, Mayer et al (2006) found continuous low level heat therapy superior to ice in preventing DOMS.

Tendinosis

Contrary to popular belief, research has shown that most chronic tendon problems do not have an inflammatory component as was once believed (hence the more correct naming of the condition as a tendinosis rather than a tendonitis). Despite this finding, ice seems to remain a popular treatment choice (along with rest, stretching, exercises and anti-inflammatories) for tendinopathies, including those of the biceps (Churgay 2009) and the Achilles tendon (Mazzone and McCue 2002, Morelli and James 2004) as well as lateral epicondylitis (tennis elbow) (Hong et al 2004). Although there is no strong evidence base to support the use of ice, clearly there will be at least a reduction of pain and from that perspective it can be seen as useful self-help or adjunct treatment strategy.

From our own experience in the clinic, we tend to use heat on the affected muscle, to help with fascial and subsequent trigger point release, combined with ice on the painful tendon.

Using hot and cold in your massage treatments

There are two ways that hot and cold can be useful for alleviation of pain issues and both are important: through self-care advice for the client and incorporation into the treatment.

There are many ways to apply hot and cold to the body during bodywork. Heat can be applied via heat blankets and wraps, infrared lamps, hydrocollator packs, wheat bags and hot stones. Clinically, moist heat has always been recommended as superior to dry heat, yet there is no research evidence to back this up. However, moist heat does result in more rapid tissue warming (as the water conducts the heat quicker) and may be more useful in clinical situations where rapid results are required.

Cold can also be applied in a variety of ways including ice pack, vapocoolant spray, ice massage and cold-water immersion, such as a whirlpool. Different effects have been found from the different methods, e.g. ice massage seems to be quicker than an ice pack at cooling tissues (Zemke et al 1998). However, a cold whirlpool will keep the tissues colder for longer after application than both ice massage and ice pack (Myrer et al 1998). For this reason, ice massage/ice pack is better where quick recovery is desired (such as immediate return to sport), whereas a cold whirlpool would be better in situations needing long-term cooling.

In general, for static application of hot or cold we would look at applying this to the area needed for the recommended time period whilst working with other techniques elsewhere on the body (alternatively you could leave the room and do your tax return but we think most massage therapists enjoy giving top value for money). So for neck pain you could put a heating pad on the neck and work the fascia on the back while the heat is doing its job. It is also possible to actually work through some heating pads using Amma or compression techniques.

Although there are no consistent evidence-based guidelines for the use of hot and cold, the following are standard principles that we have used to good effect in our own clinics over the past 25 years.

Principles for heat application

- Formula: 20 minutes on, double the time off (40 minutes).
- Repeat pattern as often as needed.

Cautions for heat

- Never use on acute inflammation.
- Do not use on bony, thin-skinned areas.
- Always check in with your client as some people are incredibly heat sensitive. Exercise caution with any heating device where the temperature is above 45 degrees.
- With pregnancy, modulate the temperature used to avoid overheating.
- Take care with diabetes, multiple sclerosis, poor circulation and rheumatoid arthritis.

Principles for cold application

- Cold can be applied via an insulated ice pack or ice directly on the skin in anactive application (use an ice cube or freeze a small cardboard cup of water and use like a lollipop).

- **Ice massage**: with direct ice application do a patch test on the client first to ensure there is not a skin sensitivity. Use circular movements directly on the area until the skin is a rosy pink. Continue to check in with your client during the process about their comfort level. Use for a maximum of 5–10 minutes.

- **Ice packs**: always make sure there is a surface between ice and skin, such as a towel. Recommended timing: 20 minutes on and 40 minutes off.

Cautions for cold

- Take care not to apply prolonged cold application near to superficial nerves, such as the peroneal, ulnar, axillary and lateral femoral cutaneous nerves, as this can result in damage.

- Exercise caution with conditions such as Raynaud's disease, diabetes, vascular disorders, tissue welting on contact and strong aversion to cold.

Principles for contrast bathing

- Alternate the application of hot and cold in 3–5 minute intervals.

Using the stones for creative application of hot and cold

Few methods of applying thermotherapy have the unique advantage of the use of stones, i.e. that you can actually WORK with the stones while simultaneously applying wet heat or cold, thus enhancing greatly the time effectiveness of your treatment. Many therapists and clients have the misconception that stone massage is just about placing stones – which is a lovely part of the work we do, but it is only 10% of it. Most of the work is done by dynamically and specifically massaging the body with the stones as extensions of the therapist's hands.

At Jing we use the stones as a clinical tool not just for relaxation. Understanding when hot and cold stone work should be used enables you to treat different pain conditions and gives you the confidence and creativity to design unique and luxurious treatments for all your clients. Many Jing therapists have the hot and cold stones constantly to hand to use in their advanced clinical massage treatments and enjoy greatly enhanced outcomes as a result.

Reflexology: *I've only used stones with reflexology, but even in this small area they are great. I've used them on pregnant mums up the arms to remove tension and relax them. I place them between the toes and under calves, clients love this.*

Myofascial work: *I feel results are much faster with the stones than with the hands alone … . There is no getting away from HOW THE CLIENT FEELS with the warmth of the smooth stones gliding over them. They can be used without oil ... just wet and then you can put a warm towel over the area to dry it and away you go with some myofascial techniques.*

Aromatherapy: *Since doing the hot stone course with Jing and using it in my clinic alongside my aromatherapy practice, I have found in treating people with severe painful muscular complaints that the analgesic and muscle relaxant aromatherapy oils get into the client's blood stream quicker when using hot stones as opposed to traditional massage.*

This creative approach leads to confident and dynamic practice, as outlined by the comments below from students who have worked with us:

Some great stone techniques to play with for general application of hot and cold

- Large hot stones can be used over the drape to warm and relax the fascia and muscles in the area of pain for up to 20 minutes before treating the area directly (replace them if they start to cool). **See Figure 6.1, p. 82**

- Use broad effleurage strokes to warm the area of pain. **See Figures 6.2 and 6.3, p. 82**

- Use can also be made of smaller and more specific stones to strip and elongate the muscles fibres, searching for trigger points. This saves your precious thumbs and gives great relief to your client. For example, to alleviate low back pain we could treat erector spinae, quadratus lumborum, gluteal muscles and the lateral rotators with these techniques. **See Figure 6.4, p. 82**

- Cold stones can be used in a similar way for acute pain to decrease the pain and swelling.

- Cold stones are usually not used for longer than 5 minutes in any one area.

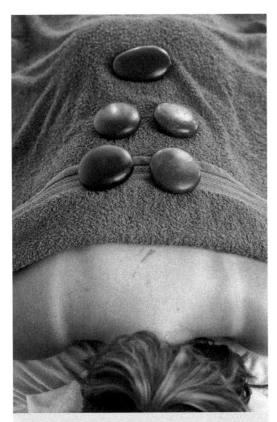

Figure 6.1
Stone placement over the drape

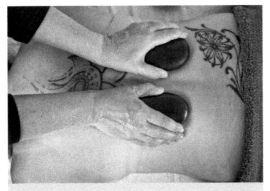

Figure 6.2
Power effleurage using stones

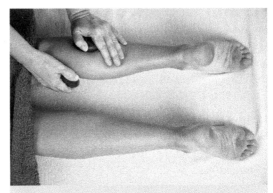

Figure 6.3
'Wringing' of calf muscles using stones

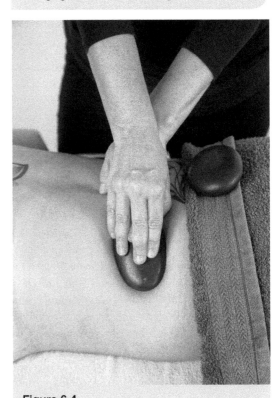

Figure 6.4
Using stones to treat quadratus lumborum for low back pain

In summary

In summary, the application of hot or cold is the cornerstone of the HFMAST protocol and, if used at the beginning of your treatment, can help to enhance your outcomes. Heat in particular lays the foundations for fascial work, trigger point work and stretching in the treatment of chronic pain.

References

Akin MD et al 2001 Continuous low-level topical heat in the treatment of dysmenorrhea. Obstetrics and Gynecology 97(3):343–349.

Bennett RM et al 2007 An internet survey of 2,596 people with fibromyalgia. BMC Musculoskeletal Disorders 8:27.

Berliner MN 1999 Thermotherapy in rheumatic diseases. Zeitschrift für ärztliche Fortbildung und Qualitatssicherung 93:331–334.

Bleakley C et al 2004 The use of ice in the treatment of acute soft-tissue injury: a systematic review of randomized controlled trials. The American Journal of Sports Medicine 32(1):251–261.

Bleakley C et al 2012 Cold-water immersion (cryotherapy) for preventing and treating muscle soreness after exercise. The Cochrane Database of Systematic Reviews 2:CD008262.

Bleakley CM, Costello JT 2013 Do thermal agents affect range of movement and mechanical properties in soft tissues? A systematic review. Archives of Physical Medicine and Rehabilitation 94(1):149–163.

Bleakley CM et al 2014 Whole-body cryotherapy: empirical evidence and theoretical perspectives. Open Access Journal of Sports Medicine 5:25–36.

Block JE 2010 Cold and compression in the management of musculoskeletal injuries and orthopedic operative procedures: a narrative review. Open Access Journal of Sports Medicine 1:105–113.

Breger Stanton DE et al 2009 A systematic review of the effectiveness of contrast baths. Journal of Hand Therapy : Official Journal of the American Society of Hand Therapists 22(1):57–69.

Brosseau L et al 2003 Thermotherapy for treatment of osteoarthritis. The Cochrane Database of Systematic Reviews (4):CD004522.

Chaudhary ES et al 2013 Comparative study of myofascial release and cold pack in upper trapezius spasm. International Journal of Health Sciences and Research (IJHSR) 3(12):20–27.

Churgay CA 2009 Diagnosis and treatment of biceps tendinitis and tendinosis. American Family Physician 80:470–476.

Cochrane DJ 2004 Alternating hot and cold water immersion for athlete recovery: a review. Physical Therapy in Sport 5(1):26–32.

Collins NC 2008 Is ice right? Does cryotherapy improve outcome for acute soft tissue injury? Emergency Medicine Journal: EMJ 25(2):65–68.

Cosgray NA et al 2004 Effect of heat modalities on hamstring length: a comparison of pneumatherm, moist heat pack, and a control. The Journal of Orthopaedic and Sports Physical Therapy 34:377–384.

Cramer H et al 2012 Thermotherapy self-treatment for neck pain relief – a randomized controlled trial. European Journal of Integrative Medicine 4(4):e371–e378.

Davis KD et al 1998 Functional MRI study of thalamic and cortical activations evoked by cutaneous heat, cold, and tactile stimuli. Journal of Neurophysiology 1998;80: 1533–1546.

French SD et al 2006 Superficial heat or cold for low back pain. The Cochrane Database of Systematic Reviews 1:CD004750.

Funk D et al 2001 Efficacy of moist heat pack application over static stretching on hamstring flexibility. Journal of Strength and Conditioning Research 15:123–126.

Hammer W 2014 The fascial system is a sensory organ. ACA News April:15–20.

Hong C-Z 2002 New trends in myofascial pain syndrome. Zhonghua Yi Xue Za Zhi (Chinese Medical Journal); Free China edn 65(11):501–512.

Hong QN et al 2004 Physiotherapists' management of patients with lateral epicondylitis (extensor tendinosis): results of a provincial survey. Physiotherapy Canada 56:215.

Hubbard TJ, Denegar CR 2004 Does cryotherapy improve outcomes with soft tissue injury? Journal of Athletic Training 39:278–279.

Kitay GS et al 2009 Efficacy of combined local mechanical vibrations, continuous passive motion and thermotherapy in the management of osteoarthritis of the knee. Osteoarthritis and Cartilage 17(10):1269–1274.

Klingler W 2012 Temperature effects on fascia. Fascia: The Tensional Network of the Human Body, Oxford: Churchill Livingstone Elsevier, pp. 421–424.

Kneipp (n.d.) The life of Sebastian Kneipp. Available at: http://www.kneipp.com/kneipp_philosophy/sebastian_kneipp/the_life_of_sebstian_kneipp.html [accessed 5 August 2014].

Kurzeja R 2003 Fibromyalgia: comparison of whole-body-cryotherapy with two classical thermotherapy methods. Aktuelle Rheumatologie 28(3):158–163.

Larsen CC et al 2015 Effects of crushed ice and wetted ice on hamstring flexibility after PNF stretching. Journal of Strength and Conditioning Research 29(2):483–488.

Leung MSF, Cheing GLY 2008 Effects of deep and superficial heating in the management of frozen shoulder. Journal of Rehabilitation Medicine 40:145–150.

MacAuley D 2001 Do textbooks agree on their advice on ice? Clinical Journal of Sports Medicine 11(2):67–72.

Majlesi J, Unalan H 2010 Effect of treatment on trigger points. Current Pain and Headache Reports 14(5):353–360. Available at: http://www.ncbi.nlm.nih.gov/pubmed/20652653 [accessed 28 April 2014].

Matteini P et al 2009 Structural behavior of highly concentrated hyaluronan. Biomacromolecules 10(6): 1516–1522.

Mayer JM et al 2005 Treating acute low back pain with continuous low-level heat wrap therapy and/or exercise: a randomized controlled trial. The Spine Journal: Official Journal of the North American Spine Society 5(4):395–403.

Mayer JM et al 2006 Continuous low-level heat wrap therapy for the prevention and early phase treatment of delayed-onset muscle soreness of the low back: a randomized controlled trial. Archives of Physical Medicine and Rehabilitation 87(10):1310–1317.

Mazzone MF, McCue T 2002 Common conditions of the Achilles tendon. American Family Physician 65:1805–1810.

Michlovitz S et al 2004 Continuous low-level heat wrap therapy is effective for treating wrist pain. Archives of Physical Medicine and Rehabilitation 85:1409–1416.

Mirkin G 2014 RICE: the end of an ice age. Stone Athletic Medicine. Available at: http://stoneathleticmedicine. com/2014/04/rice-the-end-of-an-ice-age/ [accessed 19 August 2014].

Mirkin G, Hoffman M 1978 The Sportsmedicine Book, 1st edn. Boston: Little, Brown, p. 95.

Morelli V, James E 2004 Achilles tendonopathy and tendon rupture: conservative versus surgical management. Primary Care 31(4):1039–1054, x.

Myrer JW, Draper DO, Durrant E 1994 Contrast therapy and intramuscular temperature in the human leg. Journal of Athletic Training 29(4):318–322.

Myrer JW et al 1997 Cold- and hot-pack contrast therapy: subcutaneous and intramuscular temperature change. Journal of Athletic Training 32(3):238–241.

Myrer JW, Measom G, Fellingham GW 1998 Temperature change in the human leg during and after two methods of cryotherapy. Journal of Athletic Training 33:25.

Nadler SF 2004 Nonpharmacologic management of pain. The Journal of the American Osteopathic Association 104(11 Supplement 8):S6–S12.

Nadler SF et al 2002 Continuous low-level heat wrap therapy provides more efficacy than ibuprofen and acetaminophen for acute low back pain 27(10):1012–1017.

Nadler SF, Weingand K, Kruse RJ 2004 The physiologic basis and clinical applications of cryotherapy and thermotherapy for the pain practitioner. Pain Physician 7:395–399.

Nakano J et al 2012 The effect of heat applied with stretch to increase range of motion: a systematic review. Physical Therapy in Sport: Official Journal of the Association of Chartered Physiotherapists in Sports Medicine 13(3):180–188.

Riley JL et al 2007 Self-care behaviors associated with myofascial temporomandibular disorder pain. Journal of Orofacial Pain 21:194–202.

Robinson V et al 2002 Thermotherapy for treating rheumatoid arthritis. Cochrane Database of Systematic Reviews. 2:CD002826. Available at: http://onlinelibrary. wiley.com/doi/10.1002/14651858.CD002826/abstract; jsessionid=BDF942CB06F0AF16CC8A5E53F9884C86. f04t01 [accessed 31 March 2015].

Stanton DB et al 2003 Contrast baths: what do we know about their use? Journal of Hand Therapy: official journal of the American Society of Hand Therapists 16(4): 343–346.

Therapeutic Modalities (n.d.) Physiopedia, universal access to physiotherapy knowledge. Available at: http://www.physio-pedia.com/Therapeutic_Modalities [accessed 5 August 2014].

Travell J G et al 1999 Travell & Simons Myofascial Pain & Dysfunction: The Trigger Point Manual. Volume 1: Upper Half of Body, 2nd edn. Philadelphia: Williams & Wilkins.

Yasui H et al 2010 Significant correlation between autonomic nervous activity and cerebral hemodynamics during thermotherapy on the neck. Autonomic Neuroscience: Basic & Clinical 156(1–2):96–103.

Zemke JE et al 1998 Intramuscular temperature responses in the human leg to two forms of cryotherapy: ice message and ice bag. Journal of Orthopaedic and Sports Physical Therapy 27:301–307.

Dedicated followers of fascia: the background and practice of fascial therapies

After the application of heat, the next step in the HFMAST protocol is carrying out fascial techniques. At Jing we are all truly 'dedicated followers of fascia', so let's take a whistle stop tour around the highlights of this wonderful subject.

Let's start at the very beginning: what is fascia?

To understand fascial related therapies we first have to understand the nature of fascia itself. Most of us who studied anatomy and physiology on our qualifying level courses dutifully learned about all the different body systems such as the cardiovascular system, lymph system, digestive system and, of course, the musculoskeletal system. Yet very few of us were given more than a passing reference to one of the most important and prevalent interconnected systems in the body: the fascial system. Indeed fascia has traditionally been so ignored in mainstream anatomical and medical thinking that prominent fascial researcher and bodyworker, Robert Schleip, has coined it the 'Cinderella tissue'. Yet as we all know, Cinderella finally got out of her dank basement and dazzled at the ball. Currently interest in fascia is rising to such an extent that, hopefully, over the years to come a detailed knowledge of the fascial system will be a necessary part of both mainstream and complementary therapy education.

Fascia: the boffin's definition

Innocently asking 'what is fascia' is the bodywork equivalent of asking 'what is love' (which is apparently the most searched phrase in Google 2012) and can provoke just as much heated debate. Meg attended a UK conference about fascia in 2011 and was chagrined to find most of the first day was frittered away while researchers and clinicians argued about what the heck fascia is anyway.

For a nerdy definition of fascia let's turn to the International Fascial Research Congress, which is a wonderful initiative set up by pioneers in the field who

have brought together manual therapists and scientists to give us a more full understanding of how fascial therapies work:

> *Fascia is the soft tissue component of the connective tissue system that permeates the human body. It forms a whole-body continuous three-dimensional matrix of structural support. Fascia interpenetrates and surrounds all organs, muscles, bones and nerve fibers, creating a unique environment for body systems functioning. The scope of our definition of and interest in fascia extends to all fibrous connective tissues, including aponeuroses, ligaments, tendons, retinaculae, joint capsules, organ and vessel tunics, the epineurium, the meninges, the periostea, and all the endomysial and intermuscular fibers of the myofasciae.*
> FASCIACONGRESS.ORG (ND)

Fascia: the cheat sheet definition

If that definition made your eyes glaze over (my attention usually wanders off some time around 'vessel tunics' as I get distracted by a visual of an artery in medieval garb) then consider the translated 'cheat sheet'. The key phrase in the above definition is 'the soft tissue component of the connective tissue system'. Although it is true that all fasciae are connective tissues, not all connective tissues are fasciae. If you hit your anatomy books for a refresher you will find that blood is a form of connective tissue, yet is clearly not fascia. In other words fascia is the 'fibrous soft tissue' component of connective tissue that is literally found everywhere in the body. Fascia forms ligaments, tendons, the wrapping around the brain (meninges), nerves (epineurium), bones (periosteum), muscle fibres (endomysium) and bundles of muscles (myofasciae). Previously these fasciae have all been labelled as different structures (**Figure 7.1**). Yet the mind-boggling truth is that all these tissues can be considered as one fascia and are all interconnected in a gigantic silken spider's web.

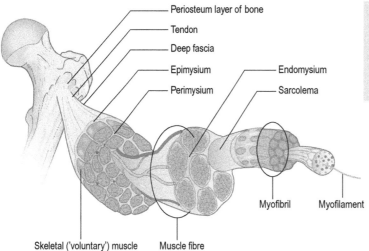

Periosteum layer of bone
Tendon
Deep fascia
Epimysium
Perimysium
Endomysium
Sarcolema
Myofibril   Myofilament
Skeletal ('voluntary') muscle   Muscle fibre

Figure 7.1
Fascial flow: ligaments, tendons, the wrapping around the bones (periosteum), muscle fibres (endomysium) and bundles of muscles (myofasciae) can all be considered to be fasciae

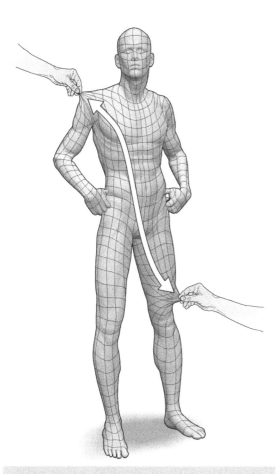

Figure 7.2
Strain in one area of the fascial 'silken body suit' can be transmitted to elsewhere in the body

The easiest way of understanding fascia is with the idea that if we had a magical substance that could dissolve everything in the body except fascia, we would still be left with a complete 3D representation of the person. Once you have this perspective of a tough silken fascia 'body suit' that permeates every structure in the body you can start to appreciate the relevance of fascia to massage. As fascia is an interconnected system, it is plausible that strain or tension in one part of the system may cause pain, lack of mobility or another dysfunction elsewhere (**Figure 7.2**). It is also likely that fascia can act as a communicating system transporting mechanical signals around the body and causing cells and tissues to act on the messages it conveys. It is impossible to put your hands on the body without in some way influencing this fascial net. As we shall see, our touch can literally be transmitted right down to the level of the cell itself through the fascia.

Fascia: the bodyworkers Holy Grail

'*The Answer to the Great Question of Life, the Universe, and Everything Is ... Forty-Two' said Deep Thought, with infinite majesty and calm. 'Forty-two!' yelled Loonquawl. 'Is that all you've got to show for seven and a half million years' work?' 'I checked it very thoroughly,' said the computer, 'and that quite definitely is the answer. I think the problem, to be quite honest with you, is that you've never actually known what the question is.'*
From Douglas Adams, The Hitchikers Guide to the Galaxy (goodreads.com (ND))

Many bodyworkers today are convinced that 'fascia is the answer'. We jokingly tell our students that if a client comes up with some strange connection ('When you press on my leg it hurts in my chest' and 'Why do I feel it in my hip when you work on my appendix scar?') they should stroke their chin knowingly and answer 'fascia'. Yet if fascia really is the answer we do need to make sure we know what the questions are.

Let's face it, fascia is just downright hot at the moment! The Cinderella tissue that was ignored for centuries is now centre stage at conferences worldwide and unites hard core scientists with new age seekers, all desperate to learn more about this gooey, gluey, connecting, transforming 'white stuff' that for years has ended up in the dissector's bin. The new Holy Grail of bodywork is enjoying its time in the sun. As Robert Schleip commented in a 2014 lecture 'Fascial research is like the gold rush. Everyone is desperate to put their name on a new fascial technique or book.'

Can it be true? Can fascia really have all of the answers? Clinical experience and recent research suggests that while it may not hold the key to 'life the universe and everything' it can certainly help us unlock a few secrets of the effects we see in massage, acupuncture and movement.

If you fall asleep in class and get asked a question, yes, the answer is invariably 'fascia'. (If you are in a Rolfing class the other plausible answers are 'the psoas' and 'gravity'.)

What is fascia made of?

If we start at the very beginning, we know the cell is the basic unit of life. Although we have a bewildering number of structures and tissues in the body, with lots of fancy sounding names, it helps to remember that there are actually only four types of cells in the body:

- Epithelial
- Neural
- Muscular
- Connective tissue.

Although all cells have multiple functions, the different types have become especially good at specific functions. Thus, nerve cells are great at conducting electrical signals, muscles are fabulous at contracting, epithelial cells are awesome at protecting and connective tissues just rock at ... well ... connecting. The novelist EM Forster summed up his humanistic philosophy to life in the epigraph for his 1910 novel (*Howards End*): 'Only connect'. This is without doubt the mantra of the connective tissues. Similar to over-anxious party hosts, fascia is destined to surround and envelop all the other structures and tissues of the body, making connections in each and every direction. Connective tissue is relentless in its quest to connect. Connecting body to brain, muscle to nerve and single muscles into top to toe chains, it weaves an endless web around the body, connecting, connecting and connecting. Similar to a good party host, in addition to connecting, the fascia also separates. Bundles of muscles are separated from other bundles of muscles or vessels by fascial sheaths and linings. Just like the Jones's must be kept away from the Smiths at the local cheese and wine party and yet the Jones's should absolutely be introduced to the Johnsons, fascia connects what needs to be connected and separates what should be kept apart.

Connective tissue is the most widespread and abundant type of tissue in the body and exists in many different forms, from very liquid to very solid, for example:

- Blood
- Fat (adipose tissue)
- Tendons
- Ligaments
- Aponeuroses (large flat tendons like thoracolumbar fascia or galea aponeurotica of the scalp)
- Cartliage
- Bone.

How can all these different tissue types be connective tissue when they are all so different?

The answer lies in the fact that they all contain the same elements: the basic connective tissue 'recipe' is essentially the same and varies only in the proportion and arrangement of the ingredients:

- **Cells**: the most common cell types are fibroblasts, which produce fibres and other intercellular materials.

- **Fibres**: the two most common types of fibre are: collagen and elastin. Collagen fibres are for strength while the elastin fibres provide tissue elasticity. There is a third fibre, reticulin, which is a form of immature collagen mainly found in the embryo.

- **Ground substance**: both the cells and the fibres are embedded in the gluey hydrophilic (water loving) intercellular substance. The consistency of this substance is highly variable from gelatin-like to a much more rigid material and consists of a watery gel of mucopolysaccharides or glycosaminoglycans (GAGs), such as chondroitin sulfate, keratin sulfate, heparan sulfate and hyaluronic acid (HA) (remember this last one as it will crop up later).

Like a cake made of the same ingredients but in different proportions, the body cleverly mixes the three constituent parts in proportion and arrangement to make many different types of structures. For example, a strong connective tissue (like the dense connective tissue found in tendons and ligaments) needs a greater proportion of the collagen fibres and fewer cells. On the other hand, a connective tissue composed of mostly cells would not be very strong, e.g. adipose connective tissue (fat). **See Figure 7.3A,B**

Harder tissues such as bone and cartilage could really be seen as dense forms of fascial tissue. Our impression of bone is based on the classroom skeleton or animal bones but this is not an accurate representation of bone in the living human being. Bones in the living body have more of the consistency of balsa wood or a hard-boiled egg. Why the difference? Bone, as with tendons, has collagen as its fibre type but the ground substance is harder consisting of mineral salts. The bones we give to the dog have had the collagen fibril part baked out of them, and are now hard and will splinter. Bone in the living human being with its collagenous network is much more pliable – especially in a child where the collagen proportion is higher leading to more tensile strength. Children's bones are literally like green branches: springy and resilient and hard to break.

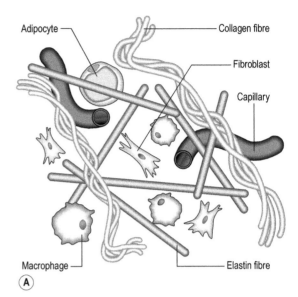

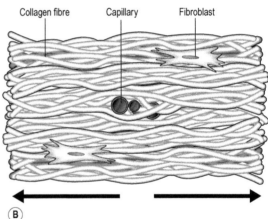

Figure 7.3A,B
All connective tissues have the same 'ingredients': cells, fibres and ground substance (A). These are arranged in different proportions to make diverse types of structures. Tendons and ligaments are also connective tissues but have more fibres and fewer cells (B)

The connective tissue recipe

In summary it's all the same 'stuff'. Our connective tissue recipe of limited ingredients (i.e. cells, fibres and ground substance) can be infinitely varied by different cell types, different fibre arrangements (e.g. arranging them regularly or irregularly, densely or loosely) or changing the ground substance from fluid to gluey, plastic or crystalline solid.

Imagine starting with some child's 'goo' (ground substance) and adding some collagen fibres (strands of leathery substance) and thin strands of elastic. That's your basic connective tissue recipe and you are not allowed to change the ingredients (apart from adding water), but you can alter their proportions and arrangement depending on where the connective tissue is needed in the body and what its job is. Thus elastic cartilage (like in the ear and skin) has more elastin, bones have a 'drier' ground substance, and tendons and ligaments have the collagen fibres arranged in lines to make them stronger.

The fascial sandwich: superficial and deep fascia

If we look at the different layers of fascia between the skin and muscle, the visual is like a fancy fascial sandwich or a super layered cake (**Figure 7.4**). So sinking from superficial to deep, the layers of the fascia are (Muscolino 2012):

- **Skin**: the outer epidermis and underlying dermis.

- **Superficial fascia**: this is also known as the subcutaneous fascia as it lies directly underneath and parallel to the skin. Superficial fascia is a fibrous layer that is connected to the skin via vertical retinacula cutis fibres. Adipose (fat) and GAG molecules are often found in loose arrangements between these retinacula cutis fibres, so subcutaneous fascia is usually described as loose or areolar fascia.

- **Retinacula cutis fibres**: superficial retinacula cutis fibres connect the superficial fascia

to the skin above and deep retinacula cutis fibres connect it to the deep fascia below.

The retinacula cutis fibres allow for sliding between the skin and the superficial and deep fascial membranes. If they get thickened, however, they can restrict motion, becoming adhesions that cause the skin and superficial fascia to stick together. This can cause pain and restrict function.

The superficial retinacula cutis fibres run vertically between the skin and the superficial fascia, while the deep retinacula cutis fibres are thinner and at a more oblique orientation between the superficial and deep fascial membrane. This means that superficial fascia is more firmly connected to the skin than to the deep fascial membrane. Under normal conditions, the deep fascia is able to move more independently of the superficial fascia and skin. However, as we know with injury or dehydration, all the fascial layers can stick together resulting in overall decreased sliding and gliding between layers.

- **Deep fascia**: the deep fascial membrane surrounds either muscle or, in areas of the body where there is no muscle, the periosteum. Lying underneath the deep fascia is a layer of HA that lubricates the layer between the deep fascia and the underlying epimysium (the outer covering of the muscle). Recent research has indicated that loss of the sliding ability of HA may be key in myofascial pain syndromes. Stay tuned as there is more on this later.

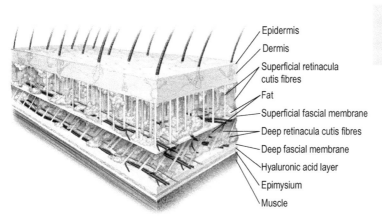

Epidermis
Dermis
Superficial retinacula cutis fibres
Fat
Superficial fascial membrane
Deep retinacula cutis fibres
Deep fascial membrane
Hyaluronic acid layer
Epimysium
Muscle

Figure 7.4
The anatomy of superficial and deep fascial layers

Towards an all new fascial anatomy

> *Once bold, the scientific culture has become increasingly timid. It seeks incremental advances. Rarely does it question the foundational concepts on which those incremental advances are based, especially those foundational concepts that show signs of having outlived their usefulness. The culture has become obedient. It bows to the regality of prevailing dogma. In so doing, it has produced mounds of data but precious little that fundamentally advances our understanding.*
> POLLACK 2013

The recent explosion of interest in fascia has brought a conundrum for those of us interested in anatomy and bodywork; namely that our received view of anatomy may be fundamentally wrong. This is obviously both a core body blow (all those notes and lectures to be thrown out) and highly exciting – which is similar to the pictogram for 'crisis' in Chinese that means both danger and opportunity.

As Pollack points out above, science over the last few decades has tended to 'tinker around the edges' of existing paradigms, rarely questioning fundamental beliefs. Anatomy is no exception. It is still widely assumed that the central tenets of our anatomical understanding are untouchable. For example:

- The body acts like a machine: bones are like levers and muscles like the pulleys that operate them.
- Muscles act over one joint or in some cases two, but NEVER three!
- When the agonist contracts, the antagonist relaxes.
- Fascia doesn't do much except stop the important structures falling out.
- Fascia is inert and doesn't contract.
- Ligaments, tendons, fascia, joint capsules and spinal meninges are all totally different structures.
- Tendons insert onto bones.
- Muscles are the prime players in movement.
- The body is constructed like a building: the skeleton and bones are like the bricks piled on top

of each other that keep the body upright. Muscles move the bones and fascia fills in the gaps.

- Joints touch. Due to the downward compressional force of gravity and because we are often 'misaligned', the joint surfaces can wear down over time.
- Properly aligned structure is key. The bones in our bodies are like a pile of bricks that need to be stacked neatly on top of each other to avoid pain and dysfunction.

Right? Wrong, wrong, wrong according to new research. One by one these sacred cows of anatomy and bodywork are crashing to the ground, yet specialist and public opinion lags far behind. It can take a bafflingly long time to change current core beliefs. (After all, the crazy notion that the world was round didn't catch on until the 17th and 18th centuries.) Hence, the status quo continues to prevail leading to corresponding errors in practice. Read on to see what the recent research tells us about these core beliefs and the new zeitgeist of a fascially based anatomy.

Our new and improved fascial anatomy

So how does our newer understanding of fascia redefine our current notions of anatomy. In short, what's hot and what's not in our anatomical fashion charts:

Single muscle theory vs trains, chains and slings

> *Your brain does not think in terms of biceps and deltoids. There is one muscle that exists in 600 fascial pockets. Ultimately, the brain creates movement in terms of large fascial networks and individual motor units, not our named muscles.*
> TOM MYERS (SMITH 2012, INTERVIEW)

- **Going down**: 'single muscle' theory.
- **Coming up**: myofascial trains, chains and slings.

It is becoming evident that our idea of one muscle operating over one joint is too simplistic. Muscles are connected in various ways via fascia to form myofascial continuities that cross several joints and can span from head to toe. Tom Myers has developed the most popular and plausible idea of how this happens with his Anatomy Trains concept (Myers 2001). Tom has delineated 12 cardinal longitudinal Anatomy Trains which are the myofascial equivalent of the song 'Dem Bones'. You know the one:

Toe bone connected to the foot bone.
Foot bone connected to the heel bone.
Heel bone connected to the ankle bone.
Ankle bone connected to the shin bone.

Tom's version goes more like, dem myofascial continuities (superficial back line verse):

Plantar fascia connected to the gastrocs
Gastrocs connected to the hamstrings
Hamstrings connected to the sacrotuberous ligament
Ligament connected to the erectors
Erectors connected to the galea aponeurotica …

Not quite as catchy I guess but you get the idea. **See Figure 7.5**

To quote Tom himself about the concept of anatomy trains:

Briefly, all our muscles have been analysed as if they were separate units within the body. This idea – that there is a separate unit like the biceps, the psoas, the latissimus – is so pervasive, that it is hard to think in any other way. But in fact all the muscle tissue is embedded within the single, ubiquitous fascial webbing of the extracellular matrix (ECM). The fibers of the ECM, especially within the myofascia where tensile pulls are regular and strong, are arranged along the same 'grain' as the muscle fibers. The muscle may end at the attachment point, but the fascia continues along its way through the ECM, linking up to other muscles in chains – a bit like a set of sausage links. The Anatomy Trains concept maps out these sets of sausage links within the body – following the grain of muscle and fascia to see what links with what.
MYERS 2006

Myers is not the only one to have come up with the idea of muscles connecting – as other bodyworkers have described similar (if slightly sinister sounding) concepts of muscle chains and slings. Moreover, as we shall see in the acupressure chapter, Chinese medicine got there before all of them with early concepts of the

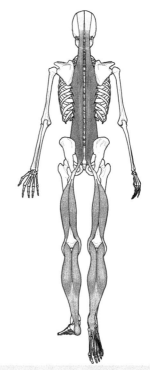

Figure 7.5
Superficial back line: Tom Myers' theory of Anatomy Trains shows how muscles are linked via fascial continuities

tendinomuscular channels that date back thousands of years.

Tendons don't insert into bone

- **Going down**: tendons insert onto bone.

- **Coming up**: tendons insert onto fascial expansions that can connect to several muscles and joints.

The nicely drawn tendons we see in textbooks are a fallacy. Instead, tendons insert into connective tissue sheets, which transmits force across joints (Van der Wal 2009).

Muscles are not the only key players in movement

- **Going down**: muscles are the prime players in movement. Fascia is inert.

- **Coming up**: fascia is just as important in movement as muscles.

Due to the fact that tendons insert onto fascial sheets rather than directly onto bones, the idea that one muscle contracts to move one bone is overly simplistic. These fascial sheets transfer the force of the muscle contraction to other muscles including synergists and – somewhat mind-bendingly – cross the joint to affect antagonists (Maas and Sandercock 2010). The idea that 'X muscle does Y movement' is therefore an outdated concept.

Gracovetsky (2008) showed that in the lumbar spine the load of movement is shared between muscles and fascia with the body moving back and forth between the two. This connection of muscles by fascial sheets means that single muscle stretches are also a mythical concept. Franklyn-Miller et al (2009) showed that a straight leg raise to produce a hamstring stretch actually resulted in 240% of the strain going to the iliotibial (IT) band, 145% to the same side lumbar fascia and 45% to the opposite lumbar fascia. Therefore, a seemingly straightforward hamstring stretch is actually stretching several other muscles as well. Crazy! Movement is clearly more complex than previously believed and fascia is mediating this sophisticated process.

Fascia can contract

- **Going down**: fascia is inert and non-contractile.
- **Coming up**: fascia can contract in a smooth muscle-like manner.

Research has shown that far from being inert, fascia contains myofibroblasts that enable it to contract in a smooth muscle-like manner (Schleip et al 2005).

Ligaments don't exist

- **Going down**: ligaments.
- **Coming up**: dynaments.

True ligaments are almost non-existent and the drawings we see in anatomy books are artefacts that are made with the anatomist's scalpel (Van der Wal 2009). Rather than non-contractile ligaments running in parallel to muscles and tendons at joints, muscles and ligaments are arranged in series to enable the transmission of forces over the joint. Van der Waal has suggested the exciting new name of dynaments for this arrangement.

Wow! So now we have upended all our traditional notions of anatomy, is there a uniting theory to bring together the strands of our new knowledge? Read on to learn about the new intellectual heir to the anatomy throne: the brilliance of biotensegrity.

The beauty of biotensegrity: from bridges to biology

> 'But the Emperor has nothing at all on!' said a little child.

Imagine if everything you had been taught about body structure was wrong, yet the new view offered seemed so thrillingly obvious you wanted to shout it from the rooftops like the child revealing the fallacy of the emperor's new clothes! This is how I felt when I learned about the brilliant concepts of biotensegrity. My visual of anatomy changed from that of a mechanistic muscle clad skeleton to the image of the body as a beautiful sea of bones floating in a tensile net of finely tuned myofascial slings and guy wires. A silken body net where force on one area automatically affects, and is spread over, the whole structure. A net where bones do not touch to form traditional joint surfaces but float apart from each other, magically held by the tension of the myofascial guy wires. A net where every building block is a smaller microcosm of the whole, so that tension or compression on any part of the structure is fed back down to the most microscopic level of the cell itself. A net where the whole is greater than the sum of the parts, where synergy is key, and where communication can travel swiftly via mechanical signals. A net that models perfectly the philosophical constructs of true holism, which Chinese medicine has been preaching for years, i.e. the interplay of opposing forces of yin and yang and integration of the whole.

This is the magical model of biotensegrity as formulated by orthopaedic surgeon Stephen Levin in the 1970s. Based on the principles of tensegrity (a composite word from tension and integrity), as originally developed by engineer Buckminster Fuller and artist Kenneth Snelson, Levin realised that this model provided a more realistic explanation for the structure of the human body than the single muscle/joint theory we are still routinely taught today. Levin's model is a true paradigm shift in our traditional anatomical map and brilliantly replaces the mechanistic viewpoint of man as machine driven by bone levers and local muscle cables. Biotensegrity captures principles of art, science, architecture and philosophy and the paradigm shift is an exciting one that reflects the reality for bodyworkers of what we feel under our hands.

From biology to bridge building, the model of tensegrity not only helps us understand the architecture of the cell but how the Brooklyn Bridge stays strong yet flexible.

To fully understand the ideas of Stephen Levin we need to start with the originator of the idea of tensegrity: the great Buckminster Fuller, affectionately known as Bucky to family and friends. Fuller was the epitome of a 'big picture' thinker and his ideas have extended into architecture, art, politics, environmentalism, and now bodywork. Bucky resisted labels preferring to call himself 'an emerging synthesis of artist, inventor, mechanic, objective economist and evolutionary strategist' (Bfi.org (n.d.)).

Big picture Bucky

During the last few years of his life, my grandfather, my grandmother, Anne and I were living together in Los Angeles, just around the corner from my mother's home. Anne lived at this house full time, while Bucky continued lecturing around Spaceship Earth, orbiting in and out of this 'west coast' base and his central office in Philadelphia. One day when I was driving him to the airport for one of his many trips he said to me 'Jaime, we have half an hour now during this drive. What is the most important thing we can be thinking about?' I don't remember specifically how I responded on that occasion but I am sure it centred on the big picture of 'making the world work for 100% of humanity.' You never caught Bucky veering from that focus – it was the 'North Star' by which he always navigated.
FULLER AND APPLEWHITE 1975

Buckminster Fuller – architect, engineer, mathematician, inventor, poet, cosmologist and holder of 25 US patents and author of 28 books – was the original big picture thinker. A man after my own heart, Buckminster Fuller was able to straddle and synthesise ideas from many disciplines and was a firm believer in the notion of synergy, i.e. the idea that 'behaviour of whole systems is unpredicted by the behaviour of their parts taken separately' (Fuller and Applewhite 1975, p. 3). Fuller contended that the scientific rationale of breaking down a subject and studying its parts separately can never lead to a comprehensive understanding of the whole. He wrote 'nature has only one department and one

language' (Fuller and Applewhite 1983, p. 234). Bucky was fundamentally concerned with making the world work for 100% of humanity and his slogan: 'More and more life support for everybody, with less and less resources' was a central principle of his practical philosophy.

Fuller turned traditional notions of architecture on their heads and instead of relying on the classical 'compression' models of construction – brick upon brick, stone upon stone – he instead looked to nature and physics for how the sun and earth stayed in mutual attraction. He came up with the idea of using tension to provide integrity in buildings (hence the coining of the word tensegrity). Fuller's tensegrity structures, such as his classic geodesic domes, were lightweight, offering 'more for less' and encompassed the inherent principle of tension rather than compression to keep component structures aligned in space. His structures are used to provide cheap affordable housing for families in Africa and exist in extreme weather conditions from tropical areas to the Arctic zone, withstanding strong winds of up to 180 mph.

Tensegrity structures are:

- Light yet strong.
- Materially and energetically efficient.
- Can move with minimum effort.
- Resilient: can dissipate stress from one part to over the whole. **See Figure 7.6**

From Fuller to fascia

But what on earth can architect Buckminster Fuller have to do with the inherent structure of the body and our particular interest in fascia?

Our journey leads us to the great mind of another big picture thinker – Dr Stephen Levin. An orthopaedic surgeon, Levin became dissatisfied with the mechanistic models of the human body he had been taught, observing that the living human body just did not act in this way. Our traditional model of structural anatomy sees the body as a hard skeleton (like a classical pillar or brick by brick building) with cables (muscles) passing over one or two joints to cause local actions. An amorphous packing material (fascia) fills in the gaps and has little function apart from lifeless support. Joints are formed where two bones touch, just as bricks do in a building.

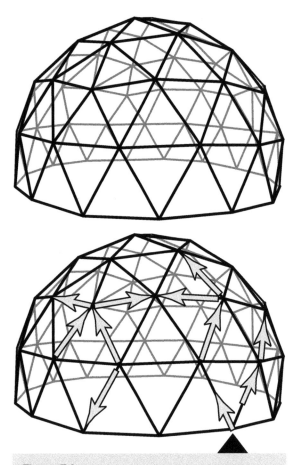

Figure 7.6
Tensegrity structures such as this geodesic dome use the concept of tension to provide strength. Any external force is transmitted in all directions to all other parts of the structure

If biologic systems conformed to [Newtonian materials physics] laws, the human bony spine would bend with less than the weight of the head on top of it and limbs will tear off with the leverage of a fly rod held in a hand. Animals larger than a lion would continually break their bones. Dinosaurs and mastodons larger than a present day elephant would have crushed under their own weight. Pterodactyls could never have flown.
LEVIN (ND)

With the audacity and clear thinking of the child pointing out the emperor was in fact naked and not wearing magical clothing, Stephen Levin convincingly argues that common sense clearly shows the fallacy of the 'stacked brick' compressional model for the human body. Without the tension of the connective tissues, the skeleton would be a heap of bones on the floor. Skeletons are unable to stand upright by themselves – they only achieve this in the classroom through supporting or hanging wires. Joint surfaces in classroom skeletons and anatomy books touch, yet Stephen Levin observed when operating on live human beings it was impossible to make any joint surface touch even when applying strong outside pressure. Like others who recognise that your own body is the greatest experimental lab, Levin even convinced a surgeon unaware of his interest in tensegrity to give him a (needed) knee operation under local anaesthetic. Under Levin's direction, the surgeon attempted to push the joint surfaces together; live camera recording showed this was impossible.

Joints wear out because we do not keep our bony 'brick columns' aligned and we end up with painful arthritis and bulging discs. We are admonished to 'sit up straight' to keep our bony columns stacked and to go to chiropractors to have our out of place bones pushed back into alignment.

Right? Wrong, thought Stephen Levin back in the 1970s, puzzled by how this model was inadequate to explain so many intricacies of the human body. The traditional view sees the body as a simple pillar being acted on by compressional forces. Yet simple reflection shows this viewpoint to be laughably inadequate and is summed up in this pithy quote from the man himself:

At no time did any of the articular surfaces ever touch; the patella seemed to be floating above the femur, and the femur seemed to float above the tibia. A visible and enterable space of 1–3 mm remained at all times.
LEVIN 2005

Poring through his textbooks to find explanations, Levin realised that traditional biomechanical views of the body were based on old fashioned concepts of 'man as machine' and stemming from Borelli's lever model in 1680. Somehow these concepts had become sacred cows, taken as fact and unquestioned for decades. Levin's own

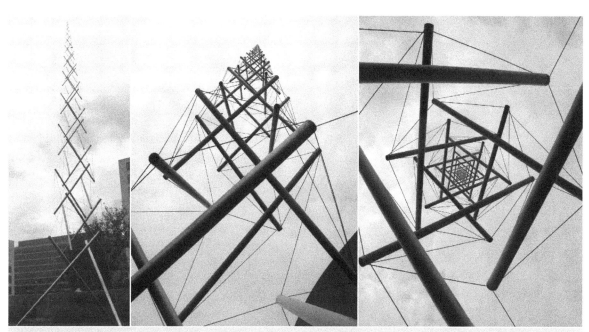

Figure 7.7
Artist Kenneth Snelson's sculpture, The Needle Tower, was the eureka moment that gave birth to Stephen Levin's theory of biotensegrity. With kind permission from Graham Scarr, *Biotensegrity: The Structural Basis of Life*, 2014

eureka moment came when observing Kenneth Snelson's needle tower sculpture and realising that, after months of frustration, 'this was it', finally a plausible model for the body, and the notion of biotensegrity was born. **See Figure 7.7**

In Levin's model, the body is a giant tensegrity structure. The bones are compressional structures and myofascial continuities act as tensional components. It is easy to see how this model of the body is light yet buoyant and that local stresses would automatically affect the whole.

Ingber and the integrins: microtensegrity at the cellular level

Yet the excitement for bodyworkers does not end at Stephen Levin's notions of 'macrotensegrity'. In another paradigm shift on a microscopic level, biologist Donald Ingber (2008) has demonstrated that this tensegrity structure is reflected right down to the level of the cell itself. Even more thrilling, mechanical signals can be transmitted to the internal environment of the cell itself via a process called mechanotransduction. Hence, tensegrity principles are key in inter- and intra-cell communication.

Ingber suggests that our notion of the cell as a water balloon with organelles floating inside is fundamentally flawed. The cell instead is structured like a tent – like its own mini-tensegrity structure – and keeps its shape via various components that both pull and push (**Figure 7.8A,B**). In the metaphor of cell as tensegrity tent we have:

- Guy wires that pull the tent surface in (contractile actomyosin filaments in the cell cytoskeleton). Indeed it is almost as if the cell is acting like its own contractile muscular system. Crazy, huh!

- Guy wires that pull the tent surface out (in a similar style to external guy wires tethered to overhead tree branches). For the cell these are represented by external tethers to the ECM via integrins. Integrins span the cell's surface meta-membrane and form multi-molecular bridges to the internal cytoskeleton of the cell.

- Tent poles that push outwards and resist compression by the tensional structures, e.g. microtubules and cross-linked actin filament bundles.

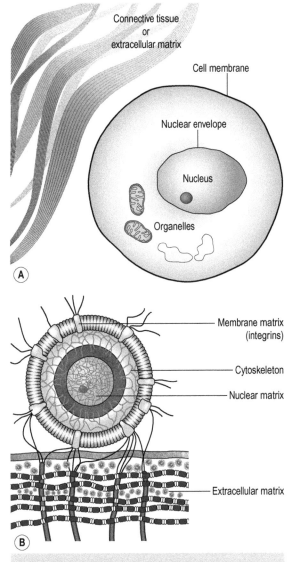

Figure 7.8A,B
Donald Ingber suggests that our notion of the cell as a water balloon containing floating organelles is flawed (A). Instead the cell is more like a mini-tensegrity structure (B)

Clearly, all these components work in sweet harmony to maintain the shape of the cell. They are an integrated system of pushing and pulling that is highly receptive to mechanical tension. Importantly, this arrangement is observed in the cytoskeleton of all cells (e.g. epithelial cells, nerve cells, immune cells, bone cells and fibroblasts) and not just in muscle cells.

Because the integrins are intimately connected to both the external and internal environment of the cell they are able to act as mechanoreceptors, sensing and transmitting mechanical information from outside to inside via the tensegrity arrangement of tensional forces. Pulls and tugs on the integrins are a much faster form of communication than chemical signals and Ingber's experiments have confirmed that mechanical stress application to surface integrin receptors results in almost immediate changes in molecular structure deep in the cytoplasm and nucleus.

What does this mean for us as bodyworkers? In a nutshell, the newsflash is that potentially any manual technique that compresses, twists or pulls on the fascia can cause changes right down to the cellular level via mechanical signals conveyed through the tensegrity structure. The cells can literally respond to signals from our hands, our body movements and stretching. I know, I know, we knew it all along! Yet it was not until this groundbreaking work by Ingber that we had a plausible scientific explanation of how manual therapy may be effective.

As Ingber puts it:

> In conclusion, physical therapies, dance, exercise and various forms of movement can indeed influence cellular activities, including cell growth, differentiation, and potentially even immune cell responses that are critical to human health. This is an obvious fact to anyone who has ever exercised regularly or has experienced the wonderful healing powers of physical therapy. Chemicals and genes are absolutely of critical importance; however, they are governed by mechanical forces, as well as chemical cues.
> INGBER 2008

The importance of biotensegrity for fascial 'aficionados'

The principles of tensegrity are important to the enquiring massage therapist as they provide us with a model for what we feel under our hands. In a healthy state, the body is strong yet light and buoyant. Our fascial work can be viewed like the ministrations of a careful puppeteer; our sensitive listening hands feel for restrictions in the net and gently work to free them. Our goal is to bring about local and global space and freedom, releasing wires that have become inadvertently stuck together or shortened, allowing bony structures to float, and restoring the integrity of the communication system. The image of a tensegrity structure helps to make sense of some of the sensations we encounter as we work within this fascial net. While working on bones and joints the sense of space and the image of 'floating bone' helps us to understand techniques such as releasing the hyoid bone, working on the patella of the knee, or releasing the scapula from where it has been plastered to the ribcage.

The principles of biotensegrity integrate nicely with Eastern philosophical notions of holism and the interplay of yin and yang, i.e. opposing forces of push and pull (compression and tension) need to be balanced in a healthy body. Tensegrity reflects Eastern notions of true strength coming from the suppleness and resilience of the whole body as exemplified in this quote explaining the principles of t'ai chi:

> *Power comes from the sinews. Strength comes from the bones. Looking at it purely physically, one who has great strength is able to carry many hundreds of pounds, but this is an externally showy action of bones and joints, a stiff strength. If on the other hand the power of your whole body is used, it may appear you are unable to lift hardly any weight at all, yet there is an internal robustness of essence and energy, and once you have achieved skill, you will seem to have something more wonderful than one who has the stiff sort of strength. Thus runs the method of physical training for self-cultivation.*
> BRENNAN 2013

In bodywork, we need to keep our focus on both global and local interventions as both are important. Tension, compression or twist on structures can initiate changes in the fascial net and our smallest touch can be reflected both down to the level of the cell and throughout the whole body. Helping our clients to understand that their bodies are tensegrity structures can initiate helpful changes in views of the self – that the spine can be strong yet flexible and is able to dynamically adapt to different positions. Necks and backs do not have to be held like ramrod vertical pillars but can bend, flex and dance in so many different planes without danger of injury. Seeing our bodies as tensegrity structures imbues us with a sense of holism, flexibility, possibility and strength.

All in all, what is there not to like about biotensegrity?

Touchy feely fascia: fascia as a sensory organ

> *Fascia provides definitely our most important perceptual organ.*
> SCHLEIP 2003a

What's the richest sensory organ in the body: ears, skin, or surely the retina of the eye with around 130 million sensory receptors? No, yet again the answer is fascia (you see it really is the answer to life the universe and everything).

Amazingly, the fascial network has TEN TIMES more sensory nerve receptors than red muscle (Schleip 2003a,b, Van der Wal 2009). Yes that's right – it seems that the brain is listening to the fascia much more than it is listening to the muscles. Fascia is riddled with sensory endings that are sensitive to different types of touch and pressure. For example, some of these nerve endings are receptive to deep touch while others respond to light stroking or changes of angle and pressure. Every time we come into contact with our clients' bodies, these receptors are responding to that touch by reporting back messages to the brain. The exotic sounding Golgi's, Pacini's and Ruffini's receptors are not dishes at your local Italian restaurant but are the names of some of these mechanoreceptors. In addition to these three, there are also thousands of unmyelinated free nerve endings known as interstitial receptors. About half of these interstitial receptors are sensitive to very light touch thus making them a likely target of certain types of fascial work, such as cranial work. **See Figure 7.9**

Clearly the fascia is intricately connected with the nervous system. This makes it likely that the formation and release of fascial restrictions is also affected by nervous system control, rather than being a purely mechanical phenomenon. There has been a long-standing debate in bodywork around the issue of how much our brains are involved in the creation and formation of soft tissue restrictions and holding patterns? Massage therapists, osteopaths, Rolfers and structural integrators have tended to see the answer as lying primarily in working on the tissues. On the other hand, movement therapists like Trager, Feldenkrais and Pilates and Alexander technique teachers have seen that directions given by the brain to the body are most important.

I love Robert Schleip's account of this intellectual standoff between the Trager and Rolfing community in the early 1990s:

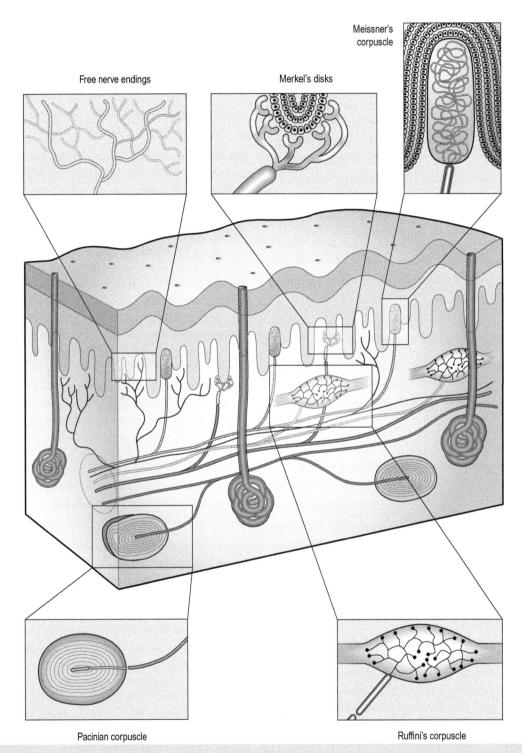

Free nerve endings

Merkel's disks

Meissner's
corpuscle

Pacinian corpuscle

Ruffini's corpuscle

Figure 7.9
Many of the mechanoreceptors sensitive to touch are found in the fascia

More than twenty years ago, I was involved in a dispute between instructors of the Feldenkrais Method of somatic education and teachers of the Rolfing Method of Structural Integration. Advocates of the second group had claimed that many postural restrictions are due to pure mechanical adhesions and restrictions within the fascial network, whereas the leading figures of the first group suggested that 'it's all in the brain', i.e., that most restrictions are due to dysfunctions in sensorimotor regulation. They cited a story by Milton Trager, which deals with an old man in a hospital whose body was very stiff and rigid. But under anaesthesia his muscle tonus got lowered and he was as limber and soft as a young baby. As soon as his consciousness returned he got stiff and rigid again. Subsequently, a small 'experiment' was set up involving several representatives of those two schools, in which three patients were undergoing orthopaedic knee surgery. I was given a consent to do some passive joint range of motion (ROM) testing with the 3 patients before and during anaesthesia. With the patient in a supine position I elevated the arms superiorly above the head and noticed the freedom of movement in this direction. With one of the patients, the elbow dropped all the way to the table above the head before the anaesthesia, and this was no different after he lost consciousness. However, with the other 2 patients I could not elevate their elbows all the way in their normal state, i.e. their elbows kept hanging somewhere in the air above the head. Five minutes later, when they had lost consciousness I again elevated their arms above the head and to my surprise, their elbows dropped all the way down to the table – no restrictions whatsoever, they just dropped! Additionally, I dorsiflexed the feet of all 3 patients. Here I could not detect any increased joint mobility during anaesthesia. (I used my subjective comparison only, without any measuring devices.) I must say that I was quite shocked by the result of my tests. From my Rolfer's point of view I had expected that remaining fascial restrictions would prevent the arms dropping all the way under anaesthesia. (I was not surprised by the unchanged mobility of the ankle joint, since none of the 3 patients seemed to have any limitations there that would concern me as a Rolfer.)Given the limited scientific rigour of this preliminary investigation, the result nevertheless convinced me that what had been perceived as mechanical tissue fixation may at least be partially due to neuromuscular regulation. The ongoing interdisciplinary dispute after this event led to a rethinking of traditional concepts of myofascial therapies, and several years later a first neurologically oriented model was published as a proposed explanatory model for the effects of myofascial manipulation
SCHLEIP 2013a

The ever adventurous Schleip also reports how doing fascial work on a fresh cut of meat is completely different from carrying out the technique on the human body. Apparently there is none of the melting type release effects commonly experienced by practitioners. An easy enough experiment to try out at home but best wait until you're alone to avoid some strange looks if you are caught fingering the family's meat and two veg.

Clearly the fascia and nervous system lie in a mutually dependent relationship and cannot and should not be separated in terms of our understanding and treatment of the human body. This is not a new concept as Andrew Taylor Still, the founder of osteopathy, neatly summarised these ideas over a hundred years ago when he wrote:

The soul of man with all the streams of pure living water seems to dwell in the fascia of the body. When you deal with the fascia. You deal and do business with the branch offices of the brain, and under the general corporation law, the same as the brain itself, and why not treat with the same degree of respect.
ANDREW TAYLOR STILL 1899 (*PHILOSOPHY OF OSTEOPATHY*)

Many of us working with the magical world of fascia would tend to agree that this work allows a unique interface for the treatment of mind and body. It is wise to remember the words of Andrew Taylor Still: that dealing with the fascia is indeed akin to dealing with the soul.

Scientist James Oschman (2003) has extended these ideas of fascia being involved in communication with his concept of a 'living matrix' encompassing superficial fascia, bone, cartilage, tendon, ligament and myofascia. Oschman has suggested that the parallel arrangement of the fibres of actin, myosin, collagen and elastin causes the myofascial system to behave like a liquid crystal enabling rapid body-wide signalling. This fascial communication system can convey signals much more quickly than the nervous system, which represents a newer invention by the body.

Proprioception, interoception and the way we feel inside

Many of these sensory receptors found in the fascia play an important part in our faculty of proprioception, i.e. our sense of bodily position and movement (Stecco et al 2006, 2011a). Meticulous dissections by the Stecco family have shown that the fascia is abundantly innervated with both free nerve endings and encapsulated Ruffini's and Pacini's corpuscles. In some locations, the fascia is more innervated than others, e.g. the flexor retinacula at the wrist has more receptors than places where the fascia inserts onto tendons such as the bicipital aponeurosis (Stecco et al 2007). This observation led Stecco to suggest that the retinaculum has more of a perceptive function whereas the tendinous expansions onto the fascia have mostly a mechanical role in the transmission of tension.

Yet the number of proprioceptors in myofascial tissue is by far outweighed, on the scale of about 7:1, by another group of receptors responsible for an under appreciated super power known as interoception (Schleip and Jager 2013). So what the heck is interoception? If you stop for a minute and tune into your inner sense of self then you are using your powers of interoception. Can you sense your heartbeat, how your belly is feeling, whether you are thirsty, or any other internal bodily sensations? It comes as no surprise to learn that this ability is intricately connected with the fascia. The receptors responsible for this sense of interoception are the unmyelinated free nerve endings that are abundant in fascial tissue. The most interesting finding about these nerve endings is that they report to the insular cortex, which is the part of the brain involved in emotional processing. By contrast, receptors for proprioception go to a totally different area of the brain called the somatosensory cortex (Berlucchi and Aglioti 2010).

Say what? Can this be true that there is a proven connection between the fascia and emotions? Could this be another 'told you so' moment for bodywork? For decades, bodyworkers have been reporting the links between emotions and fascial work. Practitioners often find in the clinic that fascial release can lead to emotional release and conversely emotional release can lead to fascial release. Several types of fascial work consciously work with both body and emotions such as the somato-emotional release practised by cranial workers and the emotional release effects of myofascial unwinding as advocated by John Barnes. The research findings certainly seem to suggest that the unmyelinated nerve endings found in fascia have a direct link with the emotional processing part of the brain, which has massive implications for our understanding and treatment of musculoskeletal dysfunctions. We do not necessarily have to be doing bodywork identified as 'fascial work' to stimulate these receptors. It seems that all pleasant and sensual touch is an interoceptive sensation that activates the insular cortex resulting in a profound sense of wellbeing (McGlone et al 2012, Olausson et al 2010). This provides scientific rationale for the long known finding of the importance of caring touch to psychological development, health and happiness (Harlow and Suomi 1970, Montagu 1971).

Moreover, the sense of interoception may be distorted in many somatoemotional disorders such as irritable bowel syndrome (IBS), post-traumatic stress disorder, anxiety, depression and drug addiction (Eisenbruch et al 2010, Naqvi and Bechara 2010, Paulus and Stein 2010, Paulus and Stewart 2014, Paulus et al 2009, Verdejo-Garcia et al 2012). In such cases individuals develop 'noisily amplified' beliefs about the interoceptive information they are sensing. This link may explain the observable positive effects of fascial work with some of these pathologies.

Mind–body interventions that develop interoceptive abilities by emphasising a more positive relationship with the inner sensations of the body may be extremely helpful in the treatment of such problems. This includes meditation and mindfulness that focus on paying attention to internal bodily states such as the breath

(Farb 2013). A host of other mind–body therapies – hypnosis, biofeedback, yoga and t'ai chi – also emphasise the importance of paying attention to the internal state and have been show to promote optimal homeostasis in the body. Such interventions have been found effective for reducing depression, insomnia, anxiety, post-traumatic stress, IBS, nausea, and acute and chronic pain, and for managing impaired circulation, diabetes and hypertension (Taylor et al 2010).

Movement or manual therapy that emphasises awareness of the body should therefore be considered a good thing. This is in contrast to competitive sports that often rely on overriding internal sensations, i.e. the 'no pain no gain' mentality. However, Schleip and Jager (2013) also state that some movement therapies or teachers emphasise proprioceptive awareness at the expense of developing interoception. For example, yoga teachers who are more concerned with the exact attainment of the perfect asana position rather than emphasising being tuned into the internal bodily state can result in students becoming what Schleip calls 'interoceptive morons'.

For bodyworkers, encouraging our clients to tune into how they feel internally while you are working can be helpful in developing interoceptive awareness. This could be achieved by verbal cues or simply thrilling touch that your client wants to pay attention to.

The importance of fascia in understanding musculoskeletal pain

Weaving fascial work into treatments can cause a huge leap in getting results for stubborn musculoskeletal conditions. We have both always seen positive results by including fascial techniques alongside the other modalities of the HFMAST approach and on occasions the results can be near miraculous. But what exactly is the role that fascia plays in pain conditions? There are some interesting findings from research that are helping shed light on this question:

1 **Fascia is highly innervated and can act as a source of nociception**: research has confirmed that the fascia may be a more important source of pain than the traditional targets of manual therapy, i.e. muscles and joints. How do we know this? Well researchers love injecting hypertonic saline into their subjects as it is known to experimentally induce musculoskeletal pain. It turns out that injecting saline into the thoracolumbar fascia causes more pain than injecting it into the muscle or directly under the skin, leading to the conclusion that the thoracolumbar fascia is 'a prime candidate to contribute to non-specific low back pain' (Schilder et al 2014). Similarly Gibson et al (2009) have shown that saline injection into the tibialis anterior of subjects with delayed onset muscle soreness (DOMS) caused more pain if it was injected under the fascia than into the muscle. Many studies have focussed on the extensive innervation in the thoracolumbar fascia and pointed to this as a potential source of nociception in low back pain (Corey et al 2011, Hoheisel et al 2011, Tesarz et al 2011, Yahia et al 1992). The study by Yahia (1992) also found that two-thirds of the sensory fibres in fascia run from the brain to the tissues. This could also help explain the influence of stressors in the development of low back pain. As we know 'top down' influences from the brain are just as important as 'bottom up' messages from the tissues.

2 **Microtearing and inflammation of the fascia can be a direct source of pain**: Schleip et al (2010) suggested that microtearing and inflammation of the fascia can be a direct source of pain, e.g. in non-specific low back pain. Liptan (2010) has extended this concept and suggested that inflammation of the fascia in this way could also be a source of peripheral nociceptive input that leads to central sensitisation in conditions such as fibromyalgia, plantar fasciitis and lateral epicondylitis (tennis elbow). Biopsy studies have indeed found increased levels of collagen and inflammatory mediators in the connective tissue of fibromyalgia patients.

It seems that this inflammation might also be reversed through fascial type therapy. A study examining the effects of whole body stretching on rats (experimenters held the rats upside down by their tails rather than dressing them in lycra and working out to '80s pop music) found that inflammation decreased with this type of static stretching (Corey et al 2012). Clearly, this is very similar to the sustained stretch induced in certain types of fascial bodywork, yoga or myofascial stretching.

3 **Sliding and gliding: stuck fascial layers can lead to pain.** A key role of fascia is to enable the sliding and gliding of adjacent tissue layers over each other (Chaitow 2014). Just like a machine, the different parts of the body need to stay 'well oiled' if they are to function effectively and loss of gliding and sliding equals increased possibility of pain. With the power of ultrasound imaging, Langevin et al (2011) has shown that patients with chronic low back pain have less sliding potential in the deeper layers of the thoracolumbar fascia. This lack of sliding and gliding seems to go hand in hand with an observable thickening of the fascia in patients with chronic pain. For example, those with chronic low back pain have fascia in the lumbar region that is 25% thicker than for those without pain (Langevin et al 2009). Similarly, Stecco et al (2013a) found that patients with chronic neck pain had increased thickness of the sternocleidomastoid and scalene fascia. Increased thickness of the Achilles tendon in tendinopathy has also been observed (Richards et al 2005, Stecco et al 2014). Stecco et al (2013a) also showed that fascial therapy was successful in decreasing both pain and the thickness of the fascial layer.

Fascinating stuff as myofascial work does indeed feel like 'unsticking layers'. Those who have received the work will be familiar with the 'rippy burny' sensations that often precede a dramatic decrease in pain and palpable softening of the tissues.

4 **The key role of hyaluronic acid (HA) in fascial pain syndromes:** a key player in the sliding and gliding potential of fascia seems to be HA – which is one of the main GAGs of the ECM. Its role is to lubricate and enable the free movement of muscles on fascia and fascia on fascia. With overuse and trauma, HA builds up in the tissues and can become fragmented and act as an irritant and 'glue' that causes restriction and inflammation. The thickening in loose connective tissue

observed in patients in pain is due to increased GAGs and HA. Due to their increased concentration, the HA molecules literally get tangled up, both with themselves and water molecules (as they are hydrophilic) (**Figure 7.10**). This causes increased viscoelasticity, tissue stiffness and decreased ROM (Matteini et al 2009). Stecco sees HA as a key player in myofascial pain syndromes (Stecco et al 2011b, 2013b). Medics have begun to recognise the role of HA in musculoskeletal pathologies and this has led to treatment with HA injections into osteoarthritic knees, ankles and frozen shoulders.

But is there a way we can disentangle these HA chains through manual therapy so that the normal gliding movements of layers can be restored? It may well be that the local pressure and heat from fascial work helps these entangled HA chains to dissolve. As the main concentration of HA is in the deep fascial layer, techniques that are aiming to work at this level would be likely to be the most successful, e.g. Rolfing/structural integration (SI), Stecco fascial manipulation and certain myofascial release (MFR) techniques all emphasise sinking down to this layer to achieve release. A brainy

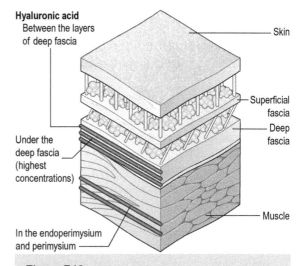

Hyaluronic acid
Between the layers of deep fascia

Skin

Superficial fascia

Deep fascia

Under the deep fascia (highest concentrations)

Muscle

In the endoperimysium and perimysium

Figure 7.10

With overuse and trauma, hyaluronic acid can become fragmented, acting as an irritant and 'glue' that causes restriction and inflammation between fascial layers

calculation by researchers (Chaudhry et al 2013, Roman et al 2013) showed that manual therapy is indeed helpful for increasing the flow of HA. The HA chains can also be disentangled by heat of over 40 degrees (Matteini et al 2009), which also confirms the role of moist heat as preparation for fascial work as advocated by the Jing HFMAST approach.

5 **Myofibroblasts and musculoskeletal pain**: until recently, fascia was thought to be a completely inert tissue devoid of any contractile properties. However, groundbreaking research (Schleip et al 2005) has shown that fascia in fact contains cells called myofibroblasts that enable it to contract in a smooth muscle-like manner. This may be the reason why fascia becomes stiff and restricted leading to pain conditions. We know, for example, that myofibroblasts are found in increased levels in conditions such as frozen shoulder, rheumatoid arthritis and Dupuytren's contracture. It also seems that certain triggers can cause long lasting fascial contractions that occur within minutes, e.g. the substances associated with wound healing and inflammation, heightened activity of the sympathetic nervous system (SNS) and alterations in pH.

6 **Stress and fascial stiffness**: have you ever noticed that some of your more stressed clients seem to have particularly tight and stiff tissues? Research has corroborated the fact that stress can indeed lead to fascial stiffness. Stimulation of the SNS leads to the production of a substance important in the immune system response known by the Star Trek type name of TGF-beta-1. Interestingly TGF-beta-1 is also a strong physiological stimulator of myofibroblast contraction; thus prolonged stress and activation of the SNS can lead directly to tissue contractures and increased fascial stiffness. Therapeutic fascial work that stimulates the mechanoreceptors – particularly Ruffini's and interstitial receptors – can inhibit this nervous system response and cause a reduction in these effects (Schleip 2011).

7 **Fascia and central sensitisation**: as with trigger points it is possible that fascial restrictions can lead to a constant nociceptive input that helps perpetuate peripheral and central sensitisation. Langevin and Sherman (2007) presented a neat theory bringing different strands of knowledge together about the multi-factorial aetiology of low back pain. They postulate that pain is due to the formation of a vicious cycle where pain-related fear leads to decreased movement, connective tissue remodelling, inflammation, nervous system sensitisation and further decreased mobility. Like the approach outlined in this book, Langevin and Sherman believe that a multidisciplinary treatment approach including direct mechanical tissue stimulation, movement re-education and psychosocial intervention is the key to treating this common condition (Langevin and Sherman 2007).

Fascia and fluid dynamics

Life is water dancing to the tune of solids.
ALBERT SZENT GYORGYI (TODAYINSCI.COM (ND))

It is easy to forget that the concentration quotients of salts in interstitial fluid and in water of an ocean are nearly identical. Our cells are, in a manner of speaking, swimming gel like structures in an ocean of interstitial fluids and we are carrying that ocean around with us.
MEERT 2013

It seems a dreamy and philosophical notion that we are just a bag of ocean water wandering around in our shoes, yet this is in fact the biological reality. We are after all two-thirds water. Given the importance of water in the body it is of great interest that one of the key areas of fascial research in recent years has been in the area of fluid dynamics. The ground substance in fascia contains substances like hyaluron that just love water and can actively draw fluid in when given free access. Normally, however, the ground substance is restrained from doing this due to the collagen fibres that are actively tensed by connective tissue cells. In other words, the ground substance is like a sponge tied up with string and is normally under hydrated.

However, with trauma to tissue the ground substance springs into action and actively absorbs fluid from the capillaries (Findley 2011).

This effect may well be of importance in our manual therapy work. Schleip et al (2012) have shown that with fascial tissue stretch, water is pushed out of the tissues, like squeezing a sponge. After a rest period, water is then sucked back in but to a greater level than before the stretch; in other words, the matrix becomes super-hydrated. This is like stepping on wet sand: with each step the water is driven out and then seeps back in. It may well be that the water getting sucked back in is different in some way and this process causes some kind of rejuvenation of the tissues.

It is plausible that the effects of our manual therapy work are due to the cells responding to the ebbs and flows of water around them; as Schleip (2013b) puts it 'speaking their primary language as some little ocean creatures'. Studies have shown fibroblasts to be highly responsive to the speed of movement of water around them and Schleip has speculated that this pushing and squeezing of fluid may well be the basis of mechanostimulation.

Having an awareness of these fluid dynamics can profoundly affect our intent while we work: having the visual of slowly squeezing and refilling tissue with fluid gives rise to a different type of bodywork than the visual of 'breaking down collagen cross links'. As Schleip says 'Speed matters.'

Becoming a fascial Ninja

So now we know all about fascia and why it may be implicated in general musculoskeletal pain conditions, lack of mobility and chronic widespread pain. That's all very well I hear you cry, but what do we DO about it. How do we actually get results with releasing fascial adhesions, restoring a full and buoyant biotensegrity to the living system and helping our clients with their problems, e.g. low back and neck and shoulder issues, temporomandibular joint (TMJ) disorders, headaches, repetitive strain injury (RSI), fibromyalgia and other stubborn pain conditions? There are so many methods of working with fascia that it can be bewildering for the massage therapist who really just wants to know 'Which are the best and most effective fascial techniques to learn?'

Unsurprisingly the approach we take to working with fascia at Jing is that of an eclectic 'fascial fusion' where we blend different fascial techniques to gain the best results, adapting the technique and the approach for the client and their pain situation. This keeps bodywork fresh, fun and creative. One of my very first massage teachers taught me that 'I have to constantly find ways to not let myself get bored with massage.' I feel that this is so true and as bodyworkers we need to make sure we don't get into a rut; to keep our bodywork alive by experimenting with different approaches, having fun with the body, constantly seeing what works and what doesn't work, blending and improvising, using technique, anatomy and intuition in equal doses.

What we have learned from research shows us that there is unlikely to be one type of fascial work that is superior to another. It is probable that different styles work through different mechanisms, e.g. the light touch of cranial work stimulates the multiple sensory receptors situated in the superficial fascia that report back to the emotional processing part of the brain, thus calming the SNS. In contrast the deeper work of Rolfing, MFR or Stecco fascial manipulation techniques may work on restoring the sliding and gliding of the HA in the deeper fascial layers.

With fascial work, all the different approaches have their own strengths and a creative combination of techniques can be incredibly powerful. Developing your skill set so you are competent in all the different branches of fascial work can be initially daunting but ultimately incredibly rewarding. In this way you become a 'fascial ninja' able to constantly adapt the technique to the situation with skill and creativity.

Overview of different approaches: your fascial toolbox

The addition of fascial techniques into your existing bodywork will, without a doubt, enable you to get better results, more clients through the door and a greater satisfaction with your work. Doing effective fascial work requires sensitivity, willingness to follow your intuition, a sense of connection with the body and the development of what we call 'listening touch'. We find these qualities usually come easily to massage therapists with good teaching and a little practice. Especially as we often work first with our hands, heart and head, and therefore it can be easier for us to adopt this approach compared with other practitioners whose training may have been more intellectually driven.

Although fascial techniques can be used as a treatment in themselves, at Jing we definitely favour the integration of techniques within a treatment as advocated in this book. Using fascial techniques at the beginning of your treatments (after application of heat) will enable your other techniques to be more effective.

In our own clinics we have successfully used fascial techniques to treat pain issues such as low back pain, sciatica, carpal tunnel syndrome, RSI, sporting injuries, rotator cuff problems, fibromyalgia, pelvic and menstrual problems, IBS, and headaches. Fascial work is an integral part of every single treatment we do and without a doubt learning fascial release techniques is an amazing investment in your career.

If we look back to our definition of fascia at the beginning of this chapter we are reminded that 'Fascia interpenetrates and surrounds all organs, muscles, bones and nerve fibres, creating a unique environment for body systems functioning' and includes 'aponeuroses, ligaments, tendons, retinaculae, joint capsules, organ and vessel tunics, epineuria, meninges, periostea, and all the endomysial and intermuscular fibers of the myofasciae'.

Wow! That's a lot of different structures to affect! It is clear from this definition that a 'full fascial toolbox' would really encompass three broad categories of techniques to address the:

1 Myofascia (fascia around and within the muscles; also the superficial fascia just below the skin)

2 Cranial fascia

3 Visceral fascia.

Other more sophisticated techniques also work more specifically on the fascia around the nerves and blood vessels.

Direct and indirect approaches to fascial release

Fascial techniques are often referred to as 'direct' or 'indirect'. In the direct method we have a clear concept of where we want the tissue to go to produce a certain effect. This is used in Rolfing and SI techniques where deep work with the fists, knuckles and elbows are used to work fascial layers, directly releasing adhesions and restrictions.

Indirect release is the term applied to releases in which the practitioner follows the direction of ease in the client's tissues rather than working directly on the 'stuck' direction of the restriction. This is similar to releasing a jammed drawer – sometimes pushing the drawer in first (direction of ease) works better than trying to pull it out directly. MFR and cranial work use this approach. In the indirect method the fascia is put on a stretch or given slight pressure to initiate a response in the tissues. The therapist then literally 'follows' where the tissue wants to go with their hands whilst keeping the stretch. After holding the stretch for between 3 and 5 minutes the tissue will eventually release in the place where it needs to. This sensation can feel literally magical and mastering the technique can require a level of practice.

I like to think of the difference between the two types of fascial work as similar to approaching two different friends with a problem. The 'direct' friend will give you good advice, telling you what you should do whereas the 'indirect' friend will just listen, giving you the space to work your way around to your own solution. Both types of friend are good to have and useful in different situations.

Some of the most well known fascial approaches are listed below.

Rolfing or structural integration (SI)

Rolfing can be like making your bed in the morning. You think you're going to get by without pulling that bed apart, so you pull up this cover and the next cover. When you get all the covers puffed up, you've got nine ridges running across the bed. Now you've got to go to a deeper layer and organize the deeper layer, and make your bed on top of that. Then you've got a made bed. Well it's the same with the body: you've got to organize those deeper layers.
IDA P. ROLF

Rolfing or SI, developed by the great Ida Rolf in the 1960s, seeks to re-establish proper vertical alignment in the body by manipulating the myofascial tissue. SI work aims to literally change the shape of the body into more optimal alignment and thereby easing pain and dysfunction caused by fascial restrictions. SI typically takes the body through a series of sessions (10 in the original 'Rolfing recipe'), starting at the feet and working up the body to achieve balance and ease. SI approaches incorporate:

- Systematic body reading to identify imbalances.

- A series of deep direct fascial techniques that incorporate work with fists, fingers and forearms together with active movement by the client. This follows one of Ida Rolf's great dictums 'Put it where it belongs and call for movement.'

- Ida was a firm believer in not chasing the symptoms, believing that proper myofascial alignment of the body through the full Rolfing 10-session series was the key to physical and psychological health. She had some great quotes including 'If your symptoms get better that's your tough luck' and 'Where you think it is, it ain't.'

Other SI approaches: these include KMI (kinesis myofascial integration, as developed by Tom Myers), Hellerwork (includes dialoguing and emotional work) and many others. All of these approaches are based heavily on Rolf's original work and retain most of her original concepts and techniques. For example, KMI uses 12 sessions rather than 10 to incorporate Tom Myers' new ideas around the Anatomy Trains; however, the techniques are broadly identical to those used by Rolfers. SI practitioners from different schools share more similarities than differences in the way they work.

Myofascial release (MFR)

Originally coined by the osteopath Robert Ward, in the 1980s the term MFR was adopted by a physical therapist John Barnes to describe his method of freeing restrictions in the myofascial system. The overall intention of MFR is to relieve pain, resolve structural dysfunction, restore function and mobility and release emotional trauma. MFR techniques rely heavily on the ability of the practitioner to use the sense of 'listening touch'; to be able to tune into the tissues and follow the fascia to where restrictions are held.

Techniques taught in this approach usually include cross hand stretches, arm and leg pulls and many others. Some of the techniques taught have a cross over with those from craniosacral therapy (e.g. transverse fascial plane releases) or, in some cases, more direct approaches (Barnes 1990).

Both MFR and SI approaches focus mainly on the myofascia, i.e. the fascia running through and around the muscles ('myo'). An all round fascial practitioner would also be proficient at techniques that seek to identify and release deeper fascial restrictions, i.e. those found in the cranium and around the organs.

Visceral manipulation

Developed by the visionary French osteopath Jean-Pierre Barrall, visceral manipulation sees fascial restrictions in the viscera (organs) as primary to other types of pain including musculoskeletal pain. Crucially, as the organs have fascial connections to the spine and other structures, restrictions in the viscera can cause a myriad of musculoskeletal problems. For example, ligaments supporting the lungs connect to the middle scalene muscles and C5–C7. Thus restrictions in the lung support membranes (pleura) can cause neck strain or chronic stiff neck. Gentle visceral manipulation of the lung pleura can quickly and effectively take people out of pain.

Crucial to the theory of visceral manipulation is the idea that organs are in perpetual motion and that each internal organ rotates on a physiological axis. In order for a person to be completely healthy all of the visceral system must have proper motion. Visceral manipulation seeks to restore optimal motion through gentle and precise fascial techniques. A brilliant study has convincingly shown that visceral work in rats can both prevent and treat adhesions of the internal organs (Bove and Chapelle 2014). Rats with experimentally induced bowel adhesions were given mini-visceral manipulation and then cut open again to see the results. Lo and behold, adhesions were seen to have been successfully treated compared to a control group. As the poor old rats were 'sacrificed' (research spin meaning 'killed') for their trouble in advancing fascial research, I do hope the experimental visceral manipulation treatments were carried out in a spa with relaxing music and a facial thrown in.

Craniosacral therapy (CST)

CST began as a branch of osteopathy. In the early 1900s Dr William Sutherland challenged the accepted anatomical wisdom that the skull bones were solidly fused in adulthood. Sutherland believed that the cranial bones were able to move and cranial osteopathy techniques were devised to correct abnormal cranial bone motion at the cranial sutures.

CST as popularised by John Upledger (1997) focuses not just on the movement of the cranial bones but also on the key role of the membranes that surround the brain, the spinal cord and, particularly, the dura mater. When assisting in a spinal operation, Upledger noticed a strong pulse in the membrane that surrounded the patient's spinal cord. He determined that the pulse was coming from the cerebrospinal fluid (CSF) that bathes the brain and spinal cord and postulated that anything that blocked the flow of this fluid could cause physical and mental distress. This pulse has come to be known as the craniosacral rhythm (CSR) and has a rhythm of around 6–12 beats per minute. Through gentle techniques that work on the dura mater and other fascial membranes, craniosacral therapists evaluate dysfunction and distortion in the dura mater and harmonise the CSR.

Research has questioned the existence of the cranial rhythm, suggesting that it might be a palpatory illusion. However, whatever the mechanisms, from our own clinical experience, cranial techniques can be very effective in working with certain pain conditions, particularly those where there is a central sensitisation or emotional component.

The sensation of tissue release in fascial work

Whatever their theoretical underpinnings, most of the methods of working with fascial restrictions report a common sensation of 'tissue release'. This is a particular sensation sensed by the practitioner that seems to coincide with a general relaxation and softening of the tissues and sometimes a sudden decrease of pain by the client. If you can feel a tissue release in a certain area of the body, this is a sign to move on to somewhere else – your work here is done! Tissue release is sensed differently by different practitioners; some therapists feel it as a softening,

a perceived lengthening (although science tells us not an actual lengthening) or a feeling of increased fluid flow. I find it is best not to 'expect' a certain sensation. I remember one MFR class where my co-teacher casually mentioned that fascial release felt like 'a shoal of fish under her hands'. We then had 6 days of stressed students proclaiming anxiously that they couldn't 'feel the fish!' The point here is to tune into what YOU feel which may be totally different from what anyone else feels. Here are some of the signs that you may notice in your own practice when you sense tissue release:

- Softening
- Lengthening
- Sense of increased fluid flow in the tissue under treatment
- Sense of increased energy flow
- Feeling of heat radiating from the body region
- Client takes deep breath or sighs
- You take a deep breath (usually just before the client does).

Here are some quotes from Jing therapists about what fascial release feels like to them:

- **As a therapist**:

Feels like a melting and also like a wave that rides away from a central point.

Like a deep constant slow stroke that never wants to end.

A sensation of deep movement beneath my hands which feels huge but barely noticeable on the surface.

Current sensation on giving treatment is like being connected with the client/fascial system as though it were suspended in space & you are just following the shape as it changes, elongates, redefines itself. Almost like a mercury globule in one of those glass temperature tubes! Slow motion & weightless.

Skin rolling & focused stretching/J stroking has more of a sense of teasing matted, almost felted wool to loosen & create space within the tissue.

- **As a receiver**:

An opening, a relieving of the deepest itch that needs to be scratched.

Relaxing, unwrapping tight spots and freedom.

Feels like spaciousness being created; blockages moving through and out; a sense of cracking open sometimes, in a good way!

Lightness and expansion in my body which carries on long after treatment is over.

Receiving it feels like you've been wearing a body-suit that has shrunk & the practitioner is teasing & lengthening you back into shape!

Why do fascial release techniques work?

All the approaches to working with fascia believe that the manual forces applied during hands on therapy change the 'density, tonus, viscosity or arrangement of fascia' in a permanent or semi-permanent way (Barnes 1990). The sensation of tissue release described above is usually felt to be a key therapeutic indicator of successfully applied technique. Certainly for therapists, the magical feeling of melting and gliding through the fascial layers seems key to getting results. So what might actually be happening? Although the sensation of tissue release can feel like a lengthening and stretching of fascial tissue, research suggests that while this might be a possibility in superficial tissues, such as the superficial nasal fascia, it is unlikely that manual techniques are producing any such change in the tougher fascia tissues, such as the fascia lata and plantar fascia (Chaudhry et al 2008).

Although we are still not totally clear on what is happening in fascial therapy, a number of plausible theories have been suggested and are outlined below.

Ida's idea: thixotrophy or the gel to sol theory

Ida Rolf first proposed the theory that connective tissue is a colloid substance in which the ground substance can be influenced by the application of energy (heat or mechanical pressure from the hands) to change from a more dense gel state to a more fluid sol state. This characteristic is called thixotrophy. The type of movement required to produce this change is crucial, as it needs to be SLOW. If quick movement is applied to a thixotrophic substance it will remain solid; if slow movement is applied the substance will literally melt under your fingers. Although the thixotrophic nature of fascia has long been believed to be the reason for the efficacy of fascial techniques and the 'melting' sensation we feel beneath our hands as practitioners, research by Robert Schleip and others has questioned this assumption. Schleip points out that the thixotrophic effect is reversible (think of melted butter going back to hard) and therefore doesn't account for permanent tissue changes (Schleip 2003a,b).

Star Trek super power theory: piezoelectric forces

Other experts (Barnes 1990, Oschman 2003) have suggested that the way in which fascia can change its shape is due to a phenomenon known as piezoelectricity. Basically the idea is that pressure and stretch from the hands creates an electrical current through the tissue causing the fascia to behave like a 'liquid crystal'. The suggestion is that the electric current stimulates the fibroblasts to alter their activity in the area.

John F. Barnes describes it in the following way (Barnes 1990):

Piezoelectric behaviour is an inherent property of bone and other mineralized and nonmineralized connective tissues. Compressional stress has been suggested to create minute quantities of electrical current flow. Like untwisting a copper wire, the techniques can restore the fascia's ability to conduct bioelectricity, thus creating the environment for enhanced healing. They can also structurally eliminate the enormous pressures that fascial restrictions exert on nerves, blood vessels and muscles. Myofascial release can restore the fascia's integrity and proper alignment and, similar to the copper wire affect, can enhance the transmission of our important healing bioelectrical currents.

Schleip points out that the time cycle involved is again too slow to account for the immediate tissue changes felt by the practitioner (Schleip 2003a,b).

Schleip's suggestion: the role of the nervous system

A newer explanation proposed by Robert Schleip (2003a,b) focuses on the mechanoreceptors found in the fascia and that manual stimulation of these leads to changes in tonus of the motor units under the practitioner's hand. As we have seen, the fascial system and autonomic nervous system are closely linked leading to changes in fascial tonus and ground substance viscosity. This would explain the short-term changes that are felt beneath the practitioner's hands.

Pollack's proposal: fluid dynamics AND electricity?

The biggest buzz at the 2012 fascial conference was the talk by Gerald Pollack about the fourth phase of water. According to Pollack, water does not just exist as solid, liquid and gas but also as a gel-like state. This type of water is formed next to any hydrophilic substance and furthermore is capable of creating an electrical charge, i.e. it acts as 'liquid crystalline water'. This liquid crystalline water envelops every macromolecule in the body, including those of the fascia. It is possible that radiant energy from the hands during manual therapy builds the liquid crystalline water that is necessary for physiological healthy function (Pollack et al 2009, Pollack 2014).

Although we are not clear exactly what is happening in fascial release, both researchers and clinicians have expressed common concepts of increased fluid flow and feelings of electrical charge. It will certainly be interesting to see what the next decade of fascial research reveals.

Practical principles of good fascial work

Use no or very little lubrication

Fascial techniques just don't work with lubrication as it creates a barrier to feeling the subtle restrictions and movement of fascial tissues. Myofascial techniques also require traction on the skin as tissues are slowly and gently pulled, pushed and stretched. On some occasions, a little water-based lubricant can be used for the direct SI based approaches; a little water on the hands works just as well. For indirect approaches we recommend no lubrication at all. This is one of the reasons why in the Jing method we carry out fascial techniques at the beginning of the treatment before applying oil or wax.

The supremacy of 'listening touch'

Whatever fascial techniques you are using they all rely on a keen sense of 'listening touch', i.e. the ability to tune into the tissues, sense where fascial restrictions are and feel the delicious tissue release. Really tune into your hands when you are working, sensing every minute detail of the tissues, the temperature and the texture of the different layers of the body. When you are learning fascial work it is easy to become obsessed with 'not feeling' things, worrying that you don't 'get it' or are not feeling what you are 'supposed' to feel. The mantra here is to tune into what you do feel rather than worrying about what you don't feel. Just like learning a new language, learning palpatory excellence takes time. Do you remember learning to ride a bike as a child? None of us leapt on a two-wheeled bike and cycled off first time around. Initially we probably learned to pedal a trike, then a two-wheeled bike with stabilisers (training wheels to the Americans out there), then fell off many times before we took our first wobbly (and probably very short) trip. This is what learning fascial work is like. Don't expect to get it the first time around. Just keep practising. The slogan here is 'Hands on bodies, hands on bodies'. This is what makes the difference when learning the language of fascia. Practice 10 minutes of fascial technique on every client and your listening touch will soon start to improve. Remember, as Jean-Pierre Barrall says, 'there are no limits to sensitivity'. Every time you touch someone with focus you can work on your skills of palpation.

Be patient

The old adage suggests that patience is a virtue and this is particularly true in fascial work. First, be patient with yourself when you are learning the work. Just like learning a new language, be prepared for the process to take some time. Second, be patient with the tissues when you are carrying out the techniques. Fascial restrictions take time to release. Being still and waiting is usually one of the hardest skills for bodyworkers to learn, as we are accustomed to working so hard to get a result. Do not force your strokes – just 'hang out' until you feel the tissue changing then follow where it takes you. Calm yourself internally; tune into your client and free yourself from the notion that you are 'doing nothing'. Often the most powerful work will occur in these moments of apparent stillness. Remember – less is more.

Speed matters

Slow down! Better results are obtained with slower, more thoughtful work. Ripping through the tissues will not lead to more gain.

Good body mechanics

Good body mechanics always lie at the heart of everything we do. If your body is uncomfortable you will be unable to carry out these sophisticated skills with the subtlety they require. Make sure your Hara is pointing in the direction of your work and you are in a comfortable stance. Check back in with your body ensuring your shoulders are relaxed and your arms are straight but with a softness to them. Keep checking back into your sense of being grounded with the 'feet, breath, belly' mantra.

Follow the tissues

Fascial work relies more on being a good follower than a leader. Think of your technique as an initial 'input' and then wait and see what the tissues want to do. With direct technique you should feel the tissues almost melting before you, like the waves of the sea parting to let you through. With indirect techniques like cross hand stretches you are putting the tissues on a stretch and then waiting to tune into their inherent motion, keeping them on a tension until you feel the release. Resist the temptation to lead or force as this will not lead to a quicker or more effective result.

Energetic distance

In addition to good body mechanics you will also need to be aware of the sensation of energetic distance between you and your client. This may sound like a slightly nebulous concept but it is of prime importance in carrying out good fascial work without exhausting yourself. Observe yourself when you are working, e.g. are you aware of where you end and your client begins in an energetic sense? Are you slightly hunched over your client and feeling like you are being overly affected by how they feel emotionally? If so bring your head back, stop staring at the body, relax your shoulders and feel your own sense of groundedness and strength. This will enable you to work without becoming exhausted or overly affected by any emotional release from your client.

Know where you are in the body

Be aware of what fascial layer you are working on. Are you on the superficial fascia with a very light touch? Are you aiming to affect the deep fascial layer? Your intent, pressure and focus will be different in each case.

Using fascial work in your treatments

How can we start to combine all these different approaches into our treatments to gain optimal results? In the Jing HFMAST approach we generally incorporate fascial work at the beginning of the treatment, after the application of heat and before our trigger point work. The protocol chapters give detailed explanations of how you can incorporate basic fascial strokes into your treatments. As you become more proficient with fascial techniques you can start to be more creative. The following are a few simple principles to get you on your way with your own creative fascial fusion style.

Think of techniques as 'templates' rather than 'absolutes'

When you are first learning it is natural to get lost in the absolute detail of how to do a particular technique, i.e. how many times do I do that stroke; how exactly do I hold the arm on an arm pull. As you become more proficient you realise that techniques are actually only 'templates' that can be played with. (The dictionary defines a template as 'something that serves as a master or pattern from which other similar things can be made'.) So think of your techniques as templates rather than absolute directions: in this way you can adapt your fascial skills to integrate ideas from all the different approaches.

If one fascial technique doesn't work then use a different one

Sounds obvious but different techniques may be more or less effective depending on the tissue and the situation. If your cross hand stretch isn't working to release stuck fascia in the low back, try some direct SI techniques. If that doesn't work maybe you need to use a cranial technique to release the dural tube. The possibilities are endless and different clients will respond to different approaches.

Combine ideas from different approaches within a treatment

Don't be a slave to one particular approach. Remember that if there was just one approach or technique out there that got consistent results every time we would all be using it. Be bold, creative and curious with your learning and bodywork, and constantly seek out new and different ways to release stuck tissue.

I hope this has given you some ideas and the confidence to play with integrating different fascial approaches. Fascia work is fun, fun, fun and gets astounding results. Keep your work fresh and exciting and you will always have clients coming back for more.

References

Barnes JF 1990 Myofascial Release: The Search for Excellence. Paoli, PA: Rehabilitation Services Inc.

Berlucchi G, Aglioti SM 2010 The body in the brain revisited. Experimental Brain Research 200:25–35.

Bfi.org. (n.d.) Big Ideas. The Buckminster Fuller Institute. Available at: https://bfi.org/about-fuller/big-ideas [accessed 18 August 2014].

Bove GM, Chapelle SL 2014 Visceral mobilization can lyse and prevent peritoneal adhesions in a rat model. Journal of Bodywork and Movement Therapies 16(1):76–82.

Brennan P 2013 Explaining taiji principles (taiji fa shuo). [online] Brennan Translation. Available at: http://brennantranslation.wordpress.com/2013/09/14/explaining-taiji-principles-taiji-fa-shuo/ [accessed 18 August 2014].

Chaitow L 2014 Somatic dysfunction and fascia's gliding-potential. Journal of Bodywork and Movement Therapies 18(1):1–3.

Chaudhry H et al 2008 Three-dimensional mathematical model for deformation of human fasciae in manual therapy. The Journal of the American Osteopathic Association 108:379–390.

Chaudhry H et al 2013 Squeeze film lubrication for non-Newtonian fluids with application to manual medicine. Biorheology 50(3–4):191–202.

Corey SM et al 2011 Sensory innervation of the nonspecialized connective tissues in the low back of the rat. Cells, Tissues, Organs 194(6):521–530.

Corey SM et al 2012 Stretching of the back improves gait, mechanical sensitivity and connective tissue inflammation in a rodent model. PLoS ONE 7:e29831.

Eisenbruch S et al 2010 Patients with irritable bowel syndrome have altered emotional modulation of neural responses to visceral stimuli. Gastroenterology 139(4):1310–1319.

Farb NAS, Segal ZV, Anderson AK 2013 Mindfulness meditation training alters cortical representations of interoceptive attention. Social Cognitive and Affective Neuroscience 8:15–26.

Fasciacongress.org (n.d.) International fascia research congress – About fascia. Available at: http://www.fasciacongress.org/about.htm [accessed 18 August 2014].

Findley TW 2011 Fascia research from a clinician/scientist's perspective. International Journal of Therapeutic Massage & Bodywork: Research, Education, & Practice 4(4).

Franklyn-Miller A et al 2009 The strain patterns of the deep fascia of the lower limb. Fascial Research II: basic science and implications for conventional and complementary health care. Elsevier GmbH, Munich

Fuller R, Applewhite E 1975 Synergetics, 1st edn. New York: Macmillan.

Fuller R, Applewhite E 1983 Synergetics 2, 1st edn. New York: Macmillan.

Gibson W et al 2009 Increased pain from muscle fascia following eccentric exercise: animal and human findings. Experimental Brain Research 194(2):299–308.

Goodreads.com 2014 The Hitchhiker's Guide to the Galaxy quotes by Douglas Adams. Available at: http://www.goodreads.com/work/quotes/3078186-the-hitchhiker-s-guide-to-the-galaxy-hitchhiker-s-guide-1 [accessed 18 August 2014].

Gracovetsky S 2008 Is the lumbodorsal fascia necessary? Journal of Bodywork and Movement Therapies 12(3):194–197.

Harlow HF, Suomi SJ 1970 Nature of love: simplified. American Psychologist 25(2):161–168, doi: 10.1037/h0029383.

Hoheisel U et al 2011 Nociceptive input from the rat thoracolumbar fascia to lumbar dorsal horn neurones. European Journal of Pain (London, England) 15(8):810–815.

Ingber DE 2008 Tensegrity and mechanotransduction. Journal of Bodywork and Movement Therapies 12(3):198–200.

Langevin HM, Sherman KJ 2007 Pathophysiological model for chronic low back pain integrating connective tissue and nervous system mechanisms. Medical Hypotheses 68(1):74–80.

Langevin HM et al 2009 Ultrasound evidence of altered lumbar connective tissue structure in human subjects with chronic low back pain. BMC Musculoskeletal Disorders 10:151.

Langevin HM et al 2011 Reduced thoracolumbar fascia shear strain in human chronic low back pain. BMC Musculoskeletal Disorders 12:203.

Levin S (n.d.) The tensegrity-truss as a model for spine mechanics: Biotensegrity. [online] Biotensegrity.com. Available at: http://www.biotensegrity.com/tensegrity_truss.php [accessed 18 August 2014].

Levin S 2005 In vivo observation of articular surface contact in knee joints. Biotensegrity.com. Available at: http://www.biotensegrity.com/in_vivio_observation_of_knee_joints.php [accessed 18 August 2014].

Liptan GL 2010 Fascia: a missing link in our understanding of the pathology of fibromyalgia. Journal of Bodywork and Movement Therapies 14(1):3–12.

Maas H, Sandercock TG 2010 Force transmission between synergistic skeletal muscles through connective tissue linkages. Journal of Biomedicine & Biotechnology (2010):Article ID 575672

McGlone F et al 2012 Touching and feeling: differences in pleasant touch processing between glabrous and hairy skin in humans. European Journal of Neuroscience 35(11):1782–1788.

Matteini P et al 2009 Structural behavior of highly concentrated hyaluronan. Biomacromolecules 8;10(6):1516–1522.

Meert GF 2013 Fluid dynamics in fascial tissues. In: Schleip R, Findley T, Chaitow L, Huijing P(eds) Fascia, 1st edn. London: Elsevier Health Sciences UK. p. 177

Montagu A 1971 Touching: The Human Significance of The Skin. New York: Columbia University Press.

Muscolino JE 2012 Fascial structure. Massage Therapy Journal Spring: pp. 73–77.

Myers T 2001 Anatomy Trains, 1st edn. Edinburgh: Churchill Livingstone.

Myers T 2006 Anatomy Trains: early dissective evidence. www.sportex.net, p.15. Available at: https://www.anatomytrains.com/main/wp-content/uploads/2012/07/dissection.pdf [accessed 18 August 2014].

Naqvi NH, Bechara A 2010 The insula and drug addiction: an interoceptive view of pleasure, urges, and decision-making. Brain Structure and Function 214(5–6):1–16.

Olausson H et al 2010 The neurophysiology of unmyelinated tactile afferents. Neuroscience and Biobehavioral Reviews 34(2):185–191.

Oschman J 2003 Energy Medicine in Therapeutics and Human Performance, 1st edn. Amsterdam: Butterworth Heinemann.

Paulus MP, Stein MB 2010 Interoception in anxiety and depression. Brain Structure & Function 214(5–6):451–463.

Paulus MP, Stewart JL 2014 Interoception and drug addiction. Neuropharmacology 76(Pt B):342–350.

Paulus MP, Tapert SF, Schulteis G 2009 The role of interoception and alliesthesia in addiction. Pharmacology Biochemistry, and Behavior 94(1):1–7.

Pollack G 2013 The Fourth Phase of Water, 1st edn. Seattle, WA: Ebner & Sons, p. 331.

Pollack GH 2014 The fourth phase of water: a role in fascia? Journal of Bodywork and Movement Therapies 17(4):510–511.

Pollack GH, Figueroa X, Zhao Q 2009 Molecules, water, and radiant energy: new clues for the origin of life. International Journal of Molecular Sciences 10(4):1419–1429.

Richards PJ, Win T, Jones PW 2005 The distribution of microvascular response in Achilles tendinopathy assessed by colour and power Doppler. Skeletal Radiology 34(6):336–342.

Roman M et al 2013 Mathematical analysis of the flow of hyaluronic acid around fascia during manual therapy motions. The Journal of the American Osteopathic Association 113(8):600–610.

Schilder A et al 2014 Sensory findings after stimulation of the thoracolumbar fascia with hypertonic saline suggest its contribution to low back pain. Pain 155(2):222–231.

Schleip R 2003a Fascial plasticity – a new neurobiological explanation: Part 1. Journal of Bodywork and Movement Therapies 7:11–19.

Schleip R 2003b Fascial plasticity – a new neurobiological explanation Part 2. Journal of Bodywork and Movement Therapies 7(2):104–116.

Schleip R 2011 Fascia as a sensory organ: a target of myofascial manipulation. In: Dalton E (ed) Dynamic Body: Exploring Form, Expanding Function. Freedom from Pain Institute pp. 137–164.

Schleip R 2013a Massage research: fascia as an organ of communication. True.massage-research.com. Available at: http://true.massage-research.com/2013/01/fascia-as-organ-of-communication-by.html [accessed 18 August 2014].

Schleip R 2013b Dr. Robert Schleip's lecture at the Third International Fascia Research Congress. YouTube. Available at: http://www.youtube.com/watch?v=miIlGLLmXIc [accessed 18 August 2014].

Schleip R, Jagerh H 2013 Interoception. In: Schleip R, Findley T, Chaitow L, Huijing P (ed) Fascia, 1st edn. London: Elsevier Health Sciences UK, pp. 89–94.

Schleip R., Klingler W, Lehmann-Horn F 2005 Active fascial contractility: fascia may be able to contract in a smooth muscle-like manner and thereby influence musculoskeletal dynamics. Medical Hypotheses 65(2):273–277.

Schleip R, Zorn A, Klingler W 2010 Biomechanical properties of fascial tissues and their role as pain generators. Journal of Musculoskeletal Pain 18(4):393–395.

Schleip R, Duerselen L, Vleeming A 2012 Strain hardening of fascia: static stretching of dense fibrous connective tissues can induce a temporary stiffness increase accompanied by enhanced matrix hydration. Journal of Bodywork and Movement Therapies 16(1):94–100.

Smith E 2012 Staying fit: Yoga, Rolfing and the elusive Cinderella tissues. The Huffington Post. Available at: http://www.huffingtonpost.com/eva-norlyk-smith-phd/fascia_b_1207768.html [accessed 18 August 2014].

Stecco A et al 2013a Ultrasonography in myofascial neck pain: randomized clinical trial for diagnosis and follow-up. Surgical and Radiologic Anatomy Apr;36(3):243–253.

Stecco A et al 2013b Fascial components of the myofascial pain syndrome. Current Pain Headache Reports 17(8):352.

Stecco C et al 2006 Histological characteristics of the deep fascia of the upper limb. Italian Journal of Anatomy and Embryology 111(2):105–110.

Stecco C et al 2007 Anatomy of the deep fascia of the upper limb. Second part: study of innervation. Morphologie 91(292):38–43.

Stecco C et al 2011a The fascia: the forgotten structure. Italian Journal of Anatomy and Embryology (Archivio Italiano di Anatomia ed Embriologia) 116:127–138.

Stecco C et al 2011b Hyaluronan within fascia in the etiology of myofascial pain. Surgical and Radiologic Anatomy 33(10):891–896.

Stecco C et al 2014 The peritendinous tissues: an anatomical study of their role in the pathogenesis of tendinopathy. Surgical and Radiologic Anatomy 36(6):561–572.

Taylor AG et al 2010 Top-down and bottom-up mechanisms in mind–body medicine: development of an integrative framework for psychophysiological research. Explore (New York, NY) 6(1):29–41.

Tesarz J et al 2011 Sensory innervation of the thoracolumbar fascia in rats and humans. Neuroscience 194:302–308.

Todayinsci.com (n.d.) Albert Szent-Gyorgyi quotes – 19 Science Quotes – Dictionary of science quotations and scientist quotes. available at: http://todayinsci.com/S/ SzentGyorgyi_Albert/SzentGyorgyiAlbert-Quotations.htm [accessed 18 August 2014].

Upledger J 1997 Your inner physician and you, 1st edn. Berkeley, CA: North Atlantic Books.

Van der Wal JC 2009 The architecture of the connective tissue in the musculoskeletal system – an often overlooked functional parameter as to proprioception in the locomotor apparatus. International Journal of Therapeutic Massage & Bodywork: Research, Education, & Practice 2(4)9–23.

Verdejo-Garcia A, Clark L, Dunn BD 2012 The role of interoception in addiction: a critical review. Neuroscience and Biobehavioral Reviews 36(8):1857–1869.

Yahia L. et al 1992 Sensory innervation of human thoracolumbar fascia. an immunohistochemical study. Acta Orthopaedica Scandinavica 63:195–197.

8

Trigger happy! The art and science of trigger point therapy

Trigger points are our next stop on the HFMAST protocol. You may remember that the third step is 'M' which represents the treatment of all the muscles around the joint for trigger points.

Trigger points: the massage therapist's best friend

Learning effective trigger point work can be a seemingly magical component to add to your toolbox of manual therapy skills. Ask any therapist who has been practising precise trigger point work for a length of time and you are likely to hear a plethora of stories of wonderful results that range from the clinically satisfying to the downright miraculous. Here is an example from a Jing trained therapist:

One of my first great successes with trigger point therapy was treating a young women called Vicky with recalcitrant face and jaw pain. A student at veterinary college, Vicky was under huge amounts of stress. When she first came to me she had a trismus. Her jaw was locked closed and at her first visit, she could only open her mouth the width of two fingers. She also suffered from severe headaches.

Vicky attended for massage and trigger point therapy weekly. In the beginning we could not treat the muscles of mastication due to the severely limited access, so treatment was focused around the neck and shoulders particularly the trapezius, sub-occipitals and SCM.

After her third appointment Vicky was very pleased to report that she could now open her mouth the width of four fingers. We then continued to treat these muscles for another three weekly appointments after which Vicky reported that her jaw felt loose and comfortable and pain free and her headaches were gone. Vicky continues to have monthly maintenance treatments to help prevent

the problem returning. This story was just one in a series of success stories with this condition which set me off on my 'Trigger Point Journey'.
TRACEY KIERNAN, DENTAL NURSE AND
MASSAGE THERAPIST

My own introduction to the power of trigger point therapy was no less dramatic. At the very beginning of my massage career my father developed a debilitating pain in his low back. Generally healthy but very conventional in his approach to treatment, he consulted the local doctor who duly referred him to a specialist who pronounced the need for an epidural and spinal manipulation. At the time I was armed with very little skill but bucketloads of enthusiasm and had recently attended a weekend workshop run by a local osteopath who had expounded the theory and practice of trigger point work. I duly got Dad on the floor and prodded his back somewhat inexpertly until I found a spot that seemed to reproduce the pain he was experiencing – the 'Ahh, that's it!' moment with clients that always remains thrilling as a massage therapist. I treated the sore spot with static compression as I had been taught and instructed him in how to treat the trigger point himself. The outcome was a complete relief of pain within a few days, a cancellation of the appointment with the orthopaedic surgeon and a rather dramatic turn around in my parents' attitude to my nascent massage career (which they had previously regarded as one of my many phases that they were hoping I would grow out of). Results all round!

I now know that the sore spot was a trigger point in the quadratus lumborum muscle. Janet Travell, founder of modern trigger point therapy, describes trigger points in this muscle as one of the most commonly overlooked causes of low back pain (Travell et al 1993, p. 29) (**Figure 8.1**). Our clinical experience over the past 20 years suggests that this statement was not mere

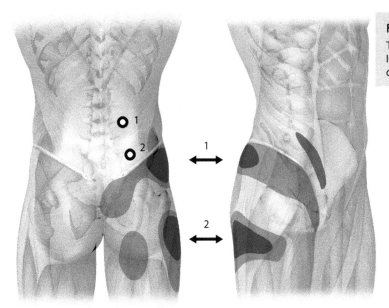

Figure 8.1
Trigger points in the quadratus lumborum muscle are one of the most overlooked causes of low back pain

hyperbole on Janet's part; certainly since that time we have both been able to help hundreds of clients attain a reduction in low back and other musculo-skeletal pain through using precise trigger point therapy as an important component of our treatment approach.

I have always been a big fan of trigger point therapy in massage treatment as it was the first advanced technique I learned that really seemed to improve my ability to obtain results with clients. There is some solid evidence behind the theory of treating trigger points for pain, and the popularity of the technique within the bodywork community strongly suggests there is something in the approach that consistently works. Trigger point therapy is a component of the toolbox of many different manual therapists, including chiropractors, osteopaths, physical therapists and massage therapists. One survey of American chiropractors showed that more than 40% used trigger point techniques on a regular basis (National Board of Chiropractic Economics 1993). Prominent bodywork authorities are also enthusiastically supportive of trigger point therapy. In *Clinical Application of Neuromuscular Techniques* co-authored with Judith DeLany, Leon Chaitow puts his academic weight firmly behind the opinion of pain researchers Melzack and Wall (1998), that trigger points are central to pain conditions:

… modern pain research has demonstrated that a feature of all chronic pain is the presence as part of etiology (often the major part) of localized areas of soft tissue dysfunction which promote pain and distress in distant structures. These are the loci that are known as trigger points.
Chaitow and DeLany 2000, p. 65

Importantly, the theory and practice of treatment of pain using trigger points is also utilised by sections of the mainstream medical community who are receptive to the scientific ideas and concepts as initially presented by the legendary Janet Travell MD, physician to President Kennedy (**Figure 8.2**). Medics use injection of trigger points with anaesthetic, saline solution or in some cases dry needling to treat a variety of musculoskeletal conditions. A 2002 medical review of the use of trigger point injections states that:

While relatively few controlled studies on trigger-point injection have been conducted, trigger-point injection and dry needling of trigger points have become widely accepted. This therapeutic approach is one of the most effective treatment options available and is cited repeatedly as a way to achieve the best results.
Alvarez and Rockwell 2002, pp. 653–661

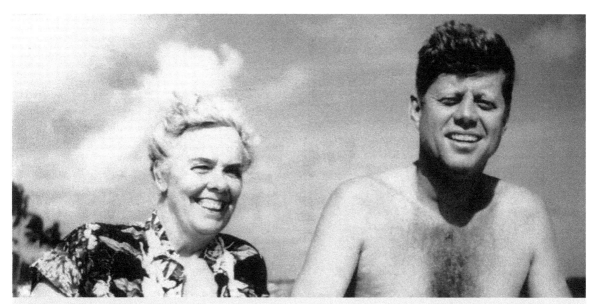

Figure 8.2
Picture of Janet Travell and President Kennedy. With kind permission from Virginia Powell Street, Janet Travell memorial website: www.janettravellmd.com

The paper goes on to note that 'Trigger-point injection can effectively inactivate trigger points and provide prompt, symptomatic relief.'

Travell's theories and meticulous clinical observations of the role of trigger points in myofascial pain are presented in two exhaustive volumes of clinical documentation, the famous 'big red books' (*Myofascial Pain and Dysfunction: The Trigger Point Manual*, Volumes 1 and 2) that are proudly displayed on any serious massage therapist's shelf! (Beware! Lugging them around can give you more than a few trigger points!) The famous quadratus lumborum muscle, site of my dad's fateful trigger point, has a full 60 pages devoted to it, just to give you an idea of the thoroughness of Travell and Simons' ideas.

Planet Janet (Figure 8.3)

Concerning your professional goals, the basic objective is: BE YOURSELF. Do not compare yourself with anyone else. No two people in the world have the same thumbprint, not even identical twins. You are unique.

It's better to wear out than to rust out.

Take care of your muscles and they will take care of you.
FAVOURITE SAYINGS OF JANET TRAVELL, WWW.
JANETTRAVELLMD.COM

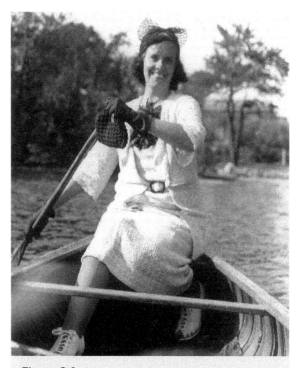

Figure 8.3
Janet Travell. With kind permission from Virginia Powell Street, Janet Travell memorial website: www.janettravellmd.com

Trigger point theory is ALL about Janet Travell. Seriously, it really is (although of course she had a little help from a few others along the way). Much of what has been theorised or written about trigger points can be directly traced back to her insights, and most of the books that have been written on the subject are condensed or simplified versions of the famous trigger point volumes co-authored with David Simons. As Clair Davies, massage therapist and author of the successful *The Trigger Point Therapy Workbook,* puts it:

> *Among those who recognize the reality and importance of myofascial pain, Janet Travell is generally recognized as the leading pioneer in diagnosis and treatment. Few would deny that she single-handedly created this branch of medicine . . . . Her revolutionary concepts about pain have improved the lives of millions of people.*
> Davies and Davies 2004, p. 15

Although there have been many other researchers over the past century who have come up with very similar concepts to those of Travell, the exhaustive clinical research carried out by Travell and Simons has earned them a place in the history books as the leading figures in this field. However, it is worth noting that, in the West the reporting of painful points that produce referred pain can be traced back as far as 1843 (Froriep 1843). In the East the documentation of painful 'ah shi' points goes back even further. Indeed, over the centuries, there are numerous examples of medics and researchers independently discovering the same phenomenon.

Accordingly there have been several different diagnostic labels given to these discoveries ranging from muscular rheumatism (Gutstein 1938), fibrositis (Gowers 1904) and, my personal favourite, myogelose (muscle gelling) (Schade 1919). Travell's own first description was called 'idiopathic myalgia' (1942) and progressed to 'trigger areas' (1957) before settling on the now currently accepted terminology of 'myofascial trigger point' (or TrP for short) in 1983 (Simons et al 1999, p. 15). Rather like the agony involved in naming a band you can imagine Travell and Simons brainstorming names late into the night, shots of whisky at hand, until they finally came up with the great 'myofascial trigger point' moniker. (Clearly whoever came up with

'myogelose' was never going to have a universally sellable concept however great their research!).

Any brief examination of the life and character of Janet shows clearly that she was a 'tour de force'; a woman of determination and will and moreover an excellent physician and healer. Balancing an intensive career with marriage and children in a pre-enlightened era, she is famous for being the first woman ever to hold the post of White House physician and Kennedy described her as a 'medical genius'. In *Kennedy,* Ted Sorensen's book, he reported that Senator Kennedy received so much relief from pain by Janet Travell's medical treatments that he had 'new hope for a life free from crutches if not from backache' (Sorensen 1965, p. 40). Although it is tempting for massage therapists to hold this up as an example of the power of manual trigger point therapy, it is worthwhile remembering that Travell's medical approach involved injecting trigger points with procaine, a drug strongly related to Novocain!

Steven and Donna Finando, authors of the book *Trigger Point Therapy for Myofascial Pain,* worked directly with Janet Travell on several occasions in the 1990s, declaring the experience to be 'the opportunity to observe a master practitioner':

> *Watching Dr. Travell treat patients was a joy. She understood what to do, where to touch, how to move, how to feel and she ultimately helped her patients. She understood what was of benefit and hypothesized about why. The concepts and approaches that she utilized simply work; they help change lives and alleviate suffering.*
> Finando and Finando 2005, p. 9

We were both lucky enough to meet Donna and Steven Finando in the summer of 2014 and enjoyed their stories about the sharp mind of Janet Travell. Steven recounted a meeting at her home, which was overflowing with multiple towering piles of research papers and academic tomes. In discussion about a particular topic, Janet mentioned a study she thought would be perfect for Steven to read. 'Go over there, young man' she said 'and look two-thirds of the way down that pile of papers and you will find what you need' (and of course he did) (**Figure 8.4**). On another occasion, Janet was lecturing

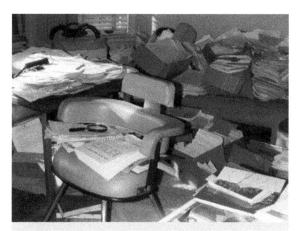

Figure 8.4
Janet Travell's study was overflowing with books and academic papers and yet she always knew exactly where everything was. With kind permission from Virginia Powell Street, Janet Travell memorial website: www.janettravellmd.com

with her colleague, John Mennell. The two worked closely together and went around the country delivering the same lecture to different groups. Mennell delivered his lecture and Janet sat in her seat taking copious notes. At the end of the lecture, Mennell addressed the audience with 'Any questions?'. Guess whose hand shot up first? Yes that's right, Janet Travell then proceeded to grill her esteemed colleague with a number of questions on a topic she had presumably heard many times before. Proof indeed of her fervent intellectual curiosity.

Undoubtedly Janet Travell had many other qualities that we should aim to emulate as therapists and not just her theoretical framework that validates applying manual pressure to sore spots of muscle tissue. Her success with clients was due to persistence, continual accumulation of a wealth of clinical experience, willingness to refine her own theories, a pursuit of scientific evidence to backup her ideas and, above all, the drive and determination to 'keep on keeping on'. Janet Travell embodied a zest and passion for her life and work as exemplified by the fact that her most famous publication, the trigger point manual volume one, was published when she was well into her 80s. As she herself famously said 'Life is like a bicycle. You don't fall off unless you stop pedalling.'

An inspirational woman with an unquenchable curiosity about the body, Travell's ideas have been highly influential in the field of musculoskeletal pain in both the orthodox and complementary medical communities. Massage therapists have as much to learn from how she lived her life as from her remarkable theories and research.

So what is a trigger point exactly?

Although the term trigger point has passed into more common usage since the publication of Travell and Simons' seminal works in the 1980s there is still a surprising amount of misinformation about what trigger points actually are (and aren't), not to mention the best way to treat them.

Let's start with the universally known classic definition from Travell and Simons themselves. You will be hard pressed to read an article or book on trigger point therapy without encountering the classic sound bite below. (This quote is ubiquitous in the same way that textbook and website explanations of fascia seem obliged to mention the hypothetical sweater with a snag in it to illuminate the 'fascia is all connected' concept.) According to 'the source', a trigger point is:

> *A hyper irritable spot in skeletal muscle that is associated with a hypersensitive palpable nodule in a taut band. The spot is painful on compression and can give rise to characteristic referred pain, referred tenderness and autonomic phenomena.*
> SIMONS ET AL 1999, P. 5

As this definition tends to make a large percentage of the population glaze over, most of your clients are likely to understand trigger points as 'muscle knots', i.e. lumps and bumps in their muscles that are responsible for their pain. Although the muscle has definitely not tied itself into a knot, the average massage therapist is well aware that clients will be seeking help for relief from these pesky 'muscle knots'. A brief Google search reveals a plethora of suitably named bodywork businesses that include 'knots' in the title. Clearly the knot analogy is a pervasive image and we all instinctively feel the urge to poke around our own bodies when we are in pain to try and find these 'hot spots'.

So if trigger points are not actually knots what are they? The key points to note are:

- They 'feel' like knots in muscle but are in fact small areas of tightly contracted muscle

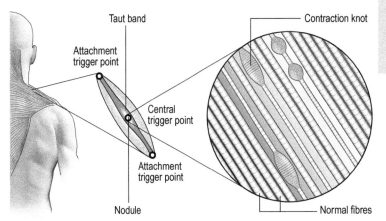

Taut band

Attachment
trigger point

Central
trigger point

Attachment
trigger point

Nodule

Contraction knot

Normal fibres

Figure 8.5

Trigger points are painful nodules found within a taut band of skeletal muscle

(NOT the same as a whole muscle spasm). **See Figure 8.5**

- They are usually found within a taut band of skeletal muscle that can be palpated.

- If you press on the trigger point it hurts.

- This is the most exciting point for therapists, the pain has a characteristic referred pain pattern. This means that the pain from trigger points often causes pain in other parts of the body distant from the trigger point itself. Good examples are the trigger points in the sternocleidomastoid muscle (SCM) that can commonly cause headaches or jaw pain. Or trigger points in the piriformis muscle that can cause a pain down the leg commonly confused with sciatica. Or trigger points in the quadratus lumborum that cause pain around the sacrum that can feel like sacroiliac pain. **See Figure 8.6**

- There is also a lesser-known, slightly mysterious part to the definition: trigger points can also cause 'autonomic referred phenomenon'. In other words trigger points can also cause symptoms you would never guess were coming from your muscles, e.g. ringing in the ears or dizziness can be caused by trigger points in the SCM.

The concept of referred pain is an important one as it means that the source of the pain can often be in a different location than where the client is feeling their discomfort. This is critical to what we do as massage therapists, as the theory of trigger point therapy suggests that if we are only treating the area of pain we are unlikely to achieve lasting results. It is likely that if the cause is myofascial trigger points and you are only in the area of pain, you will be in the wrong place 75% of the time (Chaitow and DeLany 2000, p. 69).

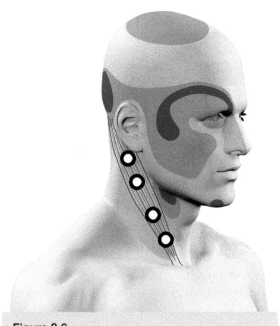

Figure 8.6

Trigger points in the sternocleidomastoid muscle (SCM) are a common cause of headaches

What are the effects of trigger points?

Pain

The bad boys of the body, trigger points are always up to no good. Travell and Simons go so far as to describe them as the 'scourge of mankind' (Travell and Simons 1999, p. 14). Many researchers have corroborated the notion that trigger points are implicated in up to 95% of chronic musculoskeletal pain (Malanga and Cruz Colon 2010), with one study suggesting that trigger points are the sole cause of such pain as much as 74% of the time (Gerwin 1995). A study of musculoskeletal disorders in Thailand found that myofascial pain syndrome was the primary diagnosis in 36% of 431 patients with recent onset pain (Chaiamnuay et al 1998).

The pain from trigger points can manifest in many different ways: it can feel like dragging, stabbing, dull, tingling, burning, superficial or deep in the joint. Trigger points can also cause weakness in the affected muscles. As there is a lack of awareness as to the concept of trigger points, the pain is often misdiagnosed as having a more serious or unknown cause leading to unnecessary medical tests or fear and hopelessness on the part of the client.

Compression of nerves and blood vessels

As nerves and blood vessels perforate the muscles at many places, the shortening of muscles caused by trigger points can lead to their entrapment with consequences of numbness, tingling (nerves) or oedema (blood vessels). I have had many cases of misdiagnosed carpal tunnel syndrome in my clinic that have been easily resolved through appropriate trigger point treatment of the scalenes or pectoralis minor muscles, both of which, when shortened by trigger points, can trap the brachial plexus (nerve bundle that runs down the arm).

Restricted movement

The taut bands that arise in connection with trigger points lead to shortening of the muscles – which in turn leads to reduced mobility and, potentially, joint dysfunction.

Autonomic effects

Autonomic effects can be found both in the area of the trigger point and in the area of referred pain. Autonomic effects include changes to skin temperature, increased sweat secretion and nausea or dizziness. Some other more bizarre cases of autonomic effects cited by Travell and Simons comprise reddening of the eyes, excessive tearing, blurred vision, a droopy eyelid, excessive salivation, persistent nasal secretion and goose bumps.

Adhesions and contractures

Persistent trigger points in muscles can lead to stiff ropy-like cords in the muscle; these are caused by fascial adhesions overlying and fixing the trigger point complex. Layers of connective tissue literally stick to each other causing hard, ropy muscles that feel like they are glued together. These are known as adhesions and severe cases can even develop into a form of contracture, similar to that seen in people with paralysis. Adhesions literally 'lock in' trigger points making them more difficult to treat and compounding problems of pain and movement. Contractures also affect the overall functioning of the muscle; the contracture is felt as hard, tight and fibrotic whereas the rest of the muscle becomes weak and atrophied (Chen et al 2006).

The great pretenders: misdiagnosis and myths attributed to trigger points

> *Muscle is an orphan organ. No medical speciality claims it. As a consequence no medical speciality is concerned with promoting funded research into the muscular causes of pain and medical students and physical therapists rarely receive adequate primary training in how to recognise and treat myofascial trigger points.*
> DAVIES AND DAVIES 2004, FOREWORD

As most primary health care providers are not specialists in musculoskeletal pain, the pain from trigger points can be a cause of medical misdiagnosis. Travll et al (1999, p. 37) list 23 common diagnoses where overlooked trigger points were the cause of symptoms. Looking down the list is similar to leafing through my client notes over the last 20 years – the conditions mentioned are common occurrences in the average massage therapist's clinic and can usually be successfully treated through trigger point therapy. The following are some examples of misdiagnosis I have encountered over the last 20 years of clinical practice:

- **Heart problems:** I was visiting my best friend in Rome when she received an emergency phone call from her mother who was experiencing persistent and frightening chest pain. A heart problem was suspected (although the presentation was not entirely typical) and she was being taken into hospital for tests and observation. My friend was beside herself with worry and arranged to immediately fly out to be with her. On the plane I explained about trigger points and literally drew a diagram on the back of a napkin showing the referral pattern of trigger points in the pectoralis major which can mimic the pain of angina. In this case, trigger points indeed turned out to be the source of the problem and a few visits to the local osteopath for treatment gave full relief.

- **Frozen shoulder:** I have had countless cases of supposed 'frozen shoulder' that have been easily resolved with appropriate trigger point therapy. Any kind of pain and restricted range of motion in the shoulder can easily be misdiagnosed as being a problem with the joint capsule when in fact the issue is clearly of a muscular origin.

- **Bursitis:** this is often used as another 'catch all' diagnosis when the practitioner is unaware of the potential effects of myofascial trigger points. I have lost count of the number of 'trochanteric bursitis' conditions that I have been able to treat through alleviating trigger points in the gluteus medius and minimus.

- **Suspected herniated cervical or lumbar disc:** disc problems are often suspected when the client experiences pain, numbness or tingling down their extremities. Again the issue can often be traced to trigger points in muscles such as the pectoralis minor or scalenes, in the case of the cervical region, or piriformis and gluteus medius, or quadratus lumborum, for the low back.

- **Osteoarthritis:** this misdiagnosis is often not the fault of the professionals but clients themselves who have a surprising ability to attribute themselves the worse possible verdict for their pain. Arthritis is a common self-imposed explanation given by many clients for their hip or knee pain. Again this is often attributable to

trigger points and can be easily resolved. Be wary of comments such as 'It's arthritis. It runs in the family. There's nothing you can do about it' and find out if this diagnosis came from a reputable health professional and whether it is backed up by adequate diagnostic tests. As a child I had a habit of reading my parents' old fashioned 'medical almanac' and self-diagnosing myself with all kinds of terrible diseases; at one point I convinced myself I had a hole in my heart and was going to die within the year. This was based on getting a bit of a chest pain after cycling too hard on my bike and reading a terrifying magazine story about a child with a hole in their heart. Clients can be just as susceptible to such conjecture and half-truths.

- **Temporomandibular joint (TMJ) disorder**: inspired by the first hand experience of one of our teachers, a former dental nurse, many of our students have enjoyed remarkable success with treatment for their TMJ disorders through trigger point work. Generally there is no problem with the joint itself, just issues with trigger points in the neck, shoulder and jaw muscles.

The sliding filaments: actin, myosin and the crowd surfing theory of muscle contraction

Scientists and researchers have spent a good amount of time examining what is going on at a microscopic level with trigger points in an attempt to explain the observed effects. To understand trigger points we need to go right down to the basic unit of the muscle cell – the sarcomere. Each individual muscle is composed of many muscle cells; these muscle cells are then in turn composed of many tubular myofibrils. Myofibrils themselves are actually repeating sections of sarcomeres.

Each sarcomere consists of a package of intertwined protein molecules; the most important two being actin (the so-called thin filament that can be remembered as actin rhymes with 'thin') and myosin (the 'thick' filament). These filaments slot in between each other. A good visual for how the actin and myosin filaments overlap each other is to put both hands in front of you, palms toward the body and slide your fingers of one hand in between those of the other.

The theory of how muscles contract – the sliding fila-ment mechanism – suggests that the myosin molecules grab onto the actin and slide them along – similar to the way a rock star does 'crowd surfing'. Normally this sarcomere activity is smoothly coordinated throughout the whole muscle to produce a contraction.

However, with trigger points this process goes a little bit awry. Research has shown that trigger points are likely to form near the motor endplate of the muscle (Travell et al 1999, p. 122) – which is the place where the nerve interacts with the muscle to give it the signal to contract. With trigger point formation a bunch of sarcomeres are stuck in contraction around the motor end plate and are unable to let go. The actin and myosin literally relentlessly grab onto each other resulting in a small area of hyper-contracted muscle, i.e. a trigger point (**Figure 8.7**).

These highly contracted sarcomeres near the motor end plate (found at the midpoint of the muscle) cause the sar-comeres on either side to be overstretched. People with trigger points often complain of their muscles feeling 'tight'. The sensation of tightness is a complicated one as it is a result of some of the sarcomeres being over-contracted and some over-stretched. Clients with trigger

points often feel the need to stretch to relieve their pain; however, stretching can be ineffective if central trigger points have not been released (Ingraham 2014).

What causes and perpetuates trigger points?

The general answer to this question is 'life!' Or certainly our average high paced, overwhelming, muscle abus-ing, prescription drug taking, fast food eating, alcohol consuming, emotionally demanding, shallow breath-ing, overly working and not enough playing modern Western type lives! Travell and Simons have credited almost every potential stressor to the body as possibly causing (or perpetuating) trigger points, including:

- **Acute sudden onset trauma**: these types of trigger points are due to one-off traumas to the body and include: car accidents, falls, fractures, sprains, dislocations or a direct blow to the muscle. These types of trigger points usually respond well to treatment if caught early enough and treated as soon as any associated soft tissue injury has healed.

- **Gradual onset**: these types of trigger points come on over time, usually in response to sustained lack of mobility (sitting at a desk for hours) or chronic overuse (endless computer work without taking a break). It is important to help the client to identify the causes of the pain as often the trigger points will not resolve until the aggravating factors are removed or modified.

- **Psychological factors**: emotional stress invariably can play a part in trigger point formation and without a doubt can perpetuate their existence beyond the practitioner's best efforts. As we have seen in Chapter 4, it is vital to treat the whole person, body and mind.

- **Nutritional factors**: Travell and Simons felt that nutritional and vitamin deficiencies were an important cause of persistent trigger points.

- **Medical factors**: several potential perpetuating medical factors have been proposed including chronic infection, allergies, chronic visceral disease, metabolic and endocrine inadequacies (such as anaemia and low thyroid function).

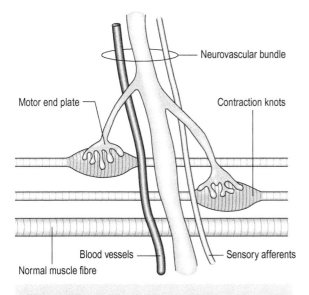

Figure 8.7
Trigger points form near the motor end plate of a muscle

An awareness of potential stressors is important because enabling clients to gain a pain-free state is NOT just about releasing trigger points during a session. Like that unwelcome relative who keeps turning up at Christmas without an invite, trigger points have a habit of coming back if the initial stressors are still in place.

Identifying these perpetuating factors is usually easier than you think if you rely on the old fashioned skills of good communication with your client and a bit of common sense. Clients are surprisingly good at coming up with their own answers if given permission; asking the simple question 'What do you think is the cause of your pain?' can be very illuminating. The stressful work environment, the dodgy office chair, the funny angle for holding the bottle to feed the new baby, the relationship problems that need addressing, the uncomfortable mattress, etc. are just some factors. Identifying the likely causes of trigger points is not always rocket science and removing these causes is a big part of enabling a permanent release from pain.

Chicken and egg: trigger points and central sensitisation

We learned in Chapter 4 about the huge part played by central sensitisation in chronic pain conditions. This is the phenomenon where there is no perceivable damage to the tissues but a huge pain response due to an over-sensitised central nervous system. It seems that trigger points and central sensitisation often go hand in hand. Yet, much like the proverbial chicken and egg conundrum, which comes first: trigger points or central sensitisation? It is likely that both may be true and in chronic musculoskeletal pain there is a self-perpetuating cycle of trigger points exacerbating central sensitisation and central sensitisation exacerbating trigger points. From a pain science perspective, trigger points are constant sources of peripheral nociceptive input that can lead to neuroplastic changes in the spinal cord and brain. This results in central sensitisation and consequent pain (Dommerholt 2011, Ge and Arendt-Nielsen 2011, Staud 2006, 2010, 2011a,b). The input from trigger points leads to hyper-excitability of central neurones that causes the terrible triad of allodynia, hyperalgesia and pain referral (Mense et al 2010). A study by Xu et al (2010) showed that painful stimulation of latent trigger points can initiate widespread central

sensitisation leading to the conclusion that trigger points are 'one of the important peripheral pain generators and initiators for central sensitisation'.

Other authors have pointed to the role of trigger points in maintaining central sensitivity in migraines (Calandre et al 2006, Giamberardino et al 2007); chronic tension-type headache (CTTH) (Fernández-de-las-Peñas et al 2007); TMJ (Fernández-de-las-Peñas et al 2010); fibromyalgia (Giamberardino et al 2011); tennis elbow (Fernández-Carnero et al 2008) and whiplash (Freeman et al 2009). Not only do trigger points contribute to central sensitivity but there is also some evidence that central sensitisation can also promote trigger point activity. The effective treatment of trigger points is as an important factor in reducing central sensitisation and pain in many chronic musculoskeletal complaints (Fernández-de-las-Peñas and Dommerholt 2014).

In terms of treatment, Fernández-de-las-Peñas and Dommerholt (2014, p. 4) recommend an approach remarkably similar to the one outlined in this book where both peripheral and central components of the pain are addressed. (Note: if you doze off at 'academic speak' skip to the digested read.)

The treatment plan should include two main components. First, peripheral and central nervous system sensitivity must be targeted by means of appropriate interventions. Second, the descending inhibitory systems must be activated. Inactivating TrP and addressing their perpetuating and promoting factors has an important function in achieving these objectives, because removing the peripheral nociceptive input from TrP will modulate the patient's central sensitivity. Clinically, when a patient presents with a pain problem mediated by predominantly peripheral sensitization mechanisms, functional activity and early and appropriate treatment of the noxious inputs should be encouraged. This may involve inactivating TrP, and mobilizing joints and nerves. For a patient with a more persistent condition mediated by predominantly central sensitization mechanisms, a multimodal therapy program is the preferred approach, which may include pharmacological and medical management, physical therapy, and cognitive behavioral or psychodynamic therapy.

Depending on the chronicity of the disorder and the associated disability, patients should receive pain neuroscience education addressing the neurobiology of pain and pain mechanisms, fear, anxiety, and other psychosocial variables. Patients need to develop different strategies for optimizing normal functional movement and to undertake active and specific or more global exercises, including aerobic exercise.
FERNÁNDEZ-DE-LAS-PEÑAS AND DOMMERHOLT 2014, P. 4

Digested read:

Treating trigger points will help with central sensitisation. If there isn't a lot of central sensitisation going on just treat the trigger points and tell 'em to keep calm and carry on. If there's loads of central sensitisation going on, still treat the trigger points but the client will have to do a heap more stuff like cognitive behaviour therapy (CBT), therapy, exercise and neuroscience education … hmmmm … someone really should write a book about that.

What are trigger points made from?

Somewhat like the nursery rhyme about little boys being made of 'slugs and snails and puppy dog tails', trigger points seem to be composed of equally noxious ingredients. In the 1980s, David Simons posited a theory of 'metabolic energy crisis' (Travell et al 1999, p. 71). In short, the hyper-contracted sarcomeres are working so hard to sustain the mini-contraction that they produce an excess of waste products that cannot be flushed away as normal (because the contracted sarcomeres are also cutting off their own blood supply). These waste products cause pain and irritation and act as a negative feedback loop that aggravates the trigger point further.

Recent research (Shah et al 2008) has backed up David Simon's hypothesis, confirming that tissue in and around active trigger points contains a biochemical milieu of irritating substances including, neuropeptides, cytokines, and catecholamines. It is this irritating chemical cocktail that sustains the mini-contracture of the trigger point, NOT electrical signals (action potentials) from the spinal cord.

Know your trigger point terminology

Reading books and articles about trigger points means seeing certain terms referenced again and again. Like learning any language it is important to understand exactly what these terms mean.

Central and attachment trigger points

Simons makes a clear distinction between central and attachment trigger points (Travell et al 1999, p. 2). Although both are involved in producing referred pain, central and attachment trigger points are caused by different processes. Luckily the names pretty much describe their locations, i.e. 'it does what it says on the tin'. Central trigger points are found near the belly of the muscle (around the motor end plate) and attachment trigger points, funnily enough, are found near muscle attachment points (either where muscles blend into tendons or at periosteal junctions).

Attachment trigger points are formed from the tensile stresses placed on the area (because of the central trigger points) and can cause inflammation, fibrosis and the deposition of calcium.

Key and satellite trigger points

I've got the key, I've got the secret.
I've got the key to another way.
URBAN COOKIE COLLECTIVE (a great song to add to your trigger point soundtrack on your iPod)

Although the Urban Cookie Collective who sang this great song were probably not referring to trigger points, it is definitely the case that in trigger point terms if 'you've got the key' you have definitely 'got the secret' to the cause of a client's pain. Key trigger points (previously referred to by Travell and Simons, in the first trigger point manual, as 'primary trigger points') are basically the main cause of the client's pain and deactivation will relieve activity in satellite trigger points (usually found in the pain reference zone of the key trigger point). For example, if you have trigger points in your trapezius this can cause referred pain around the ear where the temporalis muscle is found. Guess what happens then? Yep, satellite trigger points in the temporalis muscle develop as a result (**Figure 8.8A,B**).

If the satellites are treated but not the key, the pain is likely to return. On the other hand, if you treat the key trigger points effectively there may be no need to treat the satellite trigger points, as they will disappear of their own accord (Hong and Simons 1992). A good example of this is the treatment of TMJ pain (see Chapter 18) where debilitating jaw pain is usually resolved solely through treatment of neck and shoulder muscles, such as trapezius and SCM. Often this by itself resolves the

satellite trigger points that have formed in the masseter and other jaw muscles. The Jing approach to trigger points naturally takes into account the potential effect of key and satellite trigger points as the protocols treat all the muscles around the joint.

Active and latent trigger points

Active trigger points are busy producing pain at the moment. Active trigger points are always tender, prevent full lengthening of the muscle, weaken the muscle and refer a pain that is recognisable to the patient on direct compression.

In contrast, **latent trigger points** are lurking in muscles but not producing pain at that time. When pressed, the pain is unfamiliar to the client or is a pain they used to have but not currently. Latent trigger points can become active and start to cause pain if activated by any of the aggravating factors discussed above.

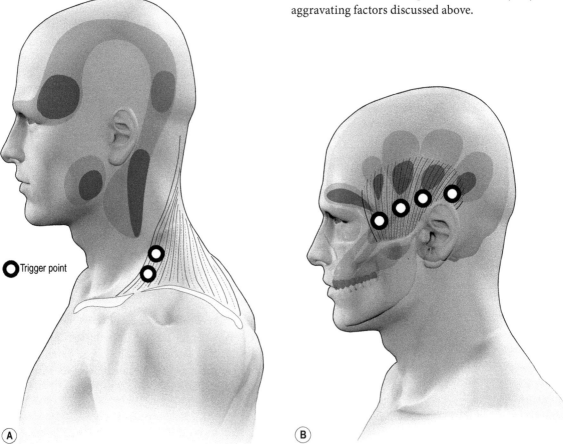

O Trigger point

(A)　　　　　(B)

Figure 8.8A,B
Key trigger points in the trapezius (A) can cause satellite trigger points in the temporalis (B)

Why do trigger points cause referred pain?

Why indeed! In a nutshell, the prevailing scientific hypothesis, the convergence projection theory (Mense 1993), suggests that the brain literally gets confused about exactly where the pain is coming from and ends up making a 'best guess' based on all the neurological information available. The confusion happens because there are more nerve endings in muscles than there are receptors in the spinal column. Therefore, signals from several different nerve endings at different locations in the muscle are passed to the same receptor (this is the 'convergence' bit). As the brain has multiple choices as to where the pain is coming from it is therefore unable to make an accurate assessment and creates a somewhat hazy image of the pain, i.e. the 'projection' or referred pain pattern.

With all due respect to the scientific boffins (of which I would definitely not include myself) this has always sounded like a bit of a 'the dog ate my homework' excuse of a theory to me. Can the carefully mapped, predictable pain patterns really boil down to 'dodgy wiring'? Although convergence projection theory may be part of the picture it doesn't really seem to explain the full effect of what is going on with referred pain. In particular, the clear correlation of referred pain patterns with both acupuncture meridians (see section below on correlation between meridians and trigger point pain referral patterns) and the 'Anatomy Trains' concepts of myofascial continuities, as developed by Tom Myers (Myers 2008), seems to offer a piece of the jigsaw puzzle that would warrant further investigation.

Are acupuncture points the same as trigger points?

The 'party line' to this question (from both camps) is usually 'no not really', but the educated reader may be narrowing their eyes in suspended disbelief at this point as anyone with a brief knowledge of acupuncture points and meridians will be seeing some clear overlaps.

Theories of trigger points and acupuncture evolved at completely different times in separate parts of the world with radically dissimilar theoretical underpinnings. Trigger points take as their basis the Western anatomical map of the body – and specifically the musculoskeletal system. Classical acupuncture points are based on the Eastern anatomical theories of meridians or energy lines, the acupuncture points being places where the qi (energy) is seen to be easily accessible to manipulation via needles or finger/thumb pressure.

Classical acupuncture points always have precise anatomical locations that are found by reference to bony landmarks and other measurements. Trigger points, by contrast, can technically be found at any place in the muscle. Although their locations, as mapped by Travell, are fairly predictable, trigger points are found by palpation, knowledge of likely locations and client feedback.

However, there are definitely convincingly strong parallels, e.g. in the 'spot the difference' illustration below of the trapezius muscle, the upper trigger point is clearly in exactly the same place as acupuncture point GB 21. Middle trigger point 6 is found in the same location as acupuncture point LI 16 (**Figure 8.9A–C**).

Moreover, the pain referral zone for the key trigger point found in the upper trapezius is very similar to the map of the Gall Bladder meridian as it traverses around the ear (**Figure 8.10, p. 129**).

Researchers corroborate this view and have found a high degree of overlap between the locations of acupuncture points and trigger points and the pathways of referral zones and meridians (Dorsher 2008, Melzack et al 1977). The Dorsher (2008) study found a 95% trigger to acupuncture point correlation and that the referred-pain patterns of myofascial trigger points accurately follow the meridian distributions of their corresponding acupuncture points in 76% of cases. He concluded that the results suggest that the theory and practice of trigger points is an independent rediscovery of ancient acupuncture concepts.

You can imagine that opinion going down well with the Western researchers who have been struggling to understand trigger points for decades. It is the academic equivalent of thumbing your nose and saying 'Yeah whatever! We thought of that centuries ago.'

The 'ouch' points

Critics of Dorsher's research suggest that a more correct interpretation of the notion of trigger points, from a Chinese medicine point of view, is through their

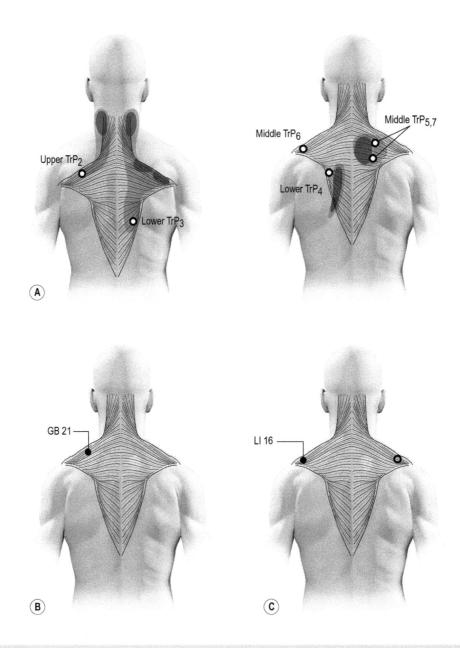

Figure 8.9A–C

Spot the difference: the location of upper trapezius trigger point (TrP2) in diagram A is exactly the same as acupressure point GB 21 in diagram B. Similarly middle TrP6 is in exactly the same location as acupressure point LI 16

correspondence with acupunctural 'ah shi' points (Birch 2003, Hong 2000).

The translation of ah shi is 'ouch!' or 'oh yes!' – which in itself seems an accurate summary of the verbal responses of clients when you hit a trigger point. Ah shi points are local areas of tenderness and are seen in Chinese medicine as areas of local qi (energy) stagnation; their locations are not predictable in the same way as classical acupuncture points but instead are found by palpation. Needling ah shi points is a well-known method

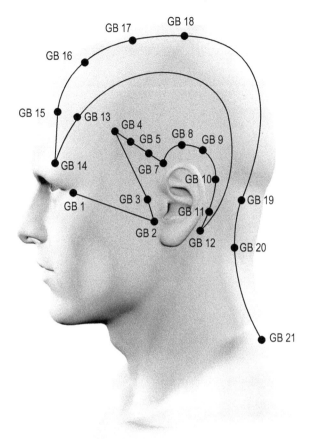

Figure 8.10
The pain referral zone for the key trigger point found in the upper trapezius is very similar to the map of the Gall Bladder meridian as it traverses around the ear

for treating musculoskeletal pain in acupuncture; the points can also be treated though Eastern-based forms of bodywork, as clearly outlined in the following text on Amma therapy (the Eastern-based bodywork system I studied during my time in New York):

> Ah shi points are used in the treatment of such conditions as sciatica, tendonitis and muscular pulls and strains. The location and tenderness of these points often indicate the nature of a disease and they can therefore be used for both diagnostic purposes and treatment. The acupuncturist palpates for tender spots on the tendino-muscle

> channels and needles these points with amazing and rapid results. ... midlevel and advanced Amma therapists also palpate for these points and apply finger pressure instead of needling the point.
> SOHN AND SOHN 1996, P. 73

In short, treatment of local tender points through manual pressure or needling is not a new concept in Chinese medicine and it is likely that trigger points and acupuncture points (in particular ah shi points) may be mediated by the same physiological mechanisms. However, ideological differences have led to a general reluctance from both sides to acknowledge these parallels; Chinese medicine is a rich philosophical system that is based on much more than local needling of tender points and adherents are keen to protect this theoretical framework. One of my Chinese medicine lecturers, at massage college years ago, told me that needling ah shi points was seen as the 'crudest form of acupuncture'. On the other hand, trigger point theory has evolved within a strict Western medical framework and some proponents wish to distinguish the ideas from those of acupuncture that are seen to have an insubstantial scientific basis.

However, it seems fairly clear to any objective outsider that there are strong correlations between the two concepts and that studying both may aid a common understanding. Through examining both systems, the case for treatment of musculoskeletal pain via local tender points seems convincing. In addition, evidence from decades of research from the Western scientific and medical community plus centuries of clinical application from the East gives a robust motive for including trigger point therapy into massage treatment.

Fascia and trigger points: the steady marriage

> The fascia and the muscles are, therefore, in immediate interrelation. They mutually induce each other to share a common fate – in both good times and bad.
> GAUTSCHI 2012, P. 237

The Roland Gautschi quote above bears a striking similarity to Frank Sinatra's conclusions about love and marriage:

> Love and marriage, love and marriage,
> Go together like a horse and carriage.
> This I tell ya, brother, you can't have one without the other.
> Try, try, try to separate them, it's an illusion.
> Try, try, try and you only come to this conclusion.
> FRANK SINATRA 1955

In a similar way, trying to separate trigger points from fascia is an illusion. Fascia dysfunction can lead to the origin and activation of trigger points whilst, conversely, trigger points can cause fascial dysfunction. Knowledge of effective treatment of both is essential for full resolution of musculoskeletal pain.

Treating trigger points

Reading the trigger point literature can be overwhelming as there are a bewildering number of treatment options both from the medical and manual therapy side. As always the questions are 'What works? And what works best?' The available evidence seems to show that trigger points exist and cause pain; however, the jury is still firmly out as to the most effective form of treatment.

From bee venom to Botox: injecting trigger points

Travell and Simons pioneered the notion of injecting trigger points to deactivate them and injection therapy remains a primary medical method of treating trigger points to this day (**Figure 8.11**). A range of substances are used including anaesthetic, saline solution, vitamin B12, steroids and, yes, even Botox and bee venom! (Dommerholt 2012, p. 300). The trigger point literature helpfully labels any type of needling method as 'invasive trigger point therapy' – just in case the consumer might think that being injected with bee venom could be a nice cuddly type of therapy for their pain! There is some evidence that injection with certain substances may be beneficial (Dommerholt and Gerwin 2010); although a 2007 review of the research evidence has concluded firmly 'The current evidence does not support the use of botulism injection in trigger points for myofascial pain'

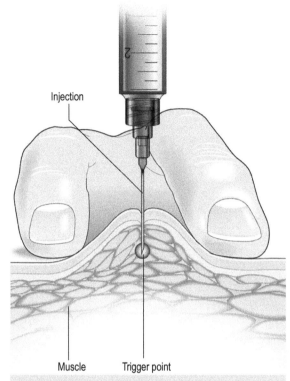

Figure 8.11

Injection therapy remains a primary medical method for treating trigger points. A range of substances is used including anaesthetic, saline solution, vitamin B12, steroids and even Botox and bee venom!

(Ho et al 2007, p. 519). Notwithstanding this clinical evidence, Botox trigger point injections are approved for migraine sufferers in both the UK and USA.

Dry needling

Despite the reluctance of some sections of the medical community to take the concepts of acupuncture on board, recent studies have shown that dry needling of trigger points is equally as effective as injections with anaesthetics (Dommerholt 2006). Another opportunity for the acupuncturists who have been successfully needling the ah shi points for centuries to sit back, stroke their chins and murmur knowingly 'I told you so!'.

Spray and stretch

Janet Travell LOVED spray and stretch! The trigger point manuals are filled with illustrations of slightly disconsolate looking patients being subjected to dramatic

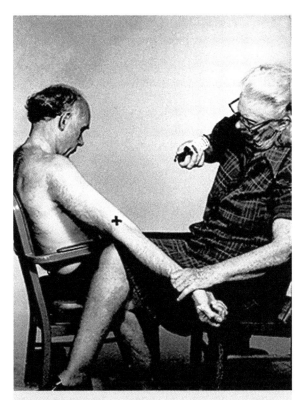

Figure 8.12
Janet Travell demonstrating her famous spray and stretch technique

spraying with what looks like a spray can used for graffiti (**Figure 8.12**). Yet despite Dr Travell's enthusiasm for the technique, it seems to be rarely practised today. This technique has a sound underlying rationale wherby the cooling spray acts as an instant pain reliever while the practitioner introduces a slow gentle stretch to the affected area to release the trigger points:

> *The operator should gently lengthen the muscle until it reaches the barrier (a rapidly increasing resistance to further movement) and then hold that degree of tension ... as the muscle 'gives up' and releases its tension, the operator smoothly takes up the slack to re-establish a new stretch position that again engages the barrier.*
> TRAVELL ET AL 1999, P. 136

Sound familiar? The description of the stretch is remarkably similar to the methods of indirect myofas-cial release as advocated by Barnes (1990) and others that we explored in Chapter 7. Techniques such as cross hand stretch, arm pulls, leg pulls and general myofascial stretching are all carried out in this way.

It is conceivable that indirect myofascial methods deactivate trigger points in a comparable way to spray and stretch techniques; therefore, warranting their inclusion in a multi-modal system as advocated in this book. Incorporating fascial techniques before specific trigger point therapy (as outlined below) can potentially release large areas of trigger points before more specific work is carried out. This is consistent with observations from our own clinical practice.

What research has to say about trigger point treatment

In general

Research has found trigger point deactivation to be useful in many conditions including low back pain (Itoh et al 2004), fibromyalgia (Giamberardino et al 2011), shoulder pain (Bron et al 2011), headaches (Alonso-Blanco et al 2012, Fernández-de-las-Peñas et al 2007), carpal tunnel syndrome (Elliott and Burkett 2013), tinnitus (Rocha and Sanchez 2007, 2012), whiplash (Freeman et al 2009) and tennis elbow (Shmushkevich and Kalichman 2013).

Manual approaches to trigger point therapy

Although skilled bodywork practitioners are fervent in their support for trigger point therapy as a powerful intervention in musculoskeletal pain conditions, it has proved difficult to consistently replicate these findings through research. Reviews have found some evidence for manual treatment for immediate pain relief at myofascial TrPs, but only limited evidence for long-term pain relief (Vernon and Schneider 2009). Part of the problem lies in the fact that identifying and treating trigger points is a skill. Those of you who do the work will know that subtle differences in pressure and accuracy make a huge difference in both locating and successfully treating trigger points. Presented with the same trapezius muscle, practitioner A may find no trigger points whereas practitioner B may be able to find and release many. The scientific method, however, is unable to take into account the variables within practitioner skills; interventions must be exact, precise and duplicable, time after time. This is a poor reflection of what actually happens in treatment where interventions are constantly flexible and changing. Many studies have suffered through poor inter-reliability in examiners actually being able to accurately locate trigger points. Findings of research studies improve if appropriate training in location of trigger points is given beforehand (Gerwin et al 1997, Sciotti et al 2001).

There also seems to be no existing consensus from the research about the best manual therapy approach to treat trigger points. Two recent reviews looked at a range of manual therapy techniques ranging from ischaemic compression, trigger point compression combined with active muscle contraction, post-isometric relaxation, fascial stretches, massage therapy, muscle energy techniques, skin rolling and strain-counter-strain (Fernández-de-las-Peñas et al 2005, Rickards 2006). Although several studies had positive results, evidencing a decrease in pain and improvement in objective measures, it was difficult for the authors to come to firm conclusions about their efficacy due to the diverse nature of techniques studied. Rickards also noted the lack of addressing contributing stressors to trigger point formation in the manual approaches used.

Some studies have shown good statistically significant results using ischaemic pressure (albeit from a tool rather than a practitioner's hand) to release trigger points (Fryer and Hodgson 2005, Gemmell et al 2008, Gulick et al 2011). The method of ischaemic compression or the more correct term of 'trigger point pressure release' is the primary approach adopted in this book. Good clinical results have been obtained using this method and particularly in conjunction with the other elements of the Jing multi-modal approach, such as the use of heat, fascial release and stretching techniques; helping clients identify and reduce potential stressors; and empowering self-care suggestions that enable clients to take their health back into their own hands. It is also possible that other techniques such as cross fibre friction may be equally as effective (Fernández-de-las-Peñas et al 2006). However, our clinical experience suggests that the approach taught here is the least painful for the client and is optimal for preventing overuse of therapists' fingers and thumbs.

Incorporating trigger point therapy into your massage treatments

In the context of the Jing multi-modal approach advocated in this book, precise trigger point therapy is the 'meat of the sandwich' and a powerful tool in its own right but even more effective when combined with the other modalities recommended.

At the point of the treatment where you are ready to carry out the precise trigger point techniques you will have already:

- Carried out an **outcome orientated consultation** that has enabled you to identify potential trigger point activating factors, including the role of emotional and psychological factors, beliefs, lifestyle and possible central sensitisation factors.

- Applied **heat** to the body to enhance the effects of fascial and trigger point release.

- Applied **fascial techniques** to release fascial adhesions and broad areas of trigger point activity.

So now you are ready to carry out the precise trigger point protocols that have served us so well in the treatment of pain for many years. Chapters 12–19 give you precise methods to treat pain in different areas of the body and these methods all rely on the same basic trigger point treatment principles as outlined below.

The method of trigger point treatment expounded here is based on principles originally taught by chiropractor Raymond Nimmo, a contemporary of Janet Travell. His approach is known as 'receptor-tonus' technique (Nimmo 1957) and has influenced several well-known manual therapy approaches to trigger point work, such as the Paul St John neuromuscular technique and modern American style neuromuscular therapy (DeLany 1999).

The method has a few distinct hallmarks that in our view make the technique highly effective and, more importantly, easy to learn:

- The method relies on treating all the muscles around the affected joint for trigger points. In this way, the practitioner is using a precise approach that logically examines all the muscles that may contain both key and satellite trigger points. The therapist does not have to rely on interpreting complicated trigger point diagrams to trace back the source of the client's pain. This massively simplifies the therapist's ability to obtain effective results with common musculoskeletal pain. For example, to treat low back pain the therapist searches for trigger points in the erector spinae, quadratus lumborum, gluteus maximus, gluteus medius, hamstrings and psoas. This is a bit of a 'no brainer' approach to trigger point treatment that is simple to learn and has effective results.

- To accurately identify trigger points, the therapist palpates the full length of the muscle being treated and encourages precise communication from the client to gain feedback on any points that reproduce their primary pain complaint. This helps to reduce one of the most common reasons for trigger point treatment failing to work, i.e. namely the inability of the therapist to find them! Engaging the client in the process enables the practitioner to develop their sense of 'listening touch' and to gain appropriate feedback about what they 'think' they feel. This eventually also builds the therapist's confidence and palpation skills.

- Key trigger points (i.e. those that reproduce the client's pain) are treated with static compression for between 8 and 12 seconds, while again engaging with the client about the nature of the pain. Key trigger points may be treated up to 3 times in a session.

- The key trigger points are treated in a similar manner (by following the same routine of treating all the muscles around the joint) on a weekly basis for up to 6 weeks. Generally a decrease in pain is noted, at the latest, at around the third weekly session at which point the time between treatments is lengthened (i.e. to once every 2 weeks).

In Chapters 12–19 the treatment protocols described provide a complete step-by-step guide through this process for each area of the body.

What do trigger points feel like?

Some trigger points are tiny and almost like a grain of rice, while others can feel like a pea or even walnut sized. They are usually found within a tighter bit of muscle (the taut band). When you first start to do this work it is likely that you will have no idea what a trigger point feels like, which is why it is crucially important to work with client communication. Over time your palpation skills will develop and you may eventually feel so confident in your ability to locate them that the client feedback can become more minimal (**Figure 8.13A–C**).

Don't sweat the 'twitch response'

Trigger point literature often refers to the 'twitch' response – which is literally a twitching response to palpation of the taut band that houses the trigger point – as this can help you identify that you are in the right place. My advice is that you shouldn't worry about it. In practice I hardly ever see it and I don't find it a helpful way to precisely identify the location of trigger points. Client communication and a good sense of listening touch are much more reliable indicators.

Communication skills in trigger point work

Good communication with your client is crucial when doing trigger point work. Agreed verbal or non-verbal feedback from your client will let you know whether you have located the trigger point accurately. It is important to educate your client as to your need for them to communicate during the treatment, as this is not something we would usually encourage during a pure relaxation massage.

Explain to your client, during the consultation, that you will be looking for 'hot spots' in their muscles that reproduce the symptoms they are experiencing. When you find one it is important that they let you know either verbally or via a prearranged non-verbal signal, i.e. wiggling the fingers of their right hand. (This can be important as when your client is in a prone position it is impossible to decipher their mumblings into the face cradle. A few frustrating rounds of 'Is that something?' and 'mwh, mwh, mwh' is enough to raise trigger point activity by itself.)

Communication can be kept to a minimum but you will need to know the following:

- Is the spot tender?

- Is there any referred pain when pressing on the point?

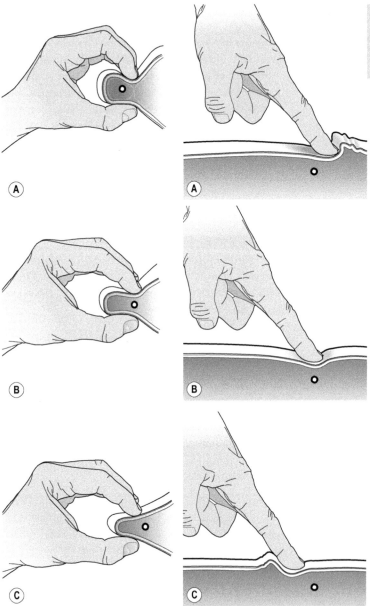

Figure 8.13A–C
Accurate location of trigger points (as in diagram B) is vital for obtaining good results

- On a pain scale of 1–10 (1 being no pain, 10 being the most) where would the client rate their 'good hurt' from the pressure. Your pressure should NEVER be causing a pain that is above a 6 on the pain scale and if it is then you should ease up. More pain does NOT mean more gain.

- Has the pain released and diminished after 8–12 seconds of pressure?

To get the best therapeutic results from your work it is important **not to cause the person pain.** You must always use a pressure that is beneath the client's pain threshold. I usually say to my clients 'If you feel like clenching your fists or teeth while I am treating you, please let me know and I will ease off the pressure.'

Treatment principles: in summary

To summarise the above, this is how the technique works in practice:

- Use the protocols described in Chapters 12–19 to locate and treat the muscles indicated in your client's pain complaint. You will be using a form of scanning palpation or pincer technique to locate trigger point nodules and taut bands of contracted muscle.

- **Scanning palpation**: this is usually carried out with supported straight fingers or thumb over thumb. The pressure is deep into the underlying tissue or bone. We recommend a few different hand positions to ensure you don't injure your thumbs:

  - Thumb over thumb with hands flat on the body. **See Figure 8.14**

  - Thumb flat on the body with added pressure from your other hand (fingers or whole hand). **See Figure 8.15**

  - Supported fingers with stacked joints (fingers, wrist, elbow and shoulder). **See Figure 8.16**

- **Pincer techniques**: the tissue and the trigger point are compressed between your fingers and thumb, e.g. commonly used with SCM or brachioradialis. **See Figure 8.17**

- With the aid of client communication, identify any active trigger points in the muscles. When you have identified a trigger point, apply firm digital pressure directly over the nodule while communicating with the patient about the:

  - intensity of local pain

  - intensity and location of any referred pain.

Remember the pain should never be more than a 6 on a 1–10 pain scale.

- Concentrate treatment on the major trigger points that reproduce the client's primary pain pattern.

- Treatment consists of 8–12 seconds of firm manual pressure applied to a trigger point. The pressure is held constant during this time and is NOT continuously increased. When you feel the tissue changing (literally melting beneath your fingertips) or your client lets you know that the pain has released/diminished you can move on.

- Release pressure and continue to palpate the length of the muscle and release any further trigger points as outlined in the protocol.

- Return to previously treated trigger points and repeat the procedure for a total of 2–3 applications per key trigger point per session. Too many applications in one visit and/or too

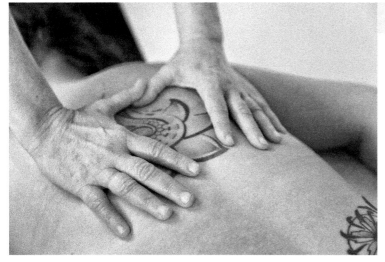

Figure 8.14

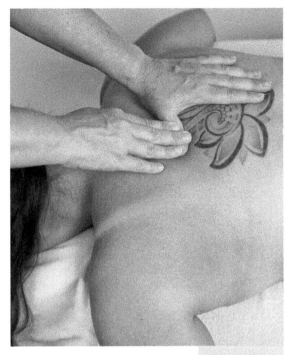

Figure 8.15

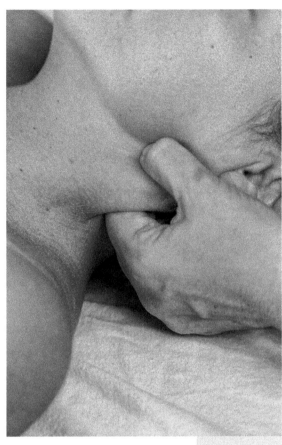

Figure 8.17

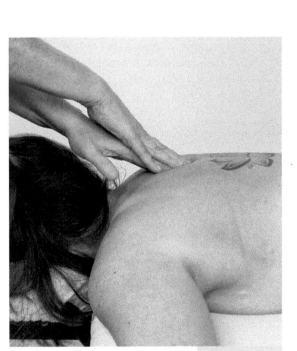

Figure 8.16

much pressure will cause the client to experience bruising or soreness post-treatment.

- Reassess the response of the trigger point and its associated taut band by palpation. If the treatment was effective you should notice an immediate change in the texture of the muscle tissue and the client will experience dramatic pain relief.

- Compression of the trigger point should always be followed by stretching of the muscle. Suitable stretches are outlined in the treatment sections.

- The trigger point work should be carried out as part of the HFMAST protocol as the other techniques in the mix will all help to reduce trigger point activity.

- Don't expect to reduce all trigger point activity in one session. Treatment frequency is once a week for up to 6 weeks. You should expect to see some reduction in pain by at least week three. Once a reduction in pain is achieved, the time between treatments can be lengthened.

References

Alonso-Blanco C, de-la-Llave-Rincón AI, Fernández-de-las-Peñas C 2012 Muscle trigger point therapy in tension-type headache. Expert Review of Neurotherapeutics 12(3): 315–322.

Alvarez J, Rockwell PG 2002 Trigger points: diagnosis and management. American Family Physician 15;65(4): 653–661.

Barnes John F 1990 Myofascial release: the search for excellence. Rehabilitation Services. Paoli, PA: Myofascial Release Seminars.

Birch S 2003 Trigger point – Acupuncture point correlations revisited. The Journal of Alternative and Complementary Medicine February 9(1):91–103.

Bron C et al 2011 Treatment of myofascial trigger points in patients with chronic shoulder pain: a randomized, controlled trial. BMC Medicine 9:8.

Calandre EP et al 2006 Trigger point evaluation in migraine patients: an indication of peripheral sensitization linked to migraine predisposition? European Journal of Neurology 13:244–249.

Chaiamnuay P et al 1998 Epidemiology of rheumatic disease in rural Thailand (a Whoilar Copcord study. Community oriented programme for the control of the rheumatic disease). Journal of Rheumatology 25: 1382–1387.

Chaitow L, DeLany JW 2000 Clinical Application of Neuromuscular Techniques: Volume 1 – The Upper Body. Edinburgh: Churchill Livingstone.

Chen CKH et al 2006 MRI diagnosis of contracture of the gluteus maximus muscle. American Journal of Roentgenology 187:W169–W174.

Davies C, Davies A 2004 The trigger point therapy workbook, 2nd edn. Oakland, CA: New Harbinger Publications.

DeLany J 1999 NMT Center – History – NeuroMuscular Therapy Training Center. Nmtcenter.com. Available at: https://www.nmtcenter.com/history/ [accessed 19 August 2014].

Dommerholt J 2011 Dry needling – peripheral and central considerations. The Journal of Manual & Manipulative Therapy 19(4):223–227.

Dommerholt J 2012 Trigger point therapy. In: Schleip R, Findley TW, Chaitow L, Huijing PA, eds Fascia: the tensional network of the human body. Edinburgh: Churchill Livingstone Elsevier, p. 300.

Dommerholt J, Gerwin RD 2010 Neurophysiological effects of trigger point needling therapies. In: Fernández-de-las-Peñas C, Arendt-Nielson L, Gerwin D (eds) Tension-type and cervicogenic headache. Sudbury, Mass: Jones and Bartlett.

Dommerholt J, Mayoral O, Grobli C 2006 Trigger point dry needling. Journal of Manual and Manipulative Therapy 14:E70–87.

Dorsher PT 2008 Can classical acupuncture points and trigger points be compared in the treatment of pain disorders? Birch's analysis revisited. Journal of Alternative and Complementary Medicine (New York, NY) 14: 353–359.

Elliott R, Burkett B 2013 Massage therapy as an effective treatment for carpal tunnel syndrome. Journal of Bodywork and Movement Therapies 17(3):332–338.

Fernández-Carnero J et al 2008 Bilateral myofascial trigger points in the forearm muscles in patients with chronic unilateral lateral epicondylalgia: a blinded, controlled study. The Clinical Journal of Pain 24(9):802–807.

Fernández-de-las-Peñas C, Dommerholt J 2014 Myofascial trigger points: peripheral or central phenomenon? Current Rheumatology Reports 16:1–6.

Fernández-de-las-Peñas C et al 2005 Manual therapies in myofascial trigger point treatment: a systematic review. Journal of Bodywork and Movement Therapies 9:27–34.

Fernández-de-las-Peñas C et al 2006 The immediate effect of ischemic compression technique and transverse friction massage on tenderness of active and latent myofascial trigger points: a pilot study. Journal of Bodywork and Movement Therapies 10(1):3–9.

Fernández-de-las-Peñas C et al 2007 Myofascial trigger points and sensitization: an updated pain model for tension-type headache. Cephalalgia: An International Journal of Headache 27(5):383–393.

Fernández-de-las-Peñas C et al 2010 Referred pain from muscle trigger points in the masticatory and neck–shoulder musculature in women with temporomandibular disorders. The Journal of Pain: Official Journal of the American Pain Society 11(12):1295–1304.

Finando D, Finando S 2005 Trigger Point Therapy for Myofascial Pain: The Practice of Informed Touch, 2nd revised edn. Rochester, VT: Healing Arts Press.

Freeman MD, Nystrom A, Centeno C 2009 Chronic whiplash and central sensitization; an evaluation of the role of a myofascial trigger points in pain modulation. Journal of Brachial Plexus and Peripheral Nerve Injury 4:2.

Froriep R 1843 Ein Beitrag zur Pathologie und Therapie des Rheumatismus. Weimar.

Fryer G, Hodgson L 2005 The effect of manual pressure release on myofascial trigger points in the upper trapezius muscle. Journal of Bodywork and Movement Therapies 9(4): 248–255.

Gautschi RU 2012 Trigger points as a fascia related disorder. In: Schleip R, Findley T, Chaitow L, Huijing P (eds) Fascia, the tensional network of the human body. London: Churchill Livingstone Elsevier, p. 237

Ge H-Y, Arendt-Nielsen L 2011 Latent myofascial trigger points. Current Pain and Headache Reports 15:386–392.

Gemmell H, Miller P, Nordstrom H 2008 Immediate effect of activator trigger point therapy and myofascial band therapy on non-specific neck pain in patients with upper trapezius trigger points compared to sham ultrasound: a randomised controlled trial. Clinical Chiropractic 11:30–36.

Gerwin RD 1995 A study of 96 subjects examined both for fibromyalgia and myofascial pain. Journal of Musculoskeletal Pain 3:121.

Gerwin RD et al 1997 Interrater reliability in myofascial trigger point examination. Pain 69(1–2):65–73.

Giamberardino MA et al 2007 Contribution of myofascial trigger points to migraine symptoms. The Journal of Pain: Official Journal of the American Pain Society 8(11): 869–878.

Giamberardino MA et al 2011 Effects of treatment of myofascial trigger points on the pain of fibromyalgia. Current Pain and Headache Reports 15(5):393–399.

Gowers WR 1904 Lumbago: its lesions and analogues. British Medical Journal 1:117–121.

Gulick DT, Palombaro K, Lattanzi JB 2011 Effect of ischemic pressure using a Backnobber II device on discomfort associated with myofascial trigger points. Journal of Bodywork & Movement Therapies 15(3):319–325.

Gutstein M 1938 Diagnosis and treatment of muscular rheumatism. British Journal of Physical Medicine 1: 302–321.

Ho K-Y et al 2007 Botulinum toxin A for myofascial trigger point injection: a qualitative systematic review. European Journal of Pain 11(5):519–527.

Hong CZ 2000 Myofascial trigger points: pathophysiology and correlation with acupuncture points. Acupuncture Medicine 18:41–47.

Hong CZ, Simons D 1992 Remote inactivation of myofascial trigger points by injection of trigger points into another muscle. Scandinavian Journal of Rheumatology 94:25.

Ingraham P 2014 Save yourself from low back pain, 1st edn. [ebook] Available at: http://saveyourself.ca/tutorials/low-back-pain.php?id=254810 [accessed 20 August 2014].

Itoh K, Katsumi Y, Kitakoji H 2004 Trigger point acupuncture treatment of chronic low back pain in elderly patients – a blinded RCT. Acupuncture In Medicine : Journal of The British Medical Acupuncture Society 22(4):170–177.

Malanga GA, Cruz Colon EJ 2010 Myofascial low back pain: a review. physical Medicine and Rehabilitation Clinics North America 21:711–724.

Melzack R, Wall P 1988 The challenge of pain. London: Penguin.

Melzack R, Stillwell DM, Fox EJ 1977 Trigger points and acupuncture points for pain: correlations and implications. Pain 3:3–23.

Mense S 1993 Neurobiological mechanisms of muscle pain referral. Schmerz (Berlin, Germany) 7(4):241– 249. Available at: http://www.ncbi.nlm.nih.gov/pubmed/18415388 [accessed 20 August 2014].

Mense S 2010 How do muscle lesions such as latent and active trigger points influence central nociceptive neurons? Journal of Musculoskeletal Pain 18:348–353.

Mense S et al 2000 Muscle Pain. Baltimore, MD: Lippincott Williams and Wilkins.

Myers TW 2008 Anatomy Trains: Myofascial Meridians for Manual and Movement Therapists, 2nd edn. Edinburgh: Churchill Livingstone.

National Board of Chiropractic Economics 1993 Chiropractic treatment procedures in job analysis of chiropractic (Table 9–11), Greelay, Colorado. Quoted in: Chaitow L, Delany JW 2000 Clinical Application of Neuromuscular Techniques: Volume 1 – The Upper Body. Edinburgh: Churchill Livingstone.

Nimmo R 1957 Receptors, effectors and tonus. Journal of the National Chiropractic Association 27(11):21.

Rickards LD 2006 The effectiveness of non-invasive treatments for active myofascial trigger point pain: a systematic review of the literature. International Journal of Osteopathic Medicine 9:120–136.

Rocha CACB, Sanchez TG 2007 Myofascial trigger points: another way of modulating tinnitus. Progress in Brain Research 166:209–214.

Rocha CB, Sanchez TG 2012 Efficacy of myofascial trigger point deactivation for tinnitus control. Brazilian Journal of Otorhinolaryngology 78(6):21–26.

Schade H 1919 Beitrage zur umgrenzung und klarung einer lehre von der erkaltung. Z Ges Exp Med 7:275–374.

Sciotti VM et al 2001Clinical precision of myofascial trigger point location in the trapezius muscle. Pain 93(3): 259–266.

Shah JP et al 2008 Biochemicals Associated with pain and inflammation are elevated in sites near to and remote from active myofascial trigger points. Archives of Physical Medicine and Rehabilitation 89:16–23.

Shmushkevich Y, Kalichman L 2013 Myofascial pain in lateral epicondylalgia: A review. Journal of Bodywork and Movement Therapies 17(4):434–439.

Simons D et al 1999 Travell & Simons' myofascial pain and dysfunction, vol 2. Baltimore: Williams and Wilkins.

Sohn T, Sohn R 1996 Amma Therapy, 1st edn. Rochester, VT: Healing Arts Press.

Sorensen TC 1965 Kennedy. New York: Harper & Row.

Staud R 2006 Are tender point injections beneficial: the role of tonic nociception in fibromyalgia. Current Pharmaceutical Design 12(1):23–27.

Staud R 2010 Is it all central sensitization? Role of peripheral tissue nociception in chronic musculoskeletal pain. Current Rheumatology Reports 12(6):448–454.

Staud R 2011a Evidence for shared pain mechanisms in osteoarthritis, low back pain, and fibromyalgia. Current Rheumatology Reports 13(6):513–520.

Staud R 2011b Peripheral pain mechanisms in chronic widespread pain. Best practice & research. Clinical rheumatology 25(2):155–164. Available at: http://www.pubmedcentral.nih.gov/articlerender.fcgi?artid=3220877&tool=pmcentrez&rendertype=abstract [accessed 14 March 2014].

Travell J, Simons D, Simons L 1993 Travell and Simons' myofascial pain and dysfunction, vol 1. Philadelphia: Lippincott, Williams and Wilkins.

Vernon H, Schneider M 2009 Chiropractic management of myofascial trigger points and myofascial pain syndrome: a systematic review of the literature. Journal of Manipulative and Physiological Therapeutics 32(1):14–24. Available at: http://www.ncbi.nlm.nih.gov/pubmed/19121461 [accessed 24 January 2014].

Xu Y-M, Ge H-Y, Arendt-Nielsen L 2010 Sustained nociceptive mechanical stimulation of latent myofascial trigger point induces central sensitization in healthy subjects. The Journal of Pain: Official Journal of the American Pain Society 11(12):1348–1355.

9

Meridian magic! Using meridians and acupressure points in massage

Eastern bodywork modalities from A–Z

There are few greater sensory experiences than receiving a two and a half hour Thai massage on a beautiful beach in South East Asia. Stretching, pulling, pushing and even bone cracking limbs with expertise in a beautiful dance that hugs, holds and encompasses body, mind and spirit. Thai massage exemplifies the skilled and truly holistic approach of many Asian bodywork therapies.

Bodywork modalities from the East (commonly now known in the US as Asian bodywork therapy or ABT) encompass well known massage styles such as shiatsu, Thai massage, Amma and tuina. More comprehensively, The American Organization for Bodywork Therapies of Asia (AOBTA) lists the following modalities on its website (Aobta.org): acupressure, Amma, AMMA Therapy®, chi nei tsang, five element shiatsu, integrative eclectic shiatsu, Japanese shiatsu, Jin Shin Do®, Bodymind Acupressure®, Jin Shou Tuina™, macrobiotic shiatsu, shiatsu, nuad bo'rarn (traditional Thai bodywork), shiatsu anma therapy, tuina, zen shiatsu, and medical qigong.

Although there are technical and theoretical differences between all of these systems (not to mention different names for similar principles), they all share a similar philosophical framework:

- Ill health results from imbalance of qi (commonly translated as 'energy' in English).

- Qi can be manipulated through manual techniques that work on energy channels or vessels through which qi flows. These are known as meridians (or sen lines in Thai massage). **See Figure 9.1A,B**

- There are points on the meridians where qi can be accessed more easily and a powerful effect can be exerted through manipulation of these points. These points are commonly known as acupressure points, acupoints or tsubos. **See Figure 9.2**

The techniques used to manipulate the meridian lines and points generally include palming, yoga type passive stretching and finger and thumb pressure. Techniques can be employed with the client clothed and are often carried out on a mat on the floor rather than using a massage table.

As the AOBTA website nicely puts it:

> Qi is the body's natural bioenergetic system that is organized in pathways related to our anatomy, physiology, associated emotions, thoughts, and psyche. The meridians form a network – like a system of roads, highways, and country lanes. Acupoints are found at the major junctions, crossroads, overpasses, bus stops, and traffic lights. The subtle art of assessment and treatment requires the selection of specific meridians and acupoints that can be used to unblock traffic jams and enhance the free flow of traffic that results in homeostasis. Freeing those energy blocks and moving towards homeostasis can help to prevent or treat both acute and chronic conditions and health concerns.

Eastern bodywork therapies have been used to good effect for thousands of years in the prevention and alleviation of common health conditions. The principles and techniques from Eastern bodywork can be creatively integrated into your treatments to great effect and, as we shall see, can have many advantages for the massage therapist.

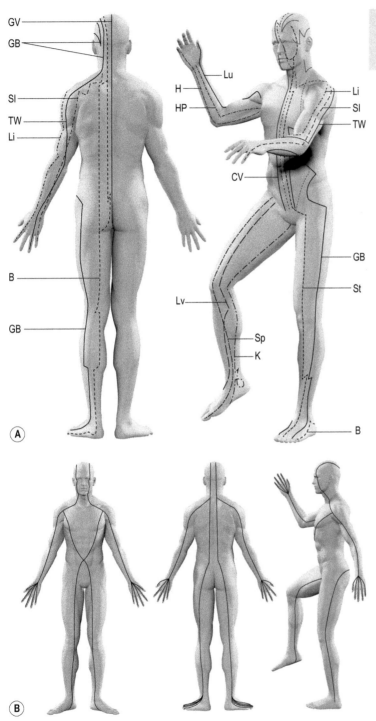

Figure 9.1A,B

(A) The principal meridians in Chinese medicine. (B) The Thai sen lines

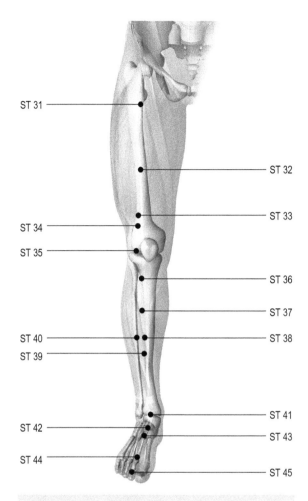

ST 31

ST 32

ST 33

ST 34

ST 35

ST 36

ST 37

ST 40

ST 38

ST 39

ST 41

ST 42

ST 43

ST 44

ST 45

Figure 9.2

Points on the meridians where qi can be accessed more easily are known as acupuncture points, acupressure points or tsubos

Why use meridians and acupressure points in massage?

Anna, one of my regular clients, staggered into my clinic looking tired and drained. Her new job involved a gruelling commute and long hours, leaving her with a sinus infection she couldn't shift. An hour later, after a thorough treatment working her Lung meridian and relevant acupressure points on her face, she was bright eyed, decongested and relieved. 'I never cease to be amazed at what massage can do' she said. A great advert for me and for massage in general.

Vivian suffers from chronic fatigue syndrome. She finds life a struggle and previous Swedish massage treatments have left her even more tired and drained. By contrast, treatments utilising acupressure and meridian techniques give her more energy and leave her feeling energetically balanced and able to cope with life.

Nicole, 3 months pregnant, was suffering terribly with morning sickness. Following her weekly massage treatment I taught her how to stimulate the acupressure point P 6 located on the wrist. The next week she came back delighted with the striking difference in her symptoms.

The above examples give you a few ideas of how incorporating meridian and acupressure principles into your massage treatments is not just good for your clients but also good for your business. Meridian based approaches have several benefits for you and your clients that can help you build the practice you desire:

- They are a great additional tool in treating conditions that do not traditionally respond to Swedish or other standard massage techniques. These include digestive complaints, colds, headaches, sleep disturbances, chronic fatigue and neck or back pain that does not respond to a muscular based approach. The research summarised at the end of this chapter shows evidence for the use of acupressure points for effective treatment of many of these conditions.

- They can be performed over light clothing that is preferable for some clients. Meridian and acupressure work can also be used successfully in on-site massage situations.

- Acupressure points can be easily integrated into the HFMAST protocol to enhance results in the treatment of common pain conditions.

- Acupressure points can be taught to clients (or caregivers) as a useful and non-invasive self-care technique.

A dynamic fusion of East and West: integrating meridian and acupressure work into your treatments

Asian bodywork styles are becoming increasingly popular in the West. Shiatsu and Thai massage are well known in the UK and the AOBTA is a well-established professional association for practitioners in the USA, with a list of 13 schools which offer their approved 500 hour entry level curriculum in Asian Bodywork Therapy (ABT). On top of this there are a plethora of continuing education programmes in various meridian based techniques. However, it is common for practitioners to keep Eastern and Western styles as separate treatments even when they are trained in both. There seems to be two main reasons for this:

1 **Conceptual:** like acupuncture, Eastern bodywork modalities are based on an entirely different theoretical system or 'map' of the body. The 'map' employed by Western manual therapy is based on more familiar notions of soft tissues, joints, nerves, blood and lymph; our goal with massage is usually to affect the muscles, fascia, tendons and ligaments (or blood and lymph flow in the case of Swedish massage or lymphatic drainage). In contrast the anatomy of the East is not muscles, joints and bones but mysterious energy vessels that make no sense within a Western framework. Qi and meridians cannot be seen or dissected out of the body – which in Western thinking means they don't exist. This theoretical separation has also led to highly similar concepts being given different names, e.g. the ah shi points of the East become the trigger points of the West with losses on both sides from not recognising that these are one and the same thing.

2 **Practical:** Eastern techniques, such as shiatsu or Thai massage, are traditionally carried out on the floor on a futon enabling the massage therapist to optimally use their body weight to apply wonderful palming compression strokes and deep stretches. This contrasts with techniques, such as Swedish massage, sports massage or fascial techniques, which again for reasons of body mechanics tend to work better with the use of a massage table.

These different theoretical and practical underpinnings have led to a belief that the two styles cannot coexist within a single treatment. This has led to a rather arbitrary division where massage therapists tend to practise one or the other of these bodywork styles without integration, even if they have training in both. I had wonderful massage training in New York where learning both Eastern and Western theory and technique was compulsory; however, integration is often frowned upon. I remember being told not to mix Swedish massage and Amma therapy as it would 'make the energy go the wrong way'. The FAQ sheet on the AOBTA website also sternly tells consumers who dare to ask the obvious question 'Isn't ABT just another form of Massage Therapy?'

No. ABT training is totally different from Massage Therapy training – which makes them separate professions . . . . The US Department of Education clearly defines ABT and Massage Therapy as separate professions with defined educational curricular differences.

Indeed, there are occasions where pure technique is appropriate but sticking too strongly to this means that we can lose out on the potential benefits for our clients of combining different styles. This is one of the hallmarks of the Jing multi-modal approach, which is a form of integrated bodywork where the practitioner is able to draw from a wide toolbox of techniques. We encourage combining styles in a creative way to give the client the best possible treatment. This is how you build a practice and how you retain clients on a week in week out basis, year after year, and most of all this is how you stop yourself getting bored with your work. You can constantly reinvent the passion that drew you to bodywork in the first place.

'The map is not the territory': integration of East and West

Two important characteristics of maps should be noticed. A map is not the territory it represents, but, if correct, it has a similar structure to the territory, which accounts for its usefulness.
ALFRED KORZBSKI

If you truly understand the essence of the different styles, East and West can easily be integrated to create a truly powerful bodywork that is unique in its own right. Although Western and Eastern massage modalities are looking at the body in a seemingly mutually exclusive way, the theoretical underpinnings are just different maps. As the great quote goes 'the map is not the territory'. Here, the body itself is the territory. Once we develop our bodywork and knowledge skills we can understand our way around it with less need for 'maps'. **See Figure 9.3**

This is a bit like trying to find your way around London or any other major city. There are many different maps of the city for different modes of transport, e.g. your smartphone app (or A–Z book if you are still living in 1983) that shows you how you can get around by foot or car; the bus map; or the map for the tube. If you don't know the city, it is much easier to use only one map to navigate your way around. But when you know the territory itself, you can start to integrate different maps. You can get to where you want to be in the most enjoyable and efficient way, hopping from the bus to the tube or deciding to get out and walk between tube and bus. It's no different with the body. This is the essence of true bodywork mastery. If you are well versed in different bodywork styles you can use whichever style will help that client most at that particular time and, in most cases, blend styles appropriately. In many situations, different bodywork techniques are achieving results by doing more or less the same thing but calling it something entirely different. As Finando and Finando (2011) point out – it is far more useful to look at what bodyworkers or acupuncturists DO to get results rather than their theoretical reasons for doing it. In other words, what we do may be incredibly useful. Our explanation for why it works may be complete rubbish.

This combined approach is exactly what we have developed at Jing. For the eclectic bodyworker, the wonderful techniques of Asian bodywork therapy can be adapted quite easily into a Western system, e.g. the compression and thumbing can be seen as working fascial septa rather than energy lines; stretches release fascia and muscles as well as balancing qi. Different point systems such as trigger, acupressure, ah shi and Stecco points have many more similarities than differences.

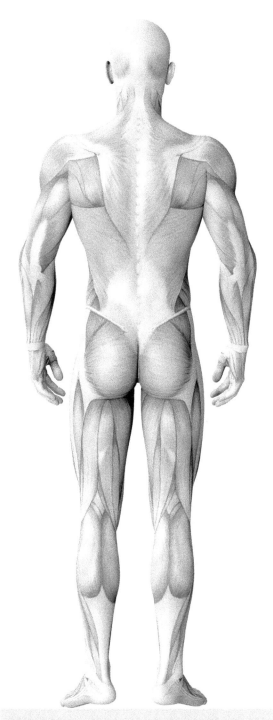

Figure 9.3

The map is not the territory: the Western 'map' of the body depicted here is based on muscles and bones rather than the invisible energy lines shown in Figure 9.1A,B

As we shall see in the next section, most excitingly, a unified theoretical framework and a firm anatomical basis for mystical Eastern notions of qi, acupoints and meridians can be found in our bodywork answer to life the, universe and everything: fascia!

Meridians meet myofascia

Lines in the body are not mystical, they are where forces balance.
Ida Rolf

Anyone who is familiar with both acupuncture meridians and Tom Myers' Anatomy Trains concepts could not have failed to notice the blinding similarities between the two. For those of you less acquainted here are a couple of 'spot the difference' pictures (**Figure 9.4A,B**).

Pretty much 'same, same', right? Tom Myers' *Anatomy Trains* book was a seminal work as it took the vague concepts of bodyworkers everywhere that 'everything is connected' and showed exactly HOW everything is connected. Muscles do not, as we previously thought, just attach to bones as single units but connect from head to toe in a series of longitudinal myofascial continuities. The first edition of Tom Myers' *Anatomy Trains* glossed over what seemed to be these potentially exciting parallels between acupuncture meridians and myofascial continuities. However, this was revised by the second edition and Tom 'Master of the Myofascia' Myers added an additional chapter on the concept stating 'In the first edition we deliberately omitted any comparison to the the acupuncture and similar meridians used in traditional Oriental medicine in order to emphasise the anatomical basis of these continuities. The close relationship between the two however is inescapable.'

Clearly there are striking parallels between the two systems that are too strong to be the result of chance. Of the 12 major meridians in Chinese medicine, nine have convincing correspondence with the fascial continuities as laid out by Myers. A brief glance at these side by side is enough to convince even the strongest sceptic that fascial continuities could indeed be the Western anatomical basis for the meridian system. As my 'spot the difference' approach is apparently not considered very scientific, the academics amongst you will

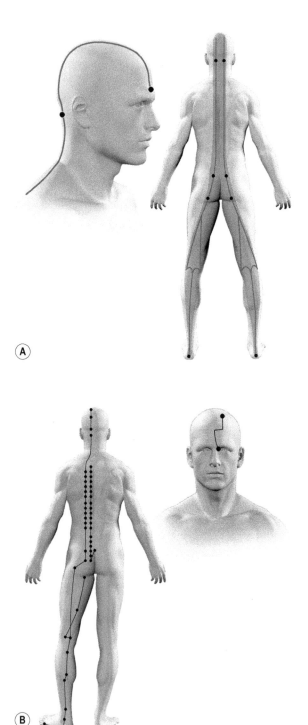

Figure 9.4A,B
The superficial back line of Tom Myers' Anatomy Trains system (A) looks remarkably similar to the Chinese Bladder meridian (B)

Table 9.1
Correspondence between Anatomy Trains and meridians

Name of Anatomy Train	Corresponding meridian
Superficial front line (SFL)	Stomach
Superficial back line (SBL)	Bladder
Lateral line (LL)	Gall Bladder
Superficial front arm line (SFAL)	Pericardium
Deep front arm line (DFAL)	Lung
Superficial back arm line (SBAL)	Triple Heater
Deep back arm line (DBAL)	Small Intestine
Deep front line (DFL)	Liver and Kidney
Spiral line (SL)	Stomach and Bladder

be pleased to hear that the correspondences have also been verified using computer software (Dorsher 2009). There was substantial overlap in the distributions of the Myers myofascial meridians with those of the acupuncture principal meridians in eight (89%) of nine comparisons, with the spiral line being a combination of two meridians (Stomach and Bladder). Dorsher concluded that 'this provides an independent, anatomic line of evidence that acupuncture principal meridians likely exist in the myofascial layer'. The correspondences are summarised in **Table 9.1.**

The lesser-spotted tendinomuscular channels

An even more convincing correlation between ancient meridians and modern Anatomy Trains can be found in the so-called tendinomuscular channels or Jingjin. The tendinomuscular channels are different in form than the primary channels as they are more solid, three-dimensional and have an intimate relationship with the 'sinews' – in other words they are three-dimensional pathways through the myofascial system (Legge 2011) (**Figure 9.5**). The Jingjin were first mentioned in the *Yellow Emperor's Inner Classic* written between 100 BCE and 100 CE, so the Yellow Emperor must be turning in his grave that Tom Myers got all the glory centuries after this first ancient

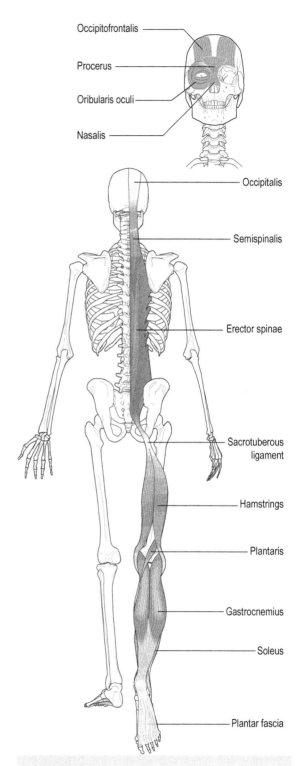

Figure 9.5
The Bladder Tendinomuscular channel

edition of 'Anatomy Trains' (clearly he needed a better publisher). The Jingjin are not very well known and are rarely used in acupuncture or Eastern bodywork which instead rely on the more well known maps of the primary channels. Robert Sohn, author of *Amma Therapy*, points out that the tendinomuscular channels are more properly the basis of Amma therapy and related oriental medical arts and that the use of primary channels has arisen due to lack of English translations of literature on traditional oriental manipulative therapy (Sohn 1996). A recent reappraisal of the channels by osteopath and acupuncturist David Legge has shown that the tendinomuscular channels were used for the treatment of musculoskeletal disorders by the needling of 'ah shi' points along their path (yes, our old friend trigger points). As Legge explains this approximates to the rationale of treating a tight myofascial train that has given way at its weakest link and is helpful in common musculoskeletal disorders such as tendinopathies, plantar fasciitis, carpal tunnel syndrome or Dupuytren's contracture.

Fascial newsflash: science confirms anatomical basis for meridians

The importance of these similarities between meridians and myofascial continuities cannot be underestimated as the lack of an anatomical correlate for the acupuncture channels had confounded Western scientists for years and caused the concepts of meridians, qi, and the basis of Asian healing modalities to be dismissed as 'unscientific hocus-pocus'.

The recent explosion in fascial research has also helped confirm the importance of the connective tissue system in understanding the mechanisms of acupuncture and Eastern bodywork. To be fair the concepts are not exactly new as ancient acupuncture texts pretty much spelled it out in references to 'fat greasy membranes, fasciae and systems of connecting membranes' through which qi is believed to flow (Dommerholt and Fernández-de-las-Peñas 2013, p. 32). Many modern leading thinkers have also commented on the possibility of the fascia as being the basis of acupuncture treatment (Finando and Finando 2012, Oschman 2000).

However, it is only over the last decade that the 'meridians are myofascia' concept has made its way to academic journals and in doing so gain needed credibility and gravitas. Several researchers have confirmed the correlation

between the meridians and the fascial system by using three-dimensional body scan data from MRIs to reconstruct the pathways of interstitial connective tissue (Bai et al 2011, Huang et al 2006). These images show that not only is the fascial system the physical representation of the meridians but that acupuncture points are often found at 'cleavages' of connective tissue planes. In other words, they are places where deeper levels of fascia can be accessed. One of the major researchers on the topic of acupuncture and fascia, Helene Langevin (Langevin and Yandow 2002), has found an 80% correspondence between the sites of acupuncture points and the location of intermuscular or intramuscular connective tissue planes in postmortem tissue sections (Langevin and Yandow 2002) (**Figure 9.6**). This finding mirrors the literal meaning for the Chinese character for acupuncture point which also means 'hole' or 'cave', i.e. a chamber to something deeper (**Figure 9.7**). Furthermore, Langevin's research showed that the meridians themselves strongly coincided with inter-muscular or intramuscular fascial planes (at least in the arm which was the area studied). Of the meridians that did not follow these inter- or intramuscular fascial planes,

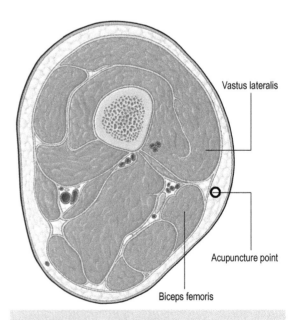

Vastus lateralis

Acupuncture point

Biceps femoris

Figure 9.6

The majority of acupuncture points are located at inter-muscular or intramuscular cleavages. The diagram shows the location of acupuncture point GB 32

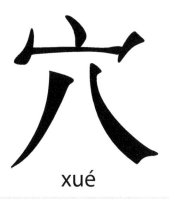

xué

Figure 9.7
The Chinese character for acupuncture point also means 'hole' or 'cave', i.e. a chamber to something deeper

there were, however, key acupuncture points along the meridian that 'clearly coincided with the intersection of multiple fascial planes'. In other words, some meridians travel along successive connective tissue planes whereas others are simply 'connecting the dots' between important acupuncture points that in themselves are holes to deeper fascial tissues. Again, this will be of little surprise to students of Asian bodywork systems who are accustomed to sensing meridians by searching for the grooves between or within muscles and palpating for points by searching for slight depressions or a sensation of yielding in the tissues. An acupuncturist colleague summed this up by saying 'qi flows in the nooks and crannies of the body, like water finding the path of least resistance. Find a groove and follow it and you are likely to be following a meridian'.

So far so good ... but so what? It seems convincing that the anatomical basis of the meridians is found in the fascial network, yet how might this help our understanding of how meridian based bodywork systems such as acupuncture, shiatsu or Thai massage actually work? As we shall see, Langevin has presented a convincing argument to demonstrate how the therapeutic effects of acupuncture may be mediated via this network of interstitial connective tissues. It does not seem too far a conceptual leap to extend this theory to the effects of Eastern bodywork in general.

Grasping the point: the 'needle grasp' phenomenon and fascial candyfloss

If you have ever been for acupuncture you may have experienced an aching sensation around the point as the needle is inserted – a pain your acupuncturist seemed secretly delighted you were experiencing. Central to the formulation of Langevin's theory was an investigation into this concept known as 'de qi' or 'obtaining qi' – which is an important central element of effective acupuncture. When inserting a needle into a point an acupuncturist often adds some kind of manipulation, i.e. either rapid rotation and/or piston pumping in an up and down motion. The acupuncturist is looking for a typical reaction known as 'needle grasp', which is literally a tug on the needle clearly described in ancient texts as 'like a fish biting on a fishing line' (Langevin et al 2002), and simultaneously the patient should experience an aching sensation in the area around the needle known as 'obtaining qi' or 'de qi'. It is common for the de qi sensation to spread along the course of a meridian. Traditional teachings place 'de qi' and 'needle grasp' as central theoretical concepts and essential to gaining a therapeutic result, i.e. literally a case of 'no pain, no gain'. Obtaining 'de qi' is also seen as important to the therapeutic efficacy of Asian bodywork as seen in this quote about stimulating tsubos (the name for acupressure points in the shiatsu system):

> When a point has been properly stimulated, a sensation called 'de qi' is experienced, which verifies that the qi of the point has been contacted. This sensation may be felt as a pain or ache accompanied by a simultaneous feeling of release; a feeling that spreads out to the affected area; a distending soreness; warmness; a tingling or numbness; or an electric sensation. If no sensation is felt, then the tsubo was not located correctly, the pressure was not applied correctly, or the client is extremely deficient in qi and xue.
> KAPKE 2004

Guess what is causing this effect? Yep, that's right, the generic answer to life, the universe and everything: 'fascia'. Langevin has convincingly shown that, in acupuncture, needle grasp is the result of the collagen and elastin fibres in connective tissue winding around the needle during needle rotation. The amazing pictures of this phenomenon have to be seen to be believed as the connective tissue gradually coils around the needle and forms a wonderful fascial candyfloss effect that gives the characteristic tugging of 'de qi' (**Figure 9.8**). Langevin has further postulated that this reaction could explain how acupuncture actually works, i.e. the winding of the fascia causes a mechanical signal to be transmitted to connective tissue cells via mechanotransduction (Langevin et al 2001). This could explain both the local and more distant effects of acupuncture, i.e. mechanical signals are transmitted via the fascia right down to the level of the cell. Presumably this is also the case with bodywork and it is interesting that many methods of stimulating acupressure points use small rotational circles which possibly have a similar effect on the fascia as the rotations of a needle. Once more we see the thrilling effects of tensegrity in action.

As we know, fascia is everywhere and these mechanotransduction effects could potentially take place wherever the needle is placed in the body. Many of the studies looking into the effectiveness of acupuncture

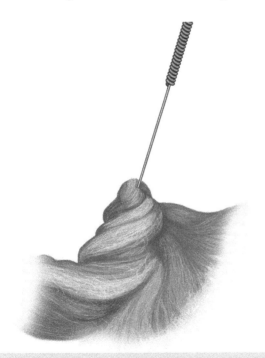

Figure 9.8
Research by Helene Langevin shows that during acupuncture, the connective tissue gradually coils around the needle, giving the characteristic tugging effect of 'de qi'

have used 'sham acupuncture' as a control group (where needles are inserted into non-acupuncture points). Interestingly, in many cases both acupuncture and sham acupuncture demonstrated significant effects by comparison to no treatment or conventional medical approaches (Finando and Finando 2011), suggesting that needle stimulation of connective tissue is a powerful mechanism wherever it is employed.

However, the work of Langevin and others would suggest that the acupuncture points are indeed special places where extra connective tissue can be accessed giving a more powerful mechanotransduction effect. If you imagine the fascia as networks of primary and secondary roads, the acupuncture points are like major intersections where several fascial pathways can be accessed. Subsequent studies by Langevin have also shown that acupuncture causes specific changes to the fibroblasts in subcutaneous connective tissue that are very similar to the changes induced by tissue stretch. In both cases the fibroblasts spread and become sheet-like and form characteristic lamellipodia (a projection on the mobile edge of the cell that can act to propel the cell along). It seems that a similar mechanotransduction effect may be happening with different therapeutic interventions such as acupuncture, fascial release, yoga or other manual therapy interventions (Langevin et al 2006).

Sing the body electric: the collagen superhighway

> *The thin red jellies within you, or within me—the bones, and the marrow in the bones,*
> *The exquisite realization of health;*
> *O I say, these are not the parts and poems of the Body only, but of the Soul,*
> *O I say now these are the Soul.*
> WALT WHITMAN 1900, THE BODY ELECTRIC

As bodyworkers the feeling that we are working with some kind of 'electrical current' is a pervasive idea; manual therapists and healers from all disciplines report the feelings of electricity, flow, and connection with their work. One of the explanations of what is happening in fascial release is the creation of a piezoelectric effect. Scientist James Oschman (2000) has long maintained that collagen is the basis of a body-wide electrical network, the existence of which could explain the effects of manual therapy and healing techniques. Similar notions are common in acupuncture and previous research studies have found that acupuncture meridians and points do in fact have lower electrical impedance than surrounding tissues (Reichmanis and Becker 1978). More recent studies by Ahn et al (2005, 2010) also provide some support to the notion that collagen may be the basis of a body-wide electrical network. Ultrasound studies found that collagenous bands are significantly associated with lower electrical impedance and that this may also account for the reduced electrical impedances previously reported at acupuncture meridians.

The fascial Holy Trinity: nerve, artery and vein

Detailed studies of the superficial fascia have also revealed the presence of numerous holes which all have a perforating triad of vein, artery and nerve. By now you have probably a sneaking suspicion that these might have something to do with acupuncture points and you are quite right, as shown by anatomist Hartmut Heine who found an 82% correspondence between the two (Heine 1995) **(Figure 9.9)**. Schleip reports research

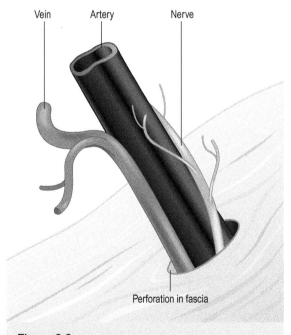

Vein   Artery   Nerve

Perforation in fascia

Figure 9.9

The superficial fascia has numerous holes where a triad of artery, nerve and vein pass through. These holes have a high correspondence with acupuncture points

that Heine carried out with German surgeon Dr Johann Bauer who found that, in patients experiencing chronic shoulder–neck or shoulder–arm pain, these perforating vessels were 'strangled' by an unusually thick ring of collagen directly on top of this perforation hole through the fascia. Microsurgery to loosen these collagen strangulations caused improvement in the pain conditions (Schleip 2011). It is obviously interesting to speculate whether bodywork and acupuncture at these points could have a similar effect to the microsurgery. Results of reduction in pain using acupressure points with chronic pain conditions would suggest that this is a strong possibility.

What is qi?

Qi is the source of all movement in the body, protects the body, is connected to harmonious transformation (metabolism), retains the body's substances and organs and warms the body.
Kaptchuk 1983

The notion of qi is central to both acupuncture and Eastern-based bodywork systems. Qi is commonly translated into English as 'energy' but, as Finando and Finando (2011) point out, this is not a direct translation and has led to misconceptions and dismissal of Eastern methods as unscientific. But with our new knowledge is it possible that when we are tuning into and balancing qi we are actually sensing the fascia? As Finando cleverly points out, in the above quote about the functions of qi, 'Fascia' can easily be substituted with no loss of meaning. So maybe the subtle fluid movements that we can tune into with our hands are really the dancing movements of the fascia.

Trigger points and Stecco points

Two more types of points are also worth looking at for their intriguing parallels with acupoints: trigger points and the points used in the Stecco fascial manipulation method. Chapter 8 has already explored the huge overlap between trigger points and acupoints both of the classical and 'ah shi' variety.

Another point-based bodywork system that has gained popularity over the past few years is the fascial manipulation (FM) method originally developed by Luigi Stecco, PT, and now carried forward by his children, Carla and Antonio, both MDs. The Stecco family are a formidable bodywork dynasty (think the Kennedys of fascial therapy) and the family are (quite rightly) current darlings of the fascial scene with their enormous contribution to research, dissection studies and application to clinical practice. The Stecco system refers to three main types of points: centres of perception (CP) are the areas where symptoms are felt while centres of coordination (CC) and centres of fusion (CF) are both points of possible densified fascial tissue that may be causing these symptoms. Points for treatment are determined via a complex assessment protocol analysing patterns of client movement (commonly taking 45 minutes to an hour); treatment is by deep friction with knuckles or elbows to the selected points. The points are found to be 'densified on palpation, tender to the patient and either in the belly of the muscle or near the retinaculum and tendons near the joint' (Hammer 2011). Stecco recognises that the CF and CC overlap with both acupuncture and trigger points. These points for treatment are also found along myofascial continuities that are very similar to Anatomy Trains (thus by extension also primary and tendinomuscular channels).

It seems that acupuncture points, trigger points and Stecco points are highly similar systems with huge overlaps. Their differences lie only in their theoretical underpinnings: a case of same thing but a different language. As they like to say in Thailand 'Same same … but different.'

Towards a fascially based explanation of Eastern bodywork

In the simplest form, Eastern bodywork and acupuncture can be viewed as an ancient fascial modality (see **Table 9.2**). The thumbing, palming and stretching techniques work on myofascial continuities known as meridians in the same way that Rolfing or KMI work on the Anatomy Trains dissected by Tom Myers. Thumb or finger pressure to acupuncture points accesses deeper fascial planes and the effects can be transmitted right down to the level of the cell via mechanotransduction. Rather than balancing the mysterious qi that makes little sense in our Western framework we could instead reconceptualise the work as tuning into and releasing fascial constrictions and abnormalities. Donna and

Table 9.2
Traditional Chinese medicine and fascial correspondence

Traditional Chinese medicine	Fascial correspondence
Acupuncture meridians	Intermuscular or intramuscular fascial planes
Acupuncture points	Cleavages within fascial planes
Qi	Sensation of palpation of fascia
Blockage of qi	Altered fascial composition (densification, areas of stuck layers, fascial adhesions)
Restoration of qi	Unsticking or releasing of fascial adhesions

Steven Finando have come to similar conclusions through their own work, also a fusion of East and West combining fascial work, trigger point work, acupuncture and Amma therapy. The Finandos must be in a unique place to have an opinion on such matters having decades of clinical work under their belts and having trained directly under the leaders in the field, including Janet Travell and Tina Sohn. In conversation with the Finandos, in the summer of 2014, we discussed the striking parallels among systems of trigger point work, fascial work and Eastern approaches. Steven commented:

> The question is what came first (treatment or theory)? The more I think about it, it seems that people thousands of years ago in the East, were paying close attention to the body and associated dysfunction and pathology. Things were showing up on the body that led to the concept of channels and points and THEN explanations for this came next. Whether these explanations reflect reality is a whole other question.

Donna then chipped in 'It reflects the reality that they understood 2000 years ago.' We can therefore conclude that the practice is solid, although the explanations may differ.

Does our client care what we are working on? Probably not. Whether we believe we are working on fascia or qi, the important point is to know where you are and what you are doing. Our ancestors in the healing world have been manipulating soft tissue via grooves and holes on the body's surface for thousands of years, gaining valid results in the treatment of pain. Combining the ancient tried and tested techniques of meridian and point work with more recent fascial understanding can only be of benefit to our clients. The key to both approaches is a sensitive palpation-led bodywork that seeks a restoration of anatomical and physiological balance. Sen lines, meridians, nadis, tsubos, acupuncture points, trigger points and Stecco points all conceptually weave and overlap with striking similarities. Millions of bodyworkers from all corners of the world have found pressing, pulling and pushing grooves and holes in the body to be of immeasurable value. That seems to me like one heck of a market research study.

What the research says

Research has shown positive results for acupressure-based systems in the treatment of numerous different conditions:

- **Pain relief:** systematic reviews of the available evidence have shown acupressure to be a viable option for pain relief in a number of situations including labour, dysmenorrhoea (menstrual pain), low back pain, chronic headache and other traumatic pains (Chen and Wang 2013, Robinson et al 2011).

- **Dysmenorrhoea (menstrual pain):** studies show that acupressure can be as effective as taking ibuprofen for the relief of period pain (Pouresmail and Ibrahimzadeh 2002). These results are also not just a quick fix as several reviews have shown positive outcomes to last at 3 and 6 month follow-ups (Cho and Hwang 2010, Chung et al 2012, Jiang et al 2013).

- **Labour pain:** a Cochrane review concluded that both acupressure and acupuncture can be useful during labour, with a role in reducing pain, increasing satisfaction with pain management and reducing use of drugs (Smith et al 2011).

- **Low back pain:** several studies have shown that Eastern bodywork modalities, including acupressure and Thai massage, can be effective

treatment for low back pain (Furlan et al 2002, Netchanok et al 2012). Hsieh et al (2006) showed that acupressure was more effective than physical therapy in reducing low back pain in terms of disability, pain scores, and functional status with a benefit that was sustained at a 6-month follow-up.

- **Chronic neck pain:** Matsubara et al (2011) looked at the use of both local and distal acupressure points for the treatment of chronic neck pain. Interestingly, both types of points were effective in reducing pain in the short term with results persisting until the next day (unfortunately there was no longer term follow-up); however, only the local points seemed to have an effect on the parasympathetic nervous system.

- **Cancer symptoms:** acupressure has been found to be a useful tool for helping to alleviate some of the symptoms of cancer treatment including fatigue (Zick et al 2011) and vomiting induced by chemotherapy (Lee and Frazier 2011).

- **Nausea and vomiting:** acupressure (in particular stimulation of point P 6 located three fingers from the wrist crease in the midline) is an effective strategy for treating nausea during pregnancy, chemotherapy or post- operatively (Lee and Frazier 2011).

- **Traumatic brain injury:** a study by McFadden et al (2011) found 4 weeks of acupressure treatment showed some improvement in working memory function for brain-injured patients compared to a control group.

- **Stroke:** meridian acupressure was helpful in improving patients function and symptoms (Kang et al 2009, Lee et al 2011).

- **Chronic obstructive pulmonary disease (COPD):** acupressure can be helpful with improving some of the distressing symptoms of COPD, including breathlessness, pulmonary function, anxiety levels and 6-minute walking distance (Wu et al 2004).

- **Improving fatigue and reducing insomnia:** several studies have shown acupressure to be an effective tool for fatigue and insomnia in a variety of patient populations (Lee et al 2011).

- **Care of the elderly:** acupressure may be a useful non-invasive treatment for helping symptom management in the care of the elderly. In an interesting study where patients served as their own control group, Yang et al (2007) showed that 15 minutes of acupressure by caregivers for 4 weeks was more effective at reducing agitated behaviour in patients with dementia than a subsequent 4-week period where the caregivers gave conversation and companionship only.

- **Help with presenting symptoms:** a survey of 633 shiatsu clients in three European countries (Austria, UK and Spain) showed improvement in presenting symptoms such as pain, stress and fatigue at 3- and 6-month follow-up. A high percentage of clients had also made lifestyle changes (diet and exercise) and reduced their reliance on conventional medicine and medication (Long 2008).

- **Fibromyalgia:** shiatsu has been shown to have positive effects in the treatment of fibromyalgia symptoms including improvement of the pain intensity, pressure pain threshold, sleep quality and symptoms impact on health (Yuan et al 2013).

Incorporating meridian and point work into your treatments

The main thrust of our argument here is that the inclusion of meridian and point work into your treatments is likely to enhance your results in the treatment of pain conditions. In clinical practice the inclusion of local point work can be key to releasing fascial restrictions effectively and suggested points for each area are included in chapters 12–19. If you know your meridians, use your knowledge to work those that are relevant to the pain condition. If you have little knowledge of Chinese medicine, then use your creativity to find the grooves, nooks and crannies of the body and work those with whatever techniques you know.

References

Ahn AC et al 2005 Electrical impedance along connective tissue planes associated with acupuncture meridians. BMC Complementary and Alternative Medicine 5:10.

Ahn AC et al 2010 Electrical impedance of acupuncture meridians: The relevance of subcutaneous collagenous bands. PLoS ONE 5.

Aobta.org 2014 Home. Available at: http://www.aobta.org [accessed 18 August 2014].

Bai Y et al 2011 Review of evidence suggesting that the fascia network could be the anatomical basis for acupoints and meridians in the human body. Evidence-Based Complementary Alternative Medicine. Article ID 260510, 6 pages. doi:10.1155/2011/260510.

Chen Y-W, Wang H-H 2014 The effectiveness of acupressure on relieving pain: a systematic review. Pain Management Nursing: Official Journal of the American Society of Pain Management Nurses 15(2):539–550.

Cho S-H, Hwang E-W 2010 Acupressure for primary dysmenorrhoea: a systematic review. Complementary Therapies in Medicine 18(1):49–56.

Chung Y-C, Chen H-H, Yeh M-L 2012 Acupoint stimulation intervention for people with primary dysmenorrhea: systematic review and meta-analysis of randomized trials. Complementary Therapies in Medicine 20(5):353–363.

Dommerholt J, Fernández-de-las-Peñas C 2013 Trigger Point Dry Needling, 1st edn. Oxford: Churchill Livingstone.

Dorsher PT 2009 Myofascial meridians as anatomical evidence of acupuncture channels. Medical Acupuncture 21(2):91–97.

Finando S, Finando D 2011 Fascia and the mechanism of acupuncture. Journal of Bodywork and Movement Therapies 15(2):168–176.

Finando S, Finando D 2012 Acupuncture, and the fascia: a reconsideration of the fundamental principles of acupuncture. The Journal of Alternative and Complementary Medicine 18:880–886.

Furlan AD et al 2002 Massage for low-back pain: a systematic review within the framework of the Cochrane Collaboration Back Review Group. Spine 27(17):1896–1910.

Hammer W 2011 What's the point? Dynamic Chiropractic 29(9).

Heine H 1995 Functional anatomy of traditional Chinese acupuncture points. Acta Anatomica 152:293.

Hsieh LL-C et al 2006 Treatment of low back pain by acupressure and physical therapy: randomised controlled trial. BMJ (Clinical Research Edn) 332:696–700.

Huang Y et al 2006 Study on the meridians and acupoints based on fasciaology: an elicitation of the study on digital human being. Zhongguo Zhen Jiu 26(11):785–788.

Jiang H-R et al 2013 Systematic Review of Randomized Clinical Trials of Acupressure Therapy for Primary Dysmenorrhea. Evidence-Based Complementary and Alternative Medicine eCAM 2013:169692.

Kang HS, Sok SR, Kang JS 2009 Effects of meridian acupressure for stroke patients in Korea. Journal of Clinical Nursing 18:2145–2152.

Kapke K (Barry) 2004 To the point: working with tsubo. Massage Therapy Articles. Massage & Bodywork Aug/Sep.

Kaptchuk T 1983 The Web that has no Weaver, 1st edn. New York: Congdon & Weed.

Langevin HM, Yandow JA 2002 Relationship of acupuncture points and meridians to connective tissue planes. The Anatomical Record 269(6):257–265.

Langevin HM, Churchill DL, Cipolla MJ 2001 Mechanical signaling through connective tissue: a mechanism for the therapeutic effect of acupuncture. The FASEB Journal 15:2275–2282.

Langevin HM et al 2002 Evidence of connective tissue involvement in acupuncture. The FASEB Journal 16:872–874.

Langevin HM et al 2006 Subcutaneous tissue fibroblast cytoskeletal remodeling induced by acupuncture: evidence for a mechanotransduction-based mechanism. Journal of Cellular Physiology 207:767–774.

Lee EJ, Frazier SK 2011 The efficacy of acupressure for symptom management: a systematic review. Journal of Pain and Symptom Management 42(4):589–603.

Lee J-S et al 2011 Acupressure for treating neurological disorders: a systematic review. The International Journal of Neuroscience 121(8):409–414.

Legge D 2011 Jing jin: a 21st century reappraisal. Journal of Chinese Medicine 95(Feb):5–8.

Long AF 2008. The effectiveness of shiatsu: findings from a cross-European, prospective observational study. Journal of Alternative and Complementary Medicine (New York, NY) 14:921–930.

McFadden KL et al 2011 Acupressure as a non-pharmacological intervention for traumatic brain injury (TBI). Journal of Neurotrauma 28:21–34.

Matsubara T et al 2011 Comparative effects of acupressure at local and distal acupuncture points on pain conditions and autonomic function in females with chronic neck pain. Evidence-Based Complementary and Alternative Medicine. Article ID 543291, 6 pages.

Netchanok S et al 2012 The effectiveness of Swedish massage and traditional Thai massage in treating chronic low back pain: a review of the literature. Complementary Therapies in Clinical Practice 18(4):227–234.

Oschman J 2000 Energy Medicine: The Scientific Basis. Edinburgh: Churchill Livingstone.

Pouresmail Z, Ibrahimzadeh R 2002 Effects of acupressure and ibuprofen on the severity of primary dysmenorrhea. Journal of Traditional Chinese Medicine Sep;22(3):205–210.

Reichmanis M, Becker RO 1978 Physiological effects of stimulation at acupuncture loci: a review. Comparative Medicine East and West 6:67–73.

Robinson N, Lorenc A, Liao X 2011 The evidence for shiatsu: a systematic review of shiatsu and acupressure. BMC Complementary and Alternative Medicine 11:88.

Schleip R 2011 Fascia as a sensory organ: a target of myofascial manipulation. In: Dalton E (ed) Dynamic Body: Exploring Form, Expanding Function. Oklahoma City, OK: Freedom from Pain Institute, pp. 137–164.

Smith CA et al 2011 Acupuncture or acupressure for pain management in labour. The Cochrane Database of Systematic Reviews (7):CD009232.

Sohn T, Sohn R 1996 Amma Therapy, 1st edn. Rochester, VT: Healing Arts Press, p. 70.

Whitman W 1900 Leaves of Grass. Philadelphia: D. McKay.

Wu H-S et al 2004 Effectiveness of acupressure in improving dyspnoea in chronic obstructive pulmonary disease. Journal of Advanced Nursing 45:252–259.

Yang M-H et al 2007 The efficacy of acupressure for decreasing agitated behaviour in dementia: a pilot study. Journal of Clinical Nursing 16:308–315.

Yuan SLK, Berssaneti AA, Marques AP 2013 Effects of shiatsu in the management of fibromyalgia symptoms: a controlled pilot study. Journal of Manipulative and Physiological Therapeutics 36(7):436–443.

Zick SM et al 2011 Relaxation acupressure reduces persistent cancer-related fatigue. Evidence-Based Complementary and Alternative Medicine. Article ID 142913, 10 pages, 2011. doi:10.1155/2011/142913.

Stretching the truth: what the new evidence tells us about stretching

Stretching is good for you, isn't it? Surely it's common wisdom that stretching makes you feel better, increases flexibility, prevents injury before sports challenges, improves athletic performance, reduces muscle soreness after exercise and alleviates the pain of a bad back (that is if you actually DID the exercises your physiotherapist prescribed). Running, cycling and health magazines promote the value of stretching for 'leaner, thinner bodies', Google harangues us with adverts for stretching-friendly Lycra clothing, and yoga has never been more popular. Stretching has become a whole industry in itself with ever-fancier names applied to the latest stretching methods. Indeed it can be dizzying to try and keep up with the current state-of-the-art stretchy technique. Stretching is 'dynamic, ballistic, proprioceptive neuromuscular facilitated (PNF), active, passive, contracty–relaxy and, above all, finger lickin' good'.

Yet, over the last decade, an explosion of academic interest into stretching has suggested that maybe stretching isn't the absolute panacea for all ills that it has been built up to be. The truth is much more complex than the simple dichotomy of 'stretching is good for you' or 'stretching is useless and a waste of time'. So let's extract the magic from the myth, hyperbole from hard facts, as we look at the academic evidence and expose the real truth about stretching.

Common wisdom about stretching

If you are at all interested in bodywork, complementary therapies or the health and fitness industry you will probably subscribe to one or more of the following beliefs about stretching:

- Stretching helps you be more flexible as it permanently lengthens short and tight muscles.
- You should stretch before you work out as it helps prevent injury.
- If you stretch before and after exercise it helps prevent and reduce muscle soreness (known in

the trade as delayed onset muscle soreness (DOMS)).

- Stretching before an event helps improve sport performance.
- Stretching makes you feel good.
- Stretching is helpful for musculoskeletal pain such as a bad back.

What the evidence says

Let's take each of these beliefs one by one and see what the research evidence has come up with.

Stretching helps you be more flexible

Well, yes it does. Numerous research studies have shown that regular stretching does indeed make us more flexible. It probably doesn't matter which technique you use as all methods show increases in range of motion (ROM). For example, if we regularly stretch our hamstrings we should be able to reach further (Decoster et al 2005). Depending on your starting place this may mean you are now able to do up your shoelaces while standing, get further into that pesky forward bend in yoga or win that circus job you have been after.

However, what is fascinating is that the reason we can stretch further is probably nothing to do with elongating the muscles permanently. A thorough systematic review of academic studies on the subject (Weppler and Magnusson 2010) proposes that any change in muscle (or connective tissue) length is transient and, in fact, the only reason we can go further on repeated exposure to stretching is due to an alteration of sensation only. In other words, we just get an increased tolerance as our brains and body just get used to stretching a little further each time, yet our resting muscle length remains exactly the same. Bad news for health and fitness magazines promising a 'longer leaner body through stretching.'

You should stretch before and after you workout as it prevents injury

Mixed news on this one. There is conflicting evidence as to whether stretching can prevent injury and the somewhat unsatisfying conclusion, when reviewing all of the evidence, is that stretching 'might prevent some injuries in some sports some of the time'.

There are several authors who have looked at all the research studies out there, e.g. a systematic review of the literature by Thacker et al (2004) concluded that 'Stretching was not significantly associated with a reduction in total injuries.' This is not particularly helpful for the athlete wondering if they should stretch or not before exercising. Thacker et al's summary of the study ends with the politician's 'we can neither confirm or deny' type of advice that:

> There is not sufficient evidence to endorse or discontinue routine stretching before or after exercise to prevent injury among competitive or recreational athletes.
> THACKER ET AL 2004

Another systematic review (Hart 2005) was less circumspect and concluded that 'Limited evidence showed stretching had no effect in reducing injuries.'

However, on closer examination of the research it seems that perhaps stretching may help to reduce injury for some sports but not others (Witvrouw et al 2004). Stretching seems to reduce injuries in sports that involve bouncing and jumping activities with a high intensity of stretch–shortening cycles (SSCs) (e.g. soccer and football if you live in the USA or football and rugby if you live in the UK). However, when the type of sports activity contains low-intensity, or limited SSCs (e.g. jogging, cycling and swimming), then stretching may not be helpful in preventing injury. This is seen in the literature, where strong evidence exists that stretching has no beneficial effect on injury prevention in these sports.

Other authors (Woods et al 2007) suggest that it has been difficult to interpret all the available research due to the number of different stretching techniques used and feels instead 'that certain techniques and protocols have shown a positive outcome on deterring injuries'. They recommend that a warm-up and stretching protocol should be implemented prior to physical activity. The routine should allow the stretching protocol to occur within the 15 minutes immediately prior to the activity in order to receive the most benefit.

Although static stretching does not reduce overall injury rates, there is preliminary evidence that it may reduce musculotendinous injuries, such as muscle strains (McHugh and Cosgrove 2010, Small et al 2008). Warm-up in general is definitely a good thing for preventing injury (Fradkin et al 2006) and most experts recommend that a warm-up routine should include stretching.

There are only a few studies on the benefits of stretching at a different time to just before exercise. However, the few that exist suggest that stretching as a regular routine is more likely to reduce injury (Shrier 2007), i.e. going to that regular yoga class may be more likely to reduce your possibility of injury than the short stretching procedure before sports.

Stretching helps prevent and reduce muscle soreness (DOMS)

The research is pretty unequivocal on this one: it doesn't help, or at best only helps a little bit. A large review of all the relevant studies (Herbert et al 2011) concluded that:

> The evidence from randomised studies suggests that muscle stretching, whether conducted before, after, or before and after exercise, does not produce clinically important reductions in delayed-onset muscle soreness in healthy adults.
> HERBERT ET AL 2011

The review cites one large study showing that stretching before and after exercise reduced peak soreness over a 1-week period but this was only by, on average, four points on a 100-point scale. Hardly something to write home about!

Stretching helps improve performance in sport

To understand the evidence from research we need to look at stretching immediately prior to an event and stretching as part of a regular training routine.

Stretching immediately prior to exercise or an event

There is a bit of a shock–horror headline about this one as recent research has suggested that not only does stretching have less impact on performance than previously thought but in some cases it actually has a negative impact. That's right, depending on the sporting event, pre-event stretching may actually cause you to under perform (Shrier 2004). This finding specifically applies to sports that require isolated force or power (such as jumping or sprinting) and in these cases stretching prior to an event can cause diminished performance. This is true whether the stretching technique used is static, ballistic or proprioceptive neuromuscular facilitation (PNF). So elite basketball players will not jump as high if they stretch immediately before playing. Maybe this was the problem in the 1990s movie *White Men Can't Jump* – perhaps the white guys were sticking too strongly to their pre-event stretching routine!

Many of the studies that show stretching to inhibit maximal muscular performance pointed the finger at static stretching (the good old traditional form of stretching where you stretch and hold) whereas dynamic stretching (swinging the body part though a full ROM without holding the stretch) did not affect performance adversely or in some studies actually improved it. This has led to static stretching being given a 'bad rap' in certain athletic circles, e.g. a review by Simic et al (2013) advised 'We conclude that the usage of static stretching as the sole activity during warm-up routine should generally be avoided.'

Some sports people have discarded stretching all together as part of a warm-up routine or use dynamic stretching instead of static. However, studies show that this may well be throwing the baby out with the bathwater as the following points should be kept in mind:

- The findings only apply to sports requiring explosive power (sprinting, jumping, etc.). Sports such as running are not affected by pre-event stretching and sports requiring high amounts of flexibility (gymnastics) would definitely benefit from static stretching pre-performance.

- A review by Kay and Blazevich (2012) found that the findings about static stretching applied only to stretches held for a longer duration of greater than 60 seconds and concluded that 'Shorter durations of stretch (less than 60 seconds) can be performed in a pre-exercise routine without compromising maximal muscle performance.'

- Static stretching only affects performance if carried out immediately before an event; if stretching is followed by other warm-up activities (such as skills practice) this potentially negative effect seems to be cancelled out (Taylor et al 2009). If a warm-up is carried out in this way then there is no difference between the effects of performance whether dynamic or static stretching is used.

- In summary, pre-event stretching and warm-up should generally be tailored to the particular sport; in this way performance can be maximised and the risk of injury minimised. So sports such as gymnastics should use short duration static stretches prior to an event whereas activities requiring explosive power benefit more from a warm up comprising of a mix of light aerobic activity, dynamic stretching and completing with dynamic activities specific to the sport in question (Behm and Chaouachi 2011).

Stretching as part of a regular exercise or training routine

Interestingly, regular stretching at other times (not immediately before an event) actually improves the results for many sporting activities including enhancing running speed (Shrier 2004). In other words, regular stretching after exercise or at a time unrelated to exercise is more beneficial than your pre-exercise stretching 'warm-up' routine. So if you want to improve general sporting performance, get to that regular stretching or yoga class!

Stretching makes you feel good

This is an easy one to personally prove or disprove as it is firmly based on the scientific foundation of what blogger Paul Ingraham (n.d.) calls the 'laboratory of me'. Does stretching make you feel good? Great, do more of it! Do you hate it? Then find another way to exercise or increase flexibility if you need to.

The potential feel-good benefits of stretching seem to have been largely overlooked in the research studies as, let's face it, academics are usually in pursuit of more 'sciencey' things to prove. Yet anecdotal evidence suggests that humans love to stretch as it helps us feel more balanced, less tired and can be an excellent form of stress relief. Stretching is the basis of spiritual practices such as yoga and the poses (asanas) help prepare the body for the contemplation of meditation afterwards. Eastern massage practices such as Thai massage and shiatsu incorporate stretching as an integral part of the art. The purpose of these stretches is not to increase flexibility but to promote balance and harmony in the meridians and energy of the body. Our ancestors may not have known how to carry out a double-blind randomised controlled trial but this does not mean that thousands of years of acute observation, as to what keeps the human race healthy and happy, should be disregarded.

One of the few studies conducted on general stretching and wellbeing took place in a Spanish workplace that implemented a short programme of stretching exercises (Montero-Marín et al 2013). Findings showed that the programme was effective for reducing levels of anxiety, bodily pain and exhaustion, and for raising levels of vitality, mental health, general health and flexibility. All in all, a great low-cost strategy for improving the wellbeing of workers.

There are also many studies testifying to the positive effects of the ultimate stretching practice – yoga – on anxiety, depression and wellbeing. There has been growing evidence of the therapeutic benefits of yoga for anxiety, depression, obsessive compulsive disorder and alcohol dependency and for improving some of the symptoms of schizophrenia (Panesar and Valachova 2011). Undoubtedly these effects are not just due to the scientific effects of stretching but the fact that, in yoga, the poses are carried out mindfully with attention to the body and the breath. As we shall see in the Self-Care Resources (available at uk.singingdragon.com/catalogue/book/9781909141230), meditation and mindfulness are excellent ways to reduce stress and chronic pain. Yoga artfully combines these principles with stretching and strengthening and is a great all round package for the self help of chronic pain.

Stretching is good for musculoskeletal pain such as a bad back

There is good news for stretching here. Many studies have demonstrated the positive effects of yoga on pain (Posadzki et al 2011). It seems that these effects may also be true for conventional stretching; as one study showed that both yoga and stretching classes were more effective (with benefits lasting several months) for improving function and reducing symptoms due to chronic low back pain than a self-care booklet (Sherman et al 2011).

So is stretching good for me or not?

As always the answer is 'it depends'. A summary of the research evidence suggests that:

- If you want to prevent injury and improve your sporting performance then regular stretching or yoga is more effective than just stretching before exercise.

- If you do a competitive sport that involves isolated force or power (sprinting and basketball) it may be wise to avoid static or PNF stretching immediately before an important event (although if you do the stretching before you carry out the rest of your warm-up routine this should not affect performance). Including dynamic stretching or active isolated stretching (AIS) should not affect performance adversely and may even improve it.

- Pre-event stretching is not a 'one size fits all' activity and should be carefully tailored to the particular sport. Stretching is only one element of an effective warm-up.

- Stretching and yoga are good if you have chronic pain such as a bad back.

- Stretching helps you feel good and can be an excellent component of an overall health and fitness regime.

● Responses to stretching are to some extent unique so your stretching routine should be designed depending on your sporting or health goals, events you compete in, individual observations of how different types of stretching feel for you and your age.

Stretching techniques for the massage therapist

There are a myriad of different types of stretching used by the bodywork therapist both within a treatment and for client self-care purposes. Stretching has always been big in manual therapy in both the East and West, e.g. Thai massage, shiatsu and tuina all feature stretching as an integral part of the therapy. Massage therapists, physiotherapists, osteopaths, chiropractors, personal trainers, Pilates teachers and yoga therapists (using yoga techniques for the treatment of pain conditions) all use stretching techniques, to varying degrees, for rehabilitation of acute and chronic pain conditions.

In addition to a range of benefits, stretching also looks and feels impressive to the client. I had one woman who came back to me solely on the basis of 'you did that stretchy thing to my neck that no one else ever did'. Our lovely Thai massage teacher Asokananda (sadly no longer with us) had a great phrase for some of the more dramatic stretches of Thai bodywork: 'show business massage'. At Jing we always use these stretches when we want to 'show off', e.g. at exhibitions a few classy stretches is enough to bring a crowd gathering! I know it's shallow but, hey, massage can be a lonely business, so take the attention when you can get it.

The names of different stretching methods can be bewildering so it is helpful to break them down into three broad categories according to how the muscle is stretched: static, dynamic and pre-contraction stretching (Page 2012). We will also discuss a couple of 'newer' forms of stretching: therapeutic stretching and fascial stretching.

1. Static stretching

This good old traditional method is still the most popular and widely known form of stretching. In static stretching the muscle is elongated to the point of a stretching sensation and held in position. This can be done in two ways:

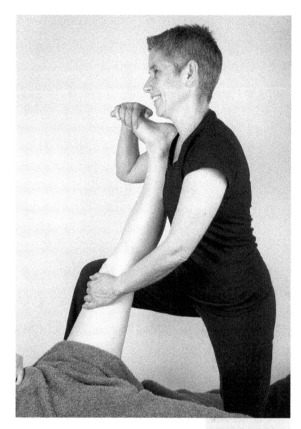

Figure 10.1

● Passively with a therapist or partner. The client lies on their back and the therapist takes the client's hamstrings to the point of stretch and holds their leg in position (**Figure 10.1**). This is also the type of stretching commonly used in shiatsu and Thai massage.

● Actively where the client is engaged in the movement. The client lies on their back and raises their leg. They then take their leg into full stretch with the assistance of a rope, a belt or their hands. This can also be achieved by the client placing their leg against the wall (**Figure 10.2**). This is the type of self-stretching used in yoga poses.

2. Dynamic stretching

Dynamic stretching can be divided into active and ballistic. It is REALLY important to understand the difference between ballistic and other forms of active stretching as they can seem similar but are actually quite different.

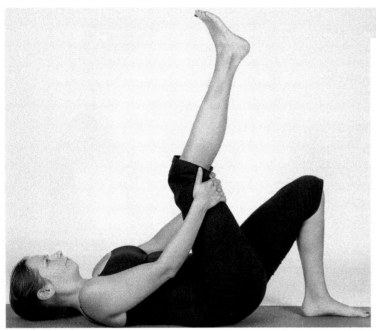

Figure 10.2

Ballistic stretching

This involves bouncing at the end range of a stretch, i.e. the good old reach for your toes and bounce up and down in the same position is a ballistic stretch for the hamstrings. PE teachers in the 1970s were big on this one as was Jane Fonda (although she apparently corrected herself in later teachings so she should not be blamed entirely for the fad that probably bumped up an entire generation's musculoskeletal injury rate).

Ballistic stretching is generally not recommended due to its potential for injury. The American Academy of Orthopedic Surgeons sternly warns on their website 'Do not bounce your stretches. Ballistic (bouncy) stretching can cause injury' (Orthoinfo.aaos.org 2014). Personally I love that the orthopaedic surgeons are using the word bouncy. Although ballistic stretching is generally not recommended for most sports people there is some new evidence suggesting that ballistic stretching significantly increases tendon elasticity and therefore, might be helpful for both preventing and treating tendon injuries (Mahieu et al 2007, Witvrouw et al 2007). Indeed ballistic stretching may well regain its place in the sun as new fascial research suggests that elastic type bouncing movements are important to build the 'silken fascial bodysuit' needed to prevent injuries to the connective

tissue. The fast, dynamic stretches included in the fascial fitness suggestions of Schleip and Müller (2013) are modified forms of ballistic stretching.

Active stretching

This type of stretching involves the client actively moving their limb through a full ROM to the end range and repeating the cycle several times. Examples of active stretching include:

- **Dynamic stretching:** a dynamic standing stretch of the hamstring involves swinging the leg back and forth to the end of the range. **See Figure 10.3**
- **Active isolated stretching:** this involves several repetitions of a movement to the end of the range followed by assistance into a short stretch either by a therapist or the client using a rope or belt. **See Figure 10.4**

It is easy to get confused between ballistic stretching (boo, hiss, bad for you) and active stretching (yay, great for you) as they both seem a bit 'bouncy'. The big difference is that in active stretching techniques you are taking the limb or body part through a full ROM each time whereas ballistic stretching involves bouncing up and down on a fully stretched muscle. If ballistic stretching is 'bouncy' then active stretching could be considered more 'swingy'. Yes, I know, highly technical language, but do keep up.

3. Pre-contraction stretches

This involves a contraction of the muscle being stretched or its agonist before stretching. PNF stretching and MET (muscle energy technique) both fall into this category. By some mysterious unknown mechanism (more on this later) these types of stretches seem to 'trick' the body into a greater stretch and are fantastic for increasing ROM, especially in the short term.

'Newer' forms of stretching are usually variations on one of the above themes. Two of our favourite new ways of working with stretching include therapeutic and myofascial stretching.

4. Therapeutic stretching

Developed by osteopath Eyal Lederman (2013), this form of stretching emphasises the functional requirements of the desired ROM increase and is based on the scientific principles of training. Lederman contends that stretching exercises used in the clinic should approximate the desired functional tasks for

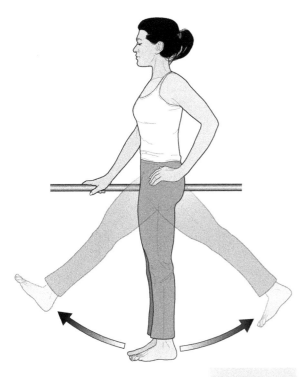

Figure 10.3

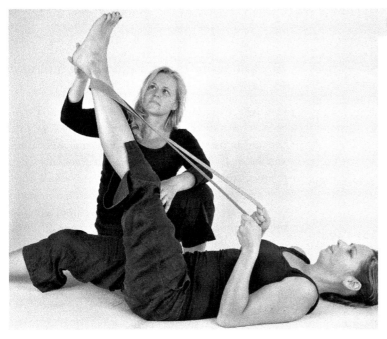

Figure 10.4

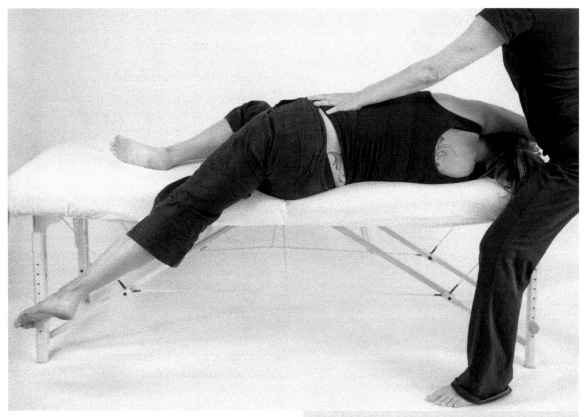

Figure 10.5
Myofascial stretching

the client and emphasises the maximal part that must be played by the client in their own self care. Lederman provides extensive academic support to back up his theories that happily all boil down to common sense principles.

5. Myofascial stretching

The fascial fitness work of Robert Schleip and Divo Müller (2013) uses two approaches:

- Fast dynamic stretching very similar to old style ballistic stretching (but carried out with a ninja type presence and focus).

- Long slow stretches that attempt to engage long fascial continuities. John Barnes also teaches long slow fascial stretching with stretches held for a minimum of 90–120 seconds. **See Figure 10.5.**

Stretching in treatment and stretching for self care

How effective is the stretching that we carry out as part of our massage treatment sessions? Is this enough by itself to create change, stimulate healing and increase ROM? After all we are generally only seeing clients once a week. The evidence would suggest that including stretching as part of a treatment is only a small part of the story. In order to maximally improve and sustain ROM increases, stretching will be most effective if part of a client's regular self-care regime. The Self-Care Resources (available at **uk.singingdragon.com/catalogue/ book/9781909141230**) show some stretches that can be carried out at home. Recommending a good yoga class will probably do the job just as well.

When prescribing stretching exercises for clients bear in mind the principles of teaching self-care exercises that are outlined in Chapter 11. Therapists often woefully shake their heads and get cross at clients who 'don't do their exercises'. We KNOW that if clients just looked after themselves and did what we told them to do for the rest of the week then they wouldn't undo our hard work. However, a moment of self-reflection will usually reveal that all our clients are doing is being just like us, i.e. finding the time, energy and motivation to do 'what's good for us' can be incredibly difficult in our fast paced overworked society.

Your job as a therapist is to find what will help your client to feel motivated to carry out any self-care exercises including stretching. As a general rule this will mean stretches that require:

- No equipment

- Are simple to carry out

- Can be performed anywhere.

Eyal Lederman (2013) suggests a graded return to functional activities is the most effective way of increasing functional ROM rather than prescribed 'exercises'. For example, if your client wants to play tennis again then they should play tennis. At the beginning this might be just a few minutes a day against a wall and then gradually increasing the different parameters of time, force, etc. In contrast, if the client wants to increase ROM so they can reach the top shelf, after an adhesive capsulitis problem, then they should practise reaching their shelves. So perhaps start by suggesting that the client rearranges items on a lower shelf, then onto the next highest shelf and so on. This approach emphasises creativity on the part of the therapist in designing functional stretching tasks that will most benefit the client as they are in alignment with their primary goals. Once you have grasped the principles, the possibilities are endless.

Principles for of all stretching methods

All stretching methods rely on increasing the distance between the attachment points of the muscle. Chapters 12–19 show specific stretches for different body parts but these all rely on the same principles:

- **Good body mechanics:** position the client (and yourself) so that you can comfortably stretch the muscle. Choose the direction of movement that will most effectively take the two attachment points further apart. This requires thinking in three-dimensions and knowing your anatomy. Visualise the location of the muscle underneath your hands as you work.

- **Good communication with the client:** it is important that you talk the client through what is going to happen to ensure their understanding and co-operation with the technique. If someone is in pain, stretching can bring up feelings of fear so it is important they understand that they remain in control and you will be working in co-operation with them. Give good clear instructions about what is going to happen and what the client needs to do at each stage.

- **Be aware of the language you use for instruction:** if you are stretching the muscle passively (as in static stretching and the first part of PNF/MET) you need your client to give you the full weight of their limb or body part. For some clients this can be really difficult. We find it is best to avoid the word 'relax' as this tends to make clients tense up even further (there is nothing guaranteed to make you feel more rigid than having a therapist bellow 'RELAX' at you accompanied by some admonishing semi-slap on the offending body part). If a client is keeping control of their limb they probably do not understand the felt body sense of what it means to fully 'let go'. This can be particularly true with vulnerable body parts such as the head. Instead give instructions such as 'I want you to make your head really heavy for me.' Monitor with your sense of listening touch whether your client is actually doing this and give them appropriate reinforcement, e.g. 'That's great' or 'That's much better, well done … now give me a little bit more weight.'

- For static stretching and PNF/MET you also need to get your client to signal when they feel the stretch. It's best to agree on a non-verbal signal such as raising the hand or wiggling the fingers, particularly if the client is in a prone position (as face cradle mumbling is guaranteed to raise the blood pressure of both therapist and client). Again watch your language and don't say

'Tell me when you have reached your limit.' Some clients will psychologically feel they don't want to have reached their limit and will endure a painful stretch beyond their natural end ROM, which could be injurious to the tissues. Instead say 'Tell me when you feel the stretch.'

- With AIS the verbal communication has a different style as the client tendency here is to become lazy and let you do the work. So the communication works better if it is more in the 'personal trainer' style, e.g. 'Come on now just a little bit further, you can do it, that's great, just a few more reps, you're doing really well.'

- **Working with the breath:** depending on the type of stretching it is usually helpful to give specific instructions for breathing (usually inhaling just before the stretch and exhaling on the stretch itself).

- **Working with listening touch**: you should always be monitoring the tissues with your sense of listening touch. Watch out for something called 'end feel' which is the end of the ROM for the client. Being sensitive with your hands can help you establish whether the client is giving you the full weight of their limb, can go a little bit further into the stretch or needs to back off a little bit as they are straining and in pain (and are reluctant to admit it!).

Different stretching methods in detail

Building on this broad overview of stretching, let's take a look at the different techniques and how they can be used during a treatment.

Static stretching

Understanding the positioning for static stretching gives you a basis for all the other methods. All of the practical chapters (see Chapters 12–19) show static stretches for particular areas of the body. These could also be easily adapted to become PNF/MET or active isolated stretches, so feel free to be creative.

Static stretching is fairly straightforward if you know your anatomy. Essentially you are just increasing the distance between two attachment points. Make sure you use good communication skills as outlined below:

- Before you take your client into the stretch, talk your client through what is going to happen, e.g. 'I am now going to stretch your hamstring muscles on the back of your leg. You can let me do the work and you don't need to help; just let me take the weight of your leg when I lift it. So when I say the word, you are going to breathe in and then breathe out as I take you into the stretch. Let me know when you feel the stretch by wiggling the fingers on your right hand. I will then be holding the position for about 30 seconds; during this time you can just breathe naturally.'

- Instruct the client to inhale as you get into a good position and take the weight of their leg in your hands.

- As your client starts to exhale take their hamstrings into a stretch by raising their straight leg, supporting it with your body weight as necessary. Take the movement slowly until you sense the 'end feel' and the client communicates that they feel the stretch. Remember to use language like 'Tell me when you feel the stretch' rather than 'Tell me when you have reached your limit.'

- Hold for 10–30 seconds and then take the stretch a little bit further if possible, working with client communication and your sense of listening touch. Most experts feel that holding a stretch for between 10–30 seconds is enough to increase flexibility (Page 2012). A static stretch held long enough (90–120 seconds) then becomes more of a myofascial stretch which can be a wonderful way of releasing long held fascial restrictions.

Pre-contraction stretching
Are you on CRAC? Different types of pre-contraction stretching

There is a great expression that the Thai people love to say to tourists: 'Same same but different' (as in the question 'Is this a real Rolex?' and the answer 'Yes sir, same same but different'). The phrase could well apply to the many different variations of PNF stretching. The bewildering list of PNF techniques includes: contract relax (CR), hold-relax (H-R), facilitated stretching, contract-relax agonist contract (CRAC), post-isometric relaxation (PIR), post-facilitation stretch (PFS) and MET. All are similar in that they use an increase in contraction of the target muscle (or in some cases the agonist) before the stretch to cause an immediately recognisable increase in ROM. They differ in factors such as how much effort is used by the client when performing the contraction (ranging from 10–100% of client effort), type of contraction used, the recommendation for when the contraction is performed (end range of muscle, close to end range or even mid-range) or whether the body part is taken into the stretch passively (traditional PNF and MET) or actively (facilitated stretching).

It is easy to get caught up in the intricacies of the different techniques in our quest to find the best and most effective method for achieving an outcome. However, it is worthwhile knowing that there is no evidence to suggest that one form of PNF stretching is superior to another. Factors such as how much effort is used or for how many seconds the stretch is held are unlikely to make a significant difference in achieving a result for your client.

The significant part seems to be the neurological 'trick' that PNF, MET and other forms of pre-contraction stretching rely on to increase ROM, i.e. if the target muscle is contracted it seems that it can then be stretched further immediately afterwards. The increase in ROM is immediately obvious to both therapist and client, which makes it a favourite in the clinic. There are few sweeter moments than having a client come in unable to turn their head and sending them out with a full ROM courtesy of some PNF trickery.

How does pre-contraction (PNF and MET) stretching work?

Short answer: we don't know. The traditional explanation was that it was due to a neurological effect known as 'autogenic inhibition', which is a short refractory period after contraction (PIR) where the muscle relaxes, thus increasing its length and the ability to be stretched further. However, electromyogram (EMG) studies have shown that this is not actually what is going on. Fascinatingly, activation in the muscle remains the same or increases after contraction rather than being silent as this theory suggested (Mitchell et al 2009, Page 2012). Again it seems that the increase in ROM may be due

to an increase in stretch tolerance as the application of MET or PNF decreases an individual's perception of muscle pain (Fryer 2011, Mitchell et al 2007). In a great party trick, Markos (1979) showed that a PNF stretch on one limb causes a similar increase on the other limb. This finding supports the feasibility of a neurological mechanism.

Treatment principles for using PNF aka MET

Any of the static stretches shown in Chapters 12–19 can be adapted to become PNF stretches by using the following steps (**Figure 10.6A–C**):

- The first stage is to take the muscle into a lengthened position, just below the 'end feel'. Use the steps described for static stretching above to take the muscle to the point just where the client starts to feel the stretch. In traditional PNF this is done passively although it is also possible to get the client to do this actively. Remember to work with client communication and the breath.

- Once the muscle is on a slight stretch, give the client a clear instruction as to how they are to now perform an isometric contraction for approximately 4–6 seconds. This usually involves telling the client to push against you or resist you in some way. In our example of the hamstrings the instruction given is 'Push against me as if you are trying to put your heel on the table. Use 20% of your strength.'

- The stretching muscle is then allowed to relax for 2 seconds and then extended further passively (with the aid of the therapist) and held in this new position for approximately 5 seconds. Staying at this muscle extension the whole process is repeated again. At least four repetitions are recommended to attain the maximum increase in ROM (Mitchell et al 2007).

Active isolated stretching (AIS; the Mattes' method)

As a practitioner you will find that you often favour one stretching technique more than another. Meg adores PNF whereas I (Rachel) am a big fan of AIS. I have found AIS to be an effective method for increasing

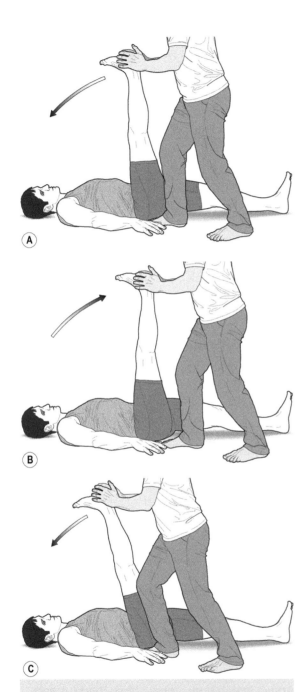

Figure 10.6A–C
Steps in PNF stretching: (A) passive stretch to ROM barrier; (B) contract against resistance for 4–6 seconds; (C) relax and repeat passive stretch to new ROM barrier

flexibility and decreasing pain, both personally and professionally. It seems, in this respect, I am in distinguished company as prominent massage therapist, teacher and author Dr Ben Benjamin (Benjamin and Haggquist 2009) described discovering AIS as the 'second major turning point of my career' and declared 'I've seen results in myself that I never thought possible.' Praise indeed from a practitioner with decades of experience in treating soft tissue injury.

AIS was developed by, massage therapist and kinesiologist, Aaron Mattes (1995) as a result of decades of research and clinical experience with thousands of clients, including Olympic champions and professional, college and high school athletes. AIS uses active movement and the theory of reciprocal inhibition to achieve greater flexibility. The amazing thing about AIS is that it combines three great physical benefits in one technique, namely:

1 **Strengthening:** as active repetitive movements are used in the stretch, this enables strengthening of the muscles that initiate the movements.

2 **Stretching:** at the same time as one set of muscles is being strengthened, the opposite muscles are being very precisely stretched.

3 **Cardiac workout:** as active movements are used, the client also enjoys the benefits of cardiac exercise.

The stretch reflex

One of the reasons that other forms of stretching can feel painful is that all muscles have an inherent 'stretch reflex' that is activated after 2 seconds in a stretched position. The stretch reflex causes the muscles to begin a slow contraction – which is the body's way of trying to protect itself from overstretching. If you continue stretching while your muscle is trying to contract it is like a tug of war – and in many cases a tug of war that can even lead to muscle damage. This is why static stretching can feel so difficult sometimes as you need to use your breath and an immense amount of patience to overcome the natural inclination of the stretch reflex (**Figure 10.7**).

One of the factors that differentiates AIS from other forms of stretching is that the stretch is only held for a maximum of 2 seconds. This means that there is no

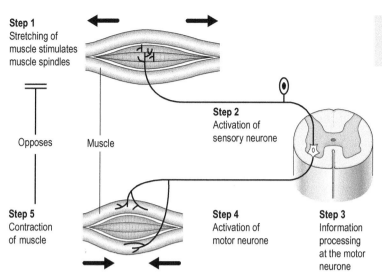

Step 1
Stretching of muscle stimulates muscle spindles

Figure 10.7
The stretch reflex

Step 2
Activation of sensory neurone

Opposes   Muscle

Step 5
Contraction of muscle

Step 4
Activation of motor neurone

Step 3
Information processing at the motor neurone

opportunity for the stretch reflex to kick in, meaning less patience and body awareness is needed to stretch the tissues and there is less possibility of damage.

Treatment principles for using AIS

All AIS follow the basic steps below:

1 Isolate the muscle to be stretched.

2 The client actively contracts the muscle opposite the target muscle (e.g. if stretching the hamstrings, contract the quadriceps).

3 The client actively lengthens the muscle to its maximum stretch, exhaling on the stretch.

4 The stretch is then taken slightly further by assistance from either a therapist or an aid such as a rope or the client's own hand. Hold the stretch for a maximum of 1.5–2 seconds then return the limb to the starting position.

5 Repeat the process 8–10 times, and 2–3 sets of 10 repetitions are usually used with alteration of limbs after each set.

AIS can be deeply satisfying as both client and therapist can see instant increases in ROM with each repetition (see **Figure 10.8**).

Tips for good AIS technique

- **Role of the assistant:** the role of the therapist is an important one as with AIS you are more of a coach

to enable the client to precisely carry out the technique rather than doing it for them (as with a passive stretch). Make sure you are encouraging the client to carry out the movement actively. It is very common for clients to get lazy and the therapist to start lifting the body part into the stretch by default. The touch you use as a therapist is for guidance only, e.g. with the hamstring stretch you are NOT lifting the leg and your touch should simply help guide the client into the right position, the client should be doing all the work. If there is serious neurological damage or the antagonist is too weak to carry out the movement you may need to use more assistance.

- **Make sure you are assisting the stretch fully:** make sure as the therapist you are taking the stretch a little further at the end of the client's active ROM. Although the stretch is short, you should be taking the stretch further than the client is able to do so on their own, whilst ensuring you are not over stretching. Also check you are holding for the full 1.5–2 seconds.

- **Good communication:** use encouraging verbal communication to keep your client going so that they are achieving maximal stretch each time.

- **Use stretches in the clinic that you will teach for self care:** Mattes recommends AIS as part of a daily routine to achieve gains in flexibility and research on stretching would back this up. It is helpful for client learning to use the same stretches as part of treatment that you are going to teach them for home use.

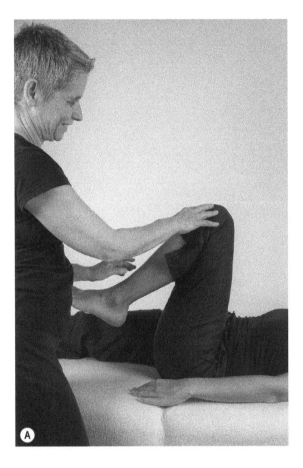

- **Draping:** the positioning and repetitive movement of AIS makes it a bit of a nightmare if you are trying to fiddle around with draping at the same time. I would generally recommend asking the client to bring something they can stretch in. Do 35–45 minutes of hands-on treatment and then let them get changed into their sporting clothes for the stretching part of the treatment.

Fascial stretching

Recent knowledge about the role of fascia has also affected traditional notions of how stretching may work. This has both given new insights into traditional forms of stretching, such as yoga, and has also led to the development of new fascially based approaches.

Crucially, traditional forms of stretching are based on the 'single unit muscle' idea where muscles are stretched by lengthening the distance between attachment points, with the notion that the neighbouring muscles are unaffected. However, our new fascial anatomy clearly shows how muscles, fascia, tendons and ligaments are linked in series rather than units that can be treated in isolation. The idea of simply being able to 'stretch a hamstring' has been shown to be a nonsense

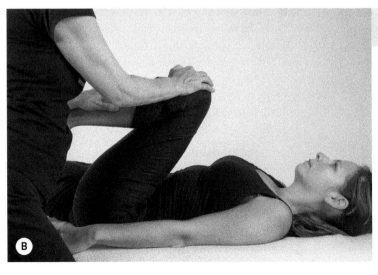

Figure 10.8A,B

with the extraordinary finding that a simple straight leg raise, aimed at stretching the hamstrings, produces 2.5 times as much stretch in the iliotibial (IT) band and an equal amount of stretch in the same side lumbar fascia (Franklyn-Miller et al 2009).

Myers and Frederick (2013) outline four potential benefits of fascial stretching:

1 Mechanical lengthening of myofascial chains

2 Tissue hydration

3 Proprioceptive stimulation

4 Direct stimulation of connective tissue cells, in particular fibroblasts.

Mechanical lengthening

Studies have shown that it is highly unlikely that fascia actually lengthens during stretching or other manual therapy procedures (Chaudhry et al 2008), although to the practitioner the wonderful gooey sensation of 'release' can really feel like lengthening. A more likely explanation for this apparent feeling of myofascial lengthening is the wholesale muscular relaxation that occurs via neurological feedback when fascial techniques including stretching are applied (Schleip 2003a,b).

One important result of fascial technique and stretching is the release of fascial layers that have literally become stuck together. Layers in the body are meant to slide smoothly over each other, yet dysfunction can arise due to the loss of serous lubrication between layers and the establishment of cross linkages that restrict movement and cause pain. Fascial stretching techniques literally unstick these layers, thus helping to reduce pain and restore ROM.

Tissue hydration

Fascial stretching can be helpful for the hydrostatic balance of tissues, reducing oedema and increasing water content to dehydrated tissues. Schleip et al (2012) showed that fascial stretching can work like a sponge. Stretching initially reduces the water content of the tissues but after rest the water content of ground substance substantially increases, surpassing the original levels and literally pumping the tissues with extra fluid. Stretching also reduces oedema.

Proprioceptive stimulation

There are 10 times as many receptor endings in the extracellular matrix (ECM) as in the muscle itself so it is likely that the effects of stretching are mediated via these nerve endings in the fascia.

Direct stimulation of connective tissue cells

It is possible that the effects of stretching are transmitted right through to the level of the cell. Standley et al (2010) took a human fibroblast cell and subjected it to 8 hours of simulated repetitive strain. Subsequently, he found that 90 seconds of stimulated myofascial stretch reduced the experimentally induced cell death caused by the repetitive strain.

New forms of fascial stretching

There are some newer forms of stretching that are principally directed to releasing the fascia.

These include:

- Myofascial stretching (as taught by John F. Barnes)

- Fascial stretch therapy (FST) (Frederick et al 2014)

- Fascial fitness (Schleip and Müller 2013).

Myofascial stretching

This uses the principles of myofascial release as developed by John F. Barnes. There are four ways in which myofascial stretching differs from normal stretching (Stedronsky Morton and Pardy 2006):

1 **Time element:** all stretches are held for a MINIMUM of 90–120 seconds to ensure full release of fascial restrictions.

2 **Active elongation:** the client actively elongates the tissues through reaching and telescoping movements until resistance is felt to the stretch. This is known as the 'fascial barrier' and is similar to the sensation felt during indirect myofascial techniques, such as cross hand stretch. The stretch is then held until a release is felt (sensation of melting and lengthening) and is then actively elongated to the next barrier until another release is felt, and so on.

3 **Mindfulness:** it is important for the client to be consciously present throughout the process, using the breath and a grounded and centred attitude to tune into the tissues and the feeling of stretch and release.

4 **Stretching and strengthening occur simultaneously:** the sustained stretching methods used cause simultaneous isometric contraction of other muscles.

Fascial stretch therapy (FST)

Developed by Anne and Chris Fredericks, FST combines joint distraction and long fascial stretches.

Fascial fitness

The fascial fitness routines developed by Müller and Schleip use both slow and dynamic stretching to build the resilience of the body-wide fascial net (Schleip and Müller 2013). This helps prevent many sports associated overload injuries (e.g. tendon injuries) that are more issues of the connective tissue than the musculoskeletal system. Müller and Schleip believe that the routines should be practised 1–2 times a week to build a 'resilient fascial bodysuit' over time (the process can take 6–24 months). Two types of stretching are employed. The first type is fast dynamic stretching which is similar to old style ballistic stretching but with an emphasis on smooth 'ninja' movements and preparatory counter movements, e.g. to stretch the hamstrings, the hip is taken into a brief extension first. The second type of fascial stretching uses slow dynamic stretches with multi-directional movements with slight changes of angle. This aims to involve the longest possible myofascial chains in the stretch.

Re-inventing the wheel? Traditional forms of fascial stretching

It is worth noting that many of the new forms of fascial stretching are variations of methods that have been around for centuries. The oldest form of stretching in the book – yoga – uses long sustained whole body stretches that affect whole body myofascial trains rather than single muscle groups. For example, downward dog is a fantastic stretch for the superficial back line (**Figure 10.9**).

Makko Ho stretches carried out as a self-healing adjunct to shiatsu focus on balancing the meridians;

in doing so they also stretch body wide fascial trains (**Figure 10.10A–C**). The gentle stretches of t'ai chi and qi gong also use many of the ninja type principles and preparatory counter movements advocated by the fascial fitness proponents.

Using stretching in treatment: insights from research

Stretching is a great tool for improving many different conditions seen in the massage therapist's clinic and has traditionally been advocated for use with chronic musculoskeletal conditions such as back pain, neck and shoulder conditions, adhesive capsulitis (frozen shoulder), muscle strains, osteoarthritis, tendinosis, muscle contractures and shortened muscles from neurological conditions such as spasticity. Self stretches are recommended for the prevention and treatment of both work related and athletics injuries. Stretching is also a popular technique in pre-event sports massage to help prepare athletes for an event.

However, not all these applications for stretching have the weight of evidence behind them. Here are some insights from research which will help determine what kind of stretching may be best for certain conditions:

- **Strains:** studies on using stretching for rehabilitation from hamstring strains have had positive results. Malliaropoulos et al (2004) found that young Greek athletes with second degree hamstring strains recovered much more quickly when using an intensive stretching programme as compared to a less intensive stretching routine. Another study found that

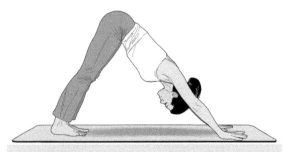

Figure 10.9
Downward dog is a fantastic stretch for the superficial back line

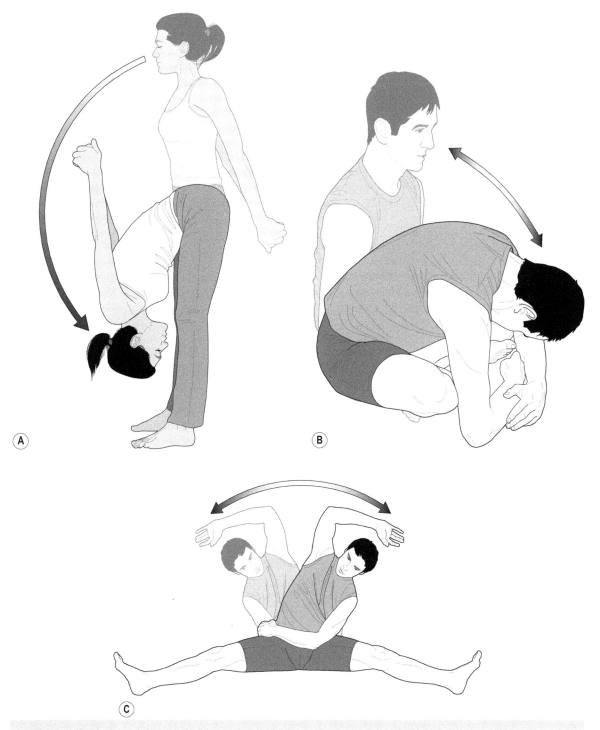

Figure 10.10A–C
Makkho stretches focus on balancing the meridians and also stretch body wide fascial trains

hamstring flexibility following a strain was more improved by using static stretching rather than dynamic stretching (O'Sullivan et al 2009).

- **Osteoarthritis:** stretching has been shown to be an effective strategy for improving function for patients with osteoarthritis (Weng et al 2009).

- **Post-surgery:** static, dynamic and PNF stretching all caused a significant increase in ROM for patients with total knee replacements, with no differences between the type of stretching used (Chow and Ng 2010).

- **Prevention of work related injury:** a review by Da Costa and Vieira (2008) found that stretching could be effective in preventing work related musculoskeletal disorders (although the quality of the studies reviewed was low). There are reports of beneficial effects from stretching programmes for computer, manufacturing and heavy workers, such as fire fighting and military recruits.

- **Prevention and treatment of contractures:** stretching is often advocated for the prevention and treatment of muscle contractures, i.e. a permanent shortening of a muscle or joint as seen in cerebral palsy or other neurological conditions. However, a large review of the evidence found that although there were some findings supporting the positive effects of a stretching session these seemed to be temporary (Bovend'Eerdt et al 2008). Katalinic et al (2010, 2011) concluded 'Regular stretch does not produce clinically important changes in joint mobility, pain, spasticity, or activity limitation in people with neurological conditions.'

- **Chronic neck pain:** 12 months of stretching is as effective as strengthening or manual therapy for clients with chronic neck pain (Hakkinen et al 2008).

- **Fibromyalgia (FM):** several studies have shown that exercise routines that include stretching are effective in helping with the symptoms of FM syndrome (Jones et al 2002, Rooks et al 2007). One study (Matsutani et al 2012) found that

stretching exercises are more effective than aerobic exercises for treating pain, number of tender points, poor sleep and depression in FM. On the other hand, the aerobic exercises seem to produce a more important effect on anxiety reduction compared to stretching exercises.

Recommendations for using stretching in treatment

- Stretching in treatment will only achieve limited results and clients should be taught self-stretching routines to supplement treatment. Stretching as part of a regular routine will be more effective both for treatment of pain and prevention of injury for athletes.

- In general, there are few differences in outcome between different methods of stretching. Type of stretching used should be chosen with outcome and individual client differences in mind.

- Stretching will be more effective if combined in the treatment after heat, fascial work and trigger point work as laid out in the HFMAST protocol.

- For pre-event massage, stretching should not be carried out immediately prior to performance especially for sports requiring a lot of jumping or explosive power. However, carrying out stretching prior to other warm-up activities should not adversely affect performance and may help to reduce musculotendinous injuries. Active stretching methods such as dynamic stretching or AIS are likely to be more effective for pre-event massage.

References

Behm DG, Chaouachi A 2011 A review of the acute effects of static and dynamic stretching on performance. European Journal of Applied Physiology 111(11):2633–2651.

Benjamin B, Haggquist J 2009 Active isolated stretching: the mattes method, part I. Massage Therapy: Everybody Deserves a Massage. Available at: http://www.massagetherapy.com/articles/index.php/article_id/1821/Active-Isolated-Stretching:-The-Mattes-Method-Part-I [accessed 19 August 2014].

Bovend'Eerdt TJ et al 2008 The effects of stretching in spasticity: a systematic review. Archives of Physical Medicine and Rehabilitation 89(7):1395–1406.

Chaudhry H et al 2008 Three-dimensional mathematical model for deformation of human fasciae in manual therapy. The Journal of the American Osteopathic Association 108:379–390.

Chow TPY, Ng GYF 2010 Active, passive and proprioceptive neuromuscular facilitation stretching are comparable in improving the knee flexion range in people with total knee replacement: a randomized controlled trial. Clinical Rehabilitation 24(10):911–918.

Da Costa BR, Vieira ER 2008 Stretching to reduce work-related musculoskeletal disorders: a systematic review. Journal of Rehabilitation Medicine: Official Journal of the UEMS European Board of Physical and Rehabilitation Medicine 40(5):321–328.

Decoster LC et al 2005 The effects of hamstring stretching on range of motion: a systematic literature review. The Journal of Orthopaedic and Sports Physical Therapy 35(6):377–387.

Fradkin AJ, Gabbe BJ, Cameron PA 2006 Does warming up prevent injury in sport? The evidence from randomised controlled trials? Journal of Science and Medicine in Sport 9(3):214–20.

Franklyn-Miller A et al 2009 The strain patterns of the deep fascia of the lower limb. Fascial Research II: Basic Science and Implications for Conventional and Complementary Health Care. Munich: Elsevier GmbH.

Frederick A, Frederick C, Myers T 2014 Fascial Stretch Therapy, 1st edn. Pencaitland, UK: Handspring Publishing.

Fryer G 2011 Muscle energy technique: an evidence-informed approach. International Journal of Osteopathic Medicine 14(1):3–9.

Hakkinen A et al 2008 Strength training and stretching versus stretching only in the treatment of patients with chronic neck pain: a randomized one-year follow-up study. Clinical Rehabilitation 22:592–600.

Hart L 2005 Effect of stretching on sport injury risk: a review. Clinical Journal of Sport Medicine: Official Journal of the Canadian Academy of Sport Medicine 15(2):113.

Herbert RD, de Noronha M, Kamper SJ 2011 Stretching to prevent or reduce muscle soreness after exercise. The Cochrane Database of Systematic Reviews (7):CD004577

Ingraham P (n.d.) Save yourself from aches, pains & injuries. SaveYourself.ca. Available at: http://saveyourself.ca [accessed 18 August 2014].

Jones KD et al 2002 A randomized controlled trial of muscle strengthening versus flexibility training in fibromyalgia. The Journal of Rheumatology 29(5):1041–1048.

Katalinic OM et al 2010 Stretch for the treatment and prevention of contractures. The Cochrane Database of Systematic Reviews 9:CD007455.

Katalinic OM, Harvey LA, Herbert RD 2011 Effectiveness of stretch for the treatment and prevention of contractures in people with neurological conditions: a systematic review. Physical Therapy 91(1):11–24.

Kay AD, Blazevich AJ 2012 Effect of acute static stretch on maximal muscle performance: a systematic review. Medicine and Science in Sports and Exercise 44(1):154–164.

Lederman E 2013 Therapeutic Stretching: towards a Functional Approach, 1st edn. London: Churchill Livingstone.

McHugh MP, Cosgrave CH 2010 To stretch or not to stretch: the role of stretching in injury prevention and performance. Scandinavian Journal of Medicine & Science in Sports 20:169–181.

Mahieu NN et al 2007 Effect of static and ballistic stretching on the muscle-tendon tissue properties. Medicine and Science in Sports and Exercise 39(3):494–501.

Malliaropoulos N et al 2004 The role of stretching in rehabilitation of hamstring injuries: 80 athletes follow-up. Medicine and Science in Sports and Exercise 36:756–759.

Markos PD 1979 Ipsilateral and contralateral effects of proprioceptive neuromuscular facilitation techniques on hip motion and electromyographic activity. Physical Therapy 59(11):1366–1373.

Matsutani LA, Assumpção A, Marques AP 2012 Stretching and aerobic exercises in the treatment of fibromyalgia: pilot study [Portuguese]. Fisioterapia em Movimento 25:411–418.

Mattes A 1995 Active isolated stretching. Sarasota, FL: Mattes.

Mitchell UH et al 2007 Acute stretch perception alteration contributes to the success of the PNF "contract-relax" stretch. Journal of Sport Rehabilitation 16:85–92.

Mitchell UH et al 2009 Neurophysiological reflex mechanisms' lack of contribution to the success of PNF stretches. Journal of Sport Rehabilitation 18:343–357.

Montero-Marín J et al 2013 Effectiveness of a stretching program on anxiety levels of workers in a logistic platform: A randomized controlled study. Atencion Primaria/ Sociedad Española de Medicina de Familia y Comunitaria 45(7):376–383.

Myers T, Frederick C 2013 Stretching and fascia. In: Schleip R, Findley T, Chaitow L, Huijing P (eds) Fascia, 1st edn. London: Elsevier Health Sciences, pp. 434–435.

Orthoinfo.aaos.org 2014 Warm up, cool down and be flexible – OrthoInfo. AAOS. Available at: http://orthoinfo.aaos.org/topic.cfm?topic=A00310 [accessed 18 August 2014].

O'Sullivan K, Murray E, Sainsbury D 2009 The effect of warm-up, static stretching and dynamic stretching on hamstring flexibility in previously injured subjects. BMC Musculoskeletal Disorders 10:37.

Page P 2012 Current concepts in muscle stretching for exercise and rehabilitation. International Journal of Sports Physical Therapy 7(1):109–119.

Panesar N, Valachova I 2011 Yoga and mental health. Australian and New Zealand Journal of Psychiatry 45:A64–A65.

Posadzki P et al 2011 Is yoga effective for pain? A systematic review of randomized clinical trials. Complementary Therapies in Medicine 19(5):281–287.

Rooks DS et al 2007 Group exercise, education, and combination self-management in women with fibromyalgia: a randomized trial. Archives of Internal Medicine 167:2192–2200.

Schleip R 2003a Fascial plasticity – A new neurobiological explanation, part 1. Journal of Bodywork and Movement Therapies 7:11–19.

Schleip R 2003b Fascial plasticity – A new neurobiological explanation, part 2. Journal of Bodywork and Movement Therapies 7(2):104–116.

Schleip R, Duerselen L, Vleeming A 2012 Strain hardening of fascia: static stretching of dense fibrous connective tissues can induce a temporary stiffness increase accompanied by enhanced matrix hydration. Journal of Bodywork and Movement Therapies 16(1): 94–100.

Schleip R, Müller DG 2013 Training principles for fascial connective tissues: scientific foundation and suggested practical applications. Journal of Bodywork and Movement Therapies 17(1):103–115.

Sherman KJ et al 2011 A randomized trial comparing yoga, stretching, and a self-care book for chronic low back pain. Archives of Internal Medicine. Malden, Mass: BMJ Books/Blackwell Pub, pp. 171(22):2019–2026.

Shrier I 2004 Does stretching improve performance? Clinical Journal of Sport Medicine 14(5):267–273.

Shrier I 2007 Does stretching help prevent injuries? In: MacAuley D, Best T, eds. Evidence Based Sports Medicine Malden, Mass: BMJ Books/Blackwell, pp. 97–116.

Simic L, Sarabon N, Markovic G 2013 Does pre-exercise static stretching inhibit maximal muscular performance? A meta-analytical review. Scandinavian Journal of Medicine & Science in Sports 23(2):131–148.

Small K, Mc Naughton L, Matthews M 2008 A systematic review into the efficacy of static stretching as part of a warm-up for the prevention of exercise-related injury. Research in Sports Medicine (Print) 16(3):213–231.

Standley PR et al 2010 In vitro modeling of repetitive motion injury and myofascial release. Journal of Bodywork & Movement Therapies 14(2):162–171.

Stedronsky Morton J, Pardy B 2006 Myofascial Stretching: A Guide to Self Treatment. Aardvark Global Publishing, LLC.

Taylor KL et al 2009 Negative effect of static stretching restored when combined with a sport specific warm-up component. Journal of Science and Medicine in Sport 12:657–661.

Thacker SB et al 2004 The impact of stretching on sports injury risk: a systematic review of the literature. Medicine and Science in Sports and Exercise 36(3):371–378.

Weng M-C et al 2009 Effects of different stretching techniques on the outcomes of isokinetic exercise in patients with knee osteoarthritis. The Kaohsiung Journal of Medical Sciences 25(6):306–315.

Weppler CH, Magnusson SP 2010 Increasing muscle extensibility: a matter of increasing length or modifying sensation? Physical Therapy 90(3):438–449.

Witvrouw E et al 2004 Stretching and injury prevention: an obscure relationship. Sports Medicine (Auckland, NZ) 34:443–449.

Witvrouw E et al 2007 The role of stretching in tendon injuries. British Journal of Sports Medicine 41(4): 224–226.

Woods K, Bishop P, Jones E 2007 Warm-up and stretching in the prevention of muscular injury. Sports Medicine (Auckland, NZ) 37(12):1089–1099.

The importance of teaching self care

The perfect man of old looked after himself before looking to help others.
Chuang Tzu
There's only one corner of the Universe you can be certain of improving and that's your own self.
Aldous Huxley

The final part of the Jing HFMAST protocol is T for teaching self-care suggestions. An emphasis on self care has always been at the heart of the complementary therapy approach. Long before the coining of the term 'biopsychosocial', complementary therapists had a core belief in holism – which is defined by the dictionary as 'The treating of the whole person, taking into account mental and social factors, rather than just the physical symptoms of a disease.' In the holistic approach, health is directly related to constitutional balance; hence, pain and disease can result from an excess or deficiency of a variety of factors including:

- Emotions

- Lack of rest

- Trauma (physical and emotional)

- Emotional stress

- Poor exercise

- Boredom and purposelessness (Sohn and Sohn 1996).

With the holistic approach, clients are seen as active agents in their path towards healing with the practitioner role being that of a facilitator towards this aim, where client and therapist work as an alliance towards mutual goals. As such it is common for therapists to give clients self-care suggestions including dietary advice, recommendations for exercise, better sleep, relaxation and meditation. For example, traditional Chinese medicine has always promoted a self-care aspect to recovery with dietary changes and t'ai chi/qi gong exercises being seen as fundamental to healing.

This paradigm contrasts with the orthodox biomedical view of medicine that became popular in the 20th century. Here the doctor is seen as 'expert', and the patient is a passive recipient of medical interventions such as medicine or surgery. Diagnoses are couched in jargon that is difficult to understand and any self-care advice is glossed over, minimised or relegated to the level of self-help booklets. The result is that the client is left feeling disempowered, out of control and helpless in the face of disabling pain. Unfortunately even some alternative health practitioners have unwittingly replicated this top-down ethos. For example, bodywork approaches that place a lot of emphasis on structural abnormality as the root of pain can leave the client once more in a position of being reliant on the 'expert'. Clients are bamboozled by practitioner's assessments of shifty pelvises, unequal leg lengths and scoliotic spines – and all they can do is be reliant on the manual therapist to put the errant structures 'back in' place. Thus, yet again we have a disempowered client reliant on the expert, white-coated therapist.

However, more recent research emphasises the need for a shift in traditional medical thinking away from this dynamic and towards a self-management and self-care approach. A UK report evaluating hundreds of research studies found that a self-management approach to persistent musculoskeletal pain can improve people's quality of life, pain levels and the way they use health care resources (De Silva 2011). Recent programmes in the UK emphasising a proactive self-management approach for chronic conditions including musculoskeletal pain and arthritis have had positive results, with participants reporting improvements in pain symptoms, confidence to manage their pain, health status, anxiety and depression (Bourne 2012).

Massage and self care

Including self-care suggestions and education into your massage sessions can improve outcomes for your clients with both acute and chronic pain conditions. For example, in sub-acute and chronic low back pain, studies have shown that massage is more effective when combined with self-care education and exercise (Furlan et al 2002). The touchy-feely positive vibe of a massage session may also mean that self-care suggestions are more likely to be taken on board especially when delivered by a supportive therapist. A study by Long (2009) made a powerful case for positive changes in health care behaviour being mediated via bodywork sessions in this way. In a 6-month study of over 600 shiatsu clients in the UK, Austria and Spain, he found that about four-fifths reported making changes to their lifestyle as a result of having shiatsu treatment, including taking more rest and relaxation or exercise, changing their diet, reducing time at work and other changes such as increased body/mind awareness and levels of confidence and resolve. Even the naysayers who see massage only as a frivolous placebo in the treatment of pain recognise it may have a place in helping to persuade clients to engage in more self management. In one review, Hurley and Bearne (2008) grumpily acknowledged that although in their view modalities such as manual therapy, electrotherapy or acupuncture are not cost effective and are largely placebo, they are popular with clients and therefore 'may have some utility in making more burdensome physiotherapeutic interventions (exercise and self-management advice) more acceptable.' In other words, manual therapy might be an effective way to get people to do their exercises. In an interesting study comparing massage, acupuncture and self care for the treatment of low back pain, Cherkin et al (2001) found that massage was superior to self-care educational materials after 10 weeks of treatment. However, after a year the self-care strategies had 'caught up' and both 10 weeks of massage and self care had equal outcomes (and both interventions were superior to acupuncture). Thus massage may be most effective at helping pain relief and improving function in the first few months, while pain relief from self care may take a while to 'kick in'. As we saw from Chapter 4, high levels of initial pain are

correlated with ensuing disability. Reducing the initial pain level through massage may thus play an important role in reducing the progression to chronicity. This idea fits nicely with the Jing combined approach emphasising both massage and self care as being important in maximising outcomes.

Locus of control and health

> *You may not control all the events that happen to you, but you can decide not to be reduced by them.*
> MAYA ANGELOU

How much do you believe you are in control of your life, health and future? Think back to when you were at school and got a poor test result. Did you hold yourself accountable for not studying enough or put the blame on your inadequate teachers, the unfair exam or the weather that day? You will know from your own experience that the world tends to be divided into two types of people: those that believe they can alter their circumstances by their actions and those who believe they are at the mercy of outside forces such as chance, fate or the whims of authority. The same is true in your practice; some of your clients will feel positive about their pain condition and eagerly take on board any self-care suggestions; others will feel at the mercy of inadequate diagnoses and harbour a general disbelief that anything can help. Psychologist Julian Rotter (1966) came up with the concept of locus of control to explain this tendency. People with an internal locus of control believe they can control events that happen to them whereas those with an external locus of control believe they are powerless to control outside events (**Figure 11.1**).

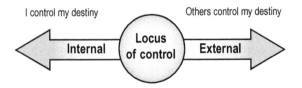

Figure 11.1

People with an internal locus of control believe they can control events that happen to them, whereas those with an external locus of control believe they are powerless to control outside events

Locus of control can be strongly correlated with health outcomes. For example, clients with a high internal locus of control have better headache treatment outcomes and less headache related disability. Conversely those who believe their headaches are more due to chance have higher levels of depression, are less likely to initiate active coping strategies, such as recognising headache triggers, and experience more headache related disability (Nicholson et al 2007). Similarly, the belief that low back pain relief is determined by factors outside of our control, such as chance or health care professionals, was related to higher levels of disability and poorer quality of life (Sengul et al 2010). Having an internal locus of control is also associated with better outcomes from treatment as patients with stronger internal beliefs gained more from an exercise-based treatment for low back pain, they also learned their exercises better and did them more frequently (Härkäpää et al 1991). Feelings of having control over your job are also predictors of absence from work due to low back pain; having high control at work, in terms of both your time and how you do things, can help prevent back pain becoming a persistent problem (Melloh et al 2012).

It is important to realise that the sense of locus of control is not fixed and can be changed with the right education and behavioural change strategies, such as those found in multi-disciplinary pain centres (Coughlin et al 2000). Clearly empowering our clients to believe they have control over their pain condition can be a crucial factor in recovery. This may already be an easier process for complementary therapists as the self-selected group who seek alternative health care are more likely to have a stronger belief in an internal health locus of control (HLC) compared to those who use Western medicine (Ono et al 2008). This means that many of your clients will be amenable to self-care suggestions and the opportunity to educate on self management should not be missed.

Components of successful self-care strategies

There are many potential components to successful self-care strategies for your clients. These include:

- Education and information about the pain condition: changing established unhelpful thoughts and behaviours that can maintain and aggravate the pain state.

- Advice on managing and returning to desired activities.

- Helping with goal setting, action planning and reviews through structured treatment plans.

- General exercise, e.g. running, cycling, swimming and walking.

- Specific exercise targeted to help the area of pain, e.g. stretching, mobilisation or rehabilitation exercises for the low back.

- Relaxation, meditation or mindfulness practices.

- Advice and referral to classes that would be helpful, e.g. yoga, Pilates or t'ai chi.

- Topical modalities for pain relief, i.e. use of hot and cold, balms, kinesio taping and splints.

- Cognitive behaviour therapy (CBT) based approaches that aim to reduce unhelpful beliefs such as catastrophising.

Crucially, it is not enough just to give your client information about what to do. You need to find the best way to motivate them to do it. Research shows that providing information is necessary but not sufficient by itself to improve health related outcomes. Information improves knowledge but not behaviour change. This is nicely exemplified by the old joke:

> Patient: 'Doctor, Doctor, what are the best exercises to do.'
> Doctor: 'The ones that you do.'

It is crucial to accept that part of your job is finding the right way to communicate and motivate your clients to involve themselves in the healing process. Therapists often get cross and complain about clients who 'Don't help themselves'; you know, those pesky people who 'Don't do their exercises.' (Totally unlike our good selves who never sit and eat cake or watch television as we are busy spending every moment in unrelenting self-improvement. Hang on a minute while I turn off the mung bean stew so I can go and meditate.) Unfortunately a tendency to 'not do what is good for us' is part of the human condition and we ourselves are no different than our clients – and the gap between knowing what is good for us and actually doing those things can be huge. For example, even though research indicates that exercise can be very helpful for decreasing pain and improving function, it is estimated that as many as 70% of physiotherapy clients do not do their prescribed exercises (Beinart et al 2013). If you get on a tube train in London there are big signs advising you to 'mind the gap' between the platform and the train; similarly, you need to 'mind the gap' between delivering information and the expectation of behaviour change. You will need to have good communication skills and a number of strategies up your sleeves to encourage your client to get involved in the process of recovery and to get across the gap between knowing what's good for them and actually initiating behaviour change.

De Silva (2011) has identified that the key features of successful self management include:

- **A sense of collaboration between client and clinician**: this is the therapeutic alliance discussed in the assessment chapter (see Chapter 5). The client needs to feel you are on their side and walking a path with them towards their goals.

- **Information and education**: many clients' feelings of helplessness are a result of incorrect or outdated information about their condition. For example, clients may hold common beliefs about the supremacy of surgical or medical interventions for musculoskeletal pain or the fear that a herniated disc will always lead to permanent disability. Through providing appropriate and targeted information you can help to change these unhelpful beliefs.

- **Behaviour change strategies such as goal setting, action planning and follow up**. Remember that information by itself is not enough to cause change. Three factors are important in behaviour change:

  - **Agenda setting**: jointly setting health goals with your client.

  - **Goal setting**: clients choosing their own small and achievable goals.

  - **Goal follow-up**: proactive follow-up is vital to maintain momentum and provide engagement and support.

Self-care strategies explored

Mindfulness and meditation

> *Breathing in I see myself as space.*
> *Breathing out I feel free.*
> THICH NHAT HANH, *PEACE IS EVERY BREATH*

The ancient practices of meditation and mindfulness have much to offer in the fast paced 21st century. Simple to learn and easy to practise and apply in every day situations, learning these effective self-help practices can transform the lives of those experiencing chronic pain. Research over the past two decades has affirmed the effectiveness of meditation and mindfulness techniques for a number of conditions including headaches, back pain, neck pain, fibromyalgia (FM), anxiety, depression and stress.

What is meditation?

When you read books about meditation, there is often a great deal of emphasis placed on different techniques such as chanting, certain practices with the breath, or visualisation. However, the most important feature of meditation is not technique but the way of being, the spirit, which is one of quiet focus and of being rather than doing. This can be a difficult concept as it is the opposite of the way we are accustomed to achieving in the West – which is usually through striving, effort and stress. At a recent meditation retreat I attended, the facilitator recommended that participants lay down during meditation rather than sitting. She explained that over-achieving Westerners even manage to make the simple act of sitting into a stressful event! Many of us have completely lost the art of totally relaxing. My European friends constantly bemoan the British and American habit of eating a plastic sandwich at their desks at lunchtime rather than a hearty meal with friends followed by a nap.

Meditation is simply a question of being, of melting, like a piece of butter left in the sun. The simplest meditation practice is to just quietly sit, to allow thoughts to come and go, without grabbing onto them. Most forms of meditation practices all place central importance on being mindful of the breath. This is a very simple process: just be aware of the breath, how it feels in your body, noticing any small movements, sounds or rhythms to which you don't usually pay attention. When you are breathing out, know that you are breathing out. When you breathe in, know that you are breathing in, without going into the usual kind of internal dialogue in which our minds endlessly engage if left to their own devices. This is so much harder than it sounds! Our 'monkey minds' are constantly aiming to stray, create noise and endless chatter.

A regular practice of meditation enables us to gradually develop our ability to be truly mindful and in the moment. There is a famous Zen saying: 'When I eat, I eat; when I sleep, I sleep.' Whatever you do, you are fully present in the act. **See Figure 11.2**

What is mindfulness?

Mindfulness is a central concept of the teachings of the Buddha and is felt to be a spiritual faculty that is of great importance in the path to enlightenment. Mindfulness is basically an attentive awareness of the reality of things (especially of the present moment). The Buddha advocated that one should establish mindfulness in one's day-to-day life maintaining, as much as possible, a calm awareness of one's bodily functions, feelings, thoughts and perceptions, and consciousness itself.

Over the last few decades, the importance of mindfulness in maintaining positive mental health and reducing stress has been recognised by modern psychology. Mindfulness practice, inherited from the Buddhist tradition, has been presented free from any religious

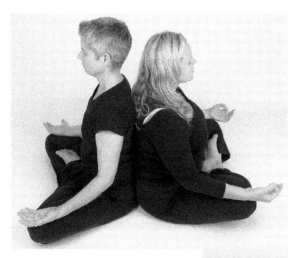

Figure 11.2

connotations and is increasingly being employed to alleviate a variety of mental and physical conditions, including chronic pain, anxiety, depression and drug dependence.

Dr Jon Kabbat-Zinn (psychologist) has been at the forefront of these developments and, in 1979, founded the Mindfulness-Based Stress Reduction (MBSR) programme at the University of Massachusetts to treat the chronically ill. His MBSR programmes (consisting of an 8-week course) have proved hugely successful in dealing with a host of physical and mental health issues.

Research basis for the use of mindfulness and meditation in the treatment of pain

A strong research base supports the use of mindfulness and meditation for effective self care in pain conditions. Systematic reviews of the evidence have found that mindfulness based interventions (MBIs) are helpful for the reduction of pain symptoms in patients with chronic pain and that reductions in pain intensity were generally well maintained over time (Chiesa and Serretti 2011, Reiner et al 2013).

The effects of mindfulness meditation are not necessarily the same for all pain conditions. Rosenzweig et al (2010) on reviewing the evidence found that MBSR techniques were most effective for those patients with arthritis, back/neck pain, or two or more pain conditions. Being a good student and doing your meditation homework also causes improvement in some outcomes but not others. Those clients who spent more time with meditation practice at home enjoyed improvements in several outcome measures, including overall psychological distress and self-rated health, but were equivalent to other clients with regard to pain and other quality of life scales.

A study of older adults with chronic low back pain found that they experienced numerous benefits from mindfulness meditation including less pain, improved attention, better sleep, enhanced wellbeing, and improved quality of life (Morone et al 2008). However, a systematic review by Cramer et al (2012) found the overall evidence for low back pain to be inconclusive, suggesting that MBSR may help improve pain acceptance although not necessarily pain intensity or disability.

Psychological wellbeing is also greatly enhanced by mindfulness and meditation, and is consistently shown to improve measures of anxiety, depression and stress (Goyal et al 2014). As we know these commonly exist in a self-perpetuating cycle in chronic pain situations, so there is definitely a great 'buy one benefit get one free' advantage for meditation here. Significantly, there seem to be strong links between increased mindfulness and reduction of catastrophising, which is known to be of extreme importance in chronic pain (Cassidy et al 2012, Schütze et al 2010).

Plews-Ogan et al (2005) advocates the use of both massage and mindfulness as useful interventions for chronic musculoskeletal pain, showing that they have different but complementary effects. Mindfulness-based stress reduction seems to be more effective and longer lasting for mood improvement, while massage is more effective for reducing pain.

Teaching mindfulness and meditation self-help concepts to your clients

> *Stop a minute, right where you are. Relax your shoulders, shake your head and spine like a dog shaking off cold water. Tell the imperious voice in your head to be still.*
> BARBARA KINGSOLVER

Teaching simple mindfulness and meditation to your clients does not have to be a complex process. A good way to introduce the concept is to first of all bring it into the bodywork session. I like to talk my clients through a short and simple mindfulness exercise at the start of their treatment. This is a great way to quieten down those clients who like to talk endlessly throughout the treatment and gives both you and your client permission to focus on their body rather than the 'monkey chatter' of their mind. Say something like:

> *Now to begin the treatment, just allow yourself to tune into your body. Gently notice the feeling of your body against the couch, sensing the texture of the towel and the warmth and pressure of my hands. And now just gently draw your attention to the breath, noticing the in breath and the out breath. Allow yourself to tune into those small movements and sounds you don't usually notice. You might be able to notice the physical sensation*

> *of the breath as it enters your nose and mouth, warming the air passages on its way to the lungs. You might be able to notice the rise and fall of the belly and the chest as you breathe in and out. You may even be able to visualise the breath like a golden or a white cloud, or whatever colour works for you.*
> *As you pay awareness to the breath you may find it start to change. Just notice the changes, don't judge or try to interpret. Allow yourself to just be. After the next breath out just notice that slight pause, the stopping and the stillness before the next breath in. Allow yourself to tune into the quality and the rhythm of that pause and notice how it feels. Then let the next breath come when it wants to without grabbing for it. You don't have to control the breath, it just happens. Notice the stillness throughout your body.*

Conclude the session by helping the client come back to their body and observe any changes:

> *So let's finish by gently drawing the attention back to the breath. Bring your mind back to the ebb and flow of the in breath and the out breath, and notice how that feels in the body. Gently tune into how your body feels and whether it feels different than at the start of the session. Notice the pause and the stopping and the stillness after the next breath out. Notice the sensations and feelings of this place …. The texture of the couch you are lying on, the feeling of my hands on your body, the smells and sounds in the room. Remember you can bring yourself back to this place at any time you need to. This sweet spot of quietness always exists inside you; you just need to notice the breath and remember that this peace always lies inside of you.*

Starting and ending the session in this way introduces the client to the format of a mindfulness of breathing session and will make it easier to teach the concept as a self-help technique. Ending the session by drawing the client's attention back to the place that they started also serves a dual function of helping them to tune into any changes you have helped to make during the session. Imprinting the memory of the feelings, sounds and

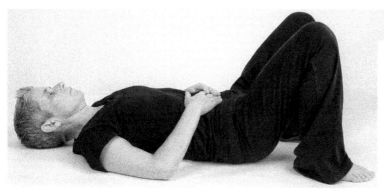

Figure 11.3

smells associated with extreme calm also serves as a helpful 'anchor point' for them to come back to in the future if they are feeling stressed or anxious (**Figure 11.3**).

Two established simple meditation exercises that I like to teach clients are the mindfulness of breathing and body scan; instructions for these can be found in the Self-Care Resources (available at uk.singingdragon.com/catalogue/book/9781909141230). Take some time to show your clients how to do one of these exercises at the end of the session and encourage them to do it daily; just 5 minutes a day will make a tremendous difference. Encourage them to build up the time as they become more familiar with the practice.

If appropriate you can encourage your client to attend a meditation or mindfulness course, which these days run in practically every town. If this is not possible, the Internet is also full of amazing resources.

Yoga as self care (Figure 11.4)

> *Yoga teaches us to cure what need not be endured and endure what cannot be cured.*
> BKS IYENGAR

Another practice with proven efficacy in the treatment of pain is the ancient art of yoga. From the hippies to the high achievers, the West has embraced yoga enthusiastically and it is now a 10-billion dollar industry in the US with over 20 million practitioners (Yogajournal.com 2012). In its dizzying rise to present day status, yoga has accrued all the trappings of Western commercialism with a proliferation of brands

from acroyoga to nude yoga to doga. (Yes, really, you can do it with your dog or naked, although presumably not both at the same time.) In this form yoga bears very little resemblance to its traditional roots as a spiritual and largely meditative practice. Ancient yoga practice places far more emphasis on the training of the mind than the physical conditioning of the body, the latter of which is more common with the Lycra clad yoga seen today. The roots of yoga reject the Cartesian duality of the West and see the mind and body as one (the word yoga comes from 'yoke' and refers literally to the yoking of mind and body). Yoga and meditation could be seen as the original pain management tools as their purpose is to train the human being to transcend the ultimate pain of life – the existential suffering of existence or 'dukkha'. Recognising the supremacy of a quiet mind to modulate the emotional and physical pain inherent in the human condition is fundamental to the yogic approach. Obviously this is now being rediscovered with modern neuroscience emphasising the importance of 'top down' messages from the brain in enabling us to moderate our pain experience. Although this central spiritual message may have been diluted in its modern day presentation, yoga still contains key components to facilitating emotional and physical health. Most yoga classes still emphasise the physical practice of the asanas as preparation for a relaxation and/or meditation at the end. I remember one of my yoga teachers getting really cross at a busy Manhattan-ite who gathered up her things to leave after the asana (yoga poses) section of the class, thus skipping the meditation at the end. The teacher said 'The asanas are not the point of class. They are just the preparation for the meditation which is the nectar, the dew drop of the practice.' That phrase about

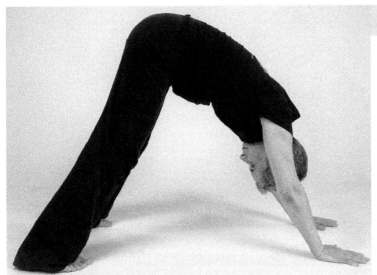

Figure 11.4

the meditation being the nectar has stayed firmly with me ever since. As a true mind–body intervention, yoga helps us still the chattering monkey mind and disengage the higher cognitions of the brain from constant focus on worries, catastrophising and rumination. As we know from the chapter on chronic pain, these 'thought viruses' are the fuel that fans the fire of persistent and self-perpetuating pain.

Yoga is an excellent self-care recommendation for your clients with musculoskeletal pain as it has many proven benefits. A systematic review found that yoga leads to a significantly greater reduction in pain than various control interventions such as standard care, self care, therapeutic exercises, touch and manipulation, or no intervention (Posadzki et al 2011). Other reviews found yoga to have positive effects on both short-term and long-term chronic low back pain (Cramer et al 2013), arthritis (Haaz and Bartlett 2011) and FM (Curtis et al 2011). Interestingly the FM study showed that yoga also had psychological benefits including reducing catastr-ophising. A systematic review of meditative movement therapies (qi gong, t'ai chi and yoga) for FM found that only yoga yielded significant effects on pain, fatigue, depression and health related quality of life (Langhorst et al 2013).

The psychological benefits of yoga are also well documented. A systematic review found evidence supporting a potential benefit from yoga for depression, as an adjunct to pharmacotherapy in schizophrenia, in children with ADHD, and in sleep complaints (Balas-ubramaniam et al 2012). Further reviews support the efficacy of yoga for depression (Pilkington et al 2005) and anxiety (Kirkwood et al 2005). Psychological benefits can be seen within a comparatively short space of time, e.g. women with anxiety who participated in a twice a week yoga class for 2 months showed significant decreases in anxiety (Javnbakht et al 2009). Most reviewers caution about jumping to extreme conclusions concerning the health benefits of yoga (Büssing et al 2012) due to the relatively small number of quality randomised controlled trials conducted overall. However, even within the rigorous world of research, yoga has gained one of the highest accolades from the academics, which is that the results are 'encouraging'. Go yoga!

In conclusion, yoga can be seen as an excellent self-help measure. With an emphasis on the body, mind and spirit, its conceptual framework lies firmly within the framework of the biopsychosocial model (Evans et al 2009).

Of course yoga classes vary greatly in their style and approach. The best way of encouraging your clients to do yoga is by personal recommendation. Network with local yoga teachers in your area to see what they offer and who you think would be right for your clients. Different styles may suit different people so it is good to have an overview of different classes and teachers so that you can refer appropriately. This is also good for business as networks with yoga teachers can be a fruitful source of clients with musculoskeletal problems.

Exercise

> *Motion is lotion and movement is medicine.*
> NOIJAM 2014

Exercise is good for you. Fact. Research, common sense and your mother are all right in that you should get up off the sofa and get some fresh air. Exercise as we all know has numerous psychological and health benefits, and can be a valuable self-help tool for your clients living with chronic musculoskeletal pain. Exercise is safe, cost-free, reduces anxiety and depression, improves physical capacity, increases function and helps you live longer. What's not to like? Yet many of us get tied up in knots about what kind of exercise is best? Running? Walking? Cycling? That funny thing that people do when they walk with ski poles (Americans look great when they do this but the British look ridiculous)? Specialist rehabilitation exercises? What about clients who hurt too much to exercise? The plethora of choices around types of exercise can be overwhelming, and frankly it's enough to make you want to go and lie on the sofa and eat crisps. So let's see if the research evidence can help us in sorting out whether toe touching, trail walking or t'ai chi is best for our clients with common pain conditions.

Aerobic exercise

Aerobic exercise usually makes you sweaty and breathless while simultaneously making you feel great. Running, cycling, walking, squash and football all fit into the category of making you red faced but radiant. Unfortunately many clients with musculoskeletal pain give up beloved aerobic exercise due to aches and pains or a belief that the activity is damaging them further. Misguided health care professionals, incorrect Internet blogs or well meaning family members can reinforce the belief that running, cycling or swimming are 'bad for your joints' and will lead to further damage and pain. In some cases aerobic activity may need to be modified but, on the whole, sweaty exercise is great

for chronic pain. Long-term benefits have been found to be improved mood, decreased pain perception and improved cardiovascular fitness (Sullivan et al 2012). There seem to be no studies on the correlation between exercise and feeling smug and virtuous, although I suspect there is a direct correlation.

If your client is fearful of exercising because it increases their pain, you will need to guide them in the graded exposure approach as described in the education section of this chapter. Set small, progressive goals of exercise duration and intensity; if a flare-up of symptoms occurs then they should decrease the time and/or intensity of exercise on the next occasion. For example, I had a very active client who had ongoing knee pain several months after a surgical intervention; she really wanted to exercise but was afraid it would cause more damage. She said she had tried to cycle but it hurt when she got into a higher gear or had to put a lot of effort in when going up hills. I firstly reassured her that exercising would not lead to further damage and established what she was actually able to do without pain – which in this case was cycling on the flat in a lower gear. I advised her to start by cycling in her lowest gear on a flat terrain and we set some incremental daily goals of increasing time spent cycling. We then gradually increased the impact on the knee by cycling in higher gears. The combination of reassurance that enjoyable exercise was not leading to damage and the feeling of control over her condition led gradually to full recovery.

Non-aerobic exercise

Non-aerobic exercises typically used for pain management and rehabilitation include strengthening, stretching and mobilisation exercises. Overall there is solid evidence supporting the effectiveness of exercise therapy for helping to relieve pain and increase function in common musculoskeletal conditions, including back pain, neck pain, FM, shoulder pain, osteoporosis, osteoarthritis, rheumatoid arthritis and ankylosing spondylitis (Hagen et al 2012). Interestingly there is no evidence that one type of exercise programme is more beneficial than another (Van Middelkoop et al 2010). For example, although strengthening exercises are often thought of as being superior, Slade and Keating (2007) showed that they were similar to McKenzie exercises or yoga for chronic low back pain. There is also no clear evidence that one-on-one sessions are superior to group sessions (Henchoz and Kai-Lik So 2008). The main message here seems to be that it is more important to be actually DOING the exercises rather than agonising over which ones are most effective.

What the evidence says about exercise

Systematic reviews of the available evidence thus far have indicated the following effects for different musculoskeletal conditions:

- **Osteoarthritis:** Fransen and McConnell (2009) found that supervised exercise programmes for osteoarthritis of the knee had similar effects on pain and function as taking anti-inflammatories. However, the effects of both were hardly something to write home about as they only reduced knee pain by 1 point on a 20-point scale. This emphasises the importance of a multi-modal approach as manual therapy may have better outcomes in the treatment of osteoarthritis. A study by Hoeksma et al (2004) found manual therapy to be superior to an exercise programme in patients with osteoarthritis of the hip.

- **Osteoporosis:** most of us are aware that exercise is important in the prevention and treatment of osteoporosis and research backs this up. There is a relatively small, but possibly important, effect of exercise on bone density compared with control groups (Howe et al 2011).

- **Rheumatoid arthritis:** based on the evidence, aerobic capacity training combined with muscle strength training is recommended as routine practice in patients with rheumatoid arthritis (Hurkmans et al 2009).

- **Ankylosing spondylitis:** a home exercise routine can give positive results compared to no exercise (Dagfinrud et al 2008).

- **Fibromyalgia syndrome (FMS):** there is strong evidence that supervised aerobic exercise decreases pain, fatigue and improves functioning in clients with FM; strengthening exercises are also beneficial (Busch et al 2007, 2011). It seems that exercise may help the 'top-down' modulation of pain by the brain and brain imaging studies suggest an association between measures of physical activity and central nervous system processing of pain (McLoughlin et al 2011). Physically active FM patients appear to maintain their ability to modulate pain while those who are less active do not.

It is recommended that exercise programmes for FMS have a variety of types of exercise included; although less supported by evidence, stretching also has a role in FMS management. One study showed that stretching exercises are more effective than the aerobic exercises on pain, number of tender points, sleep and depression in FM. However, aerobic exercises seem to produce a more important effect on anxiety reduction compared to stretching exercises, suggesting a role for a mixed exercise programme (Matsutani et al 2012). The benefits of exercise for FM patients are also enhanced when combined with targeted self-management education (Rooks et al 2007).

- **Low back pain:** many types of exercise are prescribed for low back pain. Overall exercise therapy definitely provides 'small but significant reductions in pain and disability' when compared to minimal care or no treatment for chronic low back pain (Ferreira et al 2010). Individually designed and supervised programmes containing both stretching and strengthening exercises are effective in improving both pain and function (Hayden et al 2005).

Interestingly, research shows clearly that exercise is not an appropriate recommendation for acute low back pain; in these cases it is only as effective as no intervention (Hayden et al 2005; Van Tulder et al 2000). In cases of acute low back pain, recommendations to stay active within reasonable limits are probably more beneficial than prescribing specific exercises. However, Mayer et al (2005) showed that exercise was effective for acute low back pain when combined with continuous low-level heat wrap therapy and significantly improves functional outcomes compared with either intervention alone or control.

- **Neck pain:** a systematic review of the evidence (Kay et al 2009) indicated that specific exercises may be effective for the treatment of acute and chronic neck pain, with or without headache. To be of benefit, a stretching and strengthening exercise programme should concentrate on the musculature of the cervical, shoulder–thoracic area, or both. Combining manual therapy with exercise is even more beneficial for pain reduction and improved quality of life than manual therapy alone for chronic neck pain (Miller et al 2010). This treatment combination also gives greater short-term pain reduction when compared to traditional care for acute whiplash.

- **Shoulder pain**: overall, therapeutic exercise has a positive effect on pain and function for painful shoulder conditions including rotator cuff pathology (Marinko et al 2011). Again, combining mobilisation with exercise gave additional benefits over just exercise alone (Green et al 2003).

- **Tendinosis**: for lateral and medial epicondylitis, stretching plus strengthening exercises were found to be more effective in the short term than ultrasound plus friction massage. Combining stretching with mobilisation of the wrist and forearm plus cervical/thoracic spinal manipulation gave good results in the medium term (Hoogvliet et al 2013).

What factors help clients to exercise?

This is really the million-dollar question in using exercise therapy. As we have seen from the evidence above, for most persistent pain conditions one type of exercise is pretty much as good as another. So we might need to focus less on what exercises are best for our clients and more on how we can support our clients to start integrating exercise into their daily routine. Factors that have been found to help increase participation in exercise programmes (Beinart et al 2013, Jordan et al 2010, Slade et al 2009) include the following outlined below:

- **Supervision**: this could be achieved by referring your client to a known physical trainer or activity class.

- **Graded exercise**: starting small and building up exercise works best. Use the goal setting approach to start your client on a manageable baseline of what they are able to achieve at the moment. Work with them to set incremental and manageable goals.

- **Refresher sessions**: if you have given your client home exercises take time every few sessions to check in and demonstrate them again.

- **Supplementary audio or video**: the Internet gives exciting possibilities for clients who can view reminders of exercises on computers or smartphones. You may wish to provide links to your own or other material on your website.

- **Motivational strategies**: motivate your client with goal setting and action planning, checking in regularly and praising effort. Make sure you provide the client with feedback about improvements – as often people are unable to clearly see gains for themselves, particularly if these occur over a number of weeks or months. There is an important role for what I call 'massage therapist as cheerleader'. Be your client's champion.

- **Greater health locus of control**: as discussed earlier, helping your client to feel they have a sense of control over their pain condition is key.

- **Effective communication skills**: as ever, the therapeutic alliance with the therapist is crucial to successful outcomes. Make sure you listen to your clients, remain non-judgemental and empathic.

- **Consideration of client preferences**: unsurprisingly, people are more likely to do exercises that they find fun and enjoyable. Clients prefer exercises that match their current skill and fitness levels rather than a 'one size fits all' approach. Clients are less likely to do technically complicated exercises and tend to get fearful of 'doing them incorrectly'. So salsa classes might be more effective than complex sheets of stretching exercises. **See Figure 11.5**

- **Setting**: settings that emphasise health promotion rather than rehabilitation of the sick or injured are preferred. Going to a gym

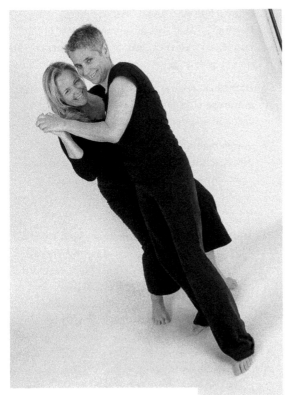

Figure 11.5

Massage therapists are in a prime position to carry out this role as they often have an intrinsic understanding of the joint role played by mind and body. This expands the potential role of massage therapist to one of health care educator and facilitator of the client taking control of their healing process.

Guidelines for client education

Educating patients about their pain conditions has been a prominent part of self-care initiatives such as the 'back schools' originally developed in Sweden in the 1960s (programmes giving practical information about back care, posture, body mechanics, back exercises, and how to prevent long-term back problems). On the whole the evidence has been promising, showing that both group and individual education approaches have positive effects on sick leave and short-term disability compared with usual care and are a credible alternative to surgical approaches, such as spinal fusion (Brox et al 2008, Engers et al 2008, Heymans et al 2005).

It seems that education plus exercise is most effective for helping pain in sub-acute and chronic pain conditions; however, for acute low back pain, just being advised to stay active has the same outcome (Liddle et al 2007).

or yoga class sends a healthier message to the brain than attending group physiotherapy sessions in a local hospital. Remember my friend with low back pain who was referred to the 'disabled hydrotherapy group!' The messages that we are sending clients are key to recovery.

The importance of education in self care

It is important to see the treatment session as a stage for client education, pain management approaches and self-care suggestions. There are simple common sense approaches that fall well within the massage therapist role that can be incredibly useful to the client. Of course, in some situations emotional or cognitive components involved in the client's pain may warrant referral to another professional (such as a CBT or other talk therapist) but in many cases a down to earth approach to the problem can be invaluable.

Studies of education for other musculoskeletal disorders has been mixed, e.g. a systematic review by Haines et al (2009) drew a big fat zero for education being effective for neck pain. This included a variety of strategies including advice to activate, advice on stress coping skills, and neck school. However, with FM the effects of exercise are enhanced when combined with education (Rooks et al 2007). There is also a credible case for educational strategies playing a role in managing acute whiplash associated disorder to prevent it becoming a chronic condition (Söderlund 2011). A recent study (Michaleff et al 2014) showed that simple advice around chronic whiplash (one session plus telephone support) was as effective as a 20-week comprehensive physiotherapy exercise programme.

But what type of education is most effective? One of the most exciting trends in recent years has been the emerging evidence around the role of neuroscience education in reducing pain and increasing function.

A neuroscience nugget a day keeps the doctors at bay

> *Of course it is happening inside your head, Harry, but why on earth should that mean that it is not real?*
> JK ROWLING (2007), *HARRY POTTER AND THE DEATHLY HALLOWS*

> *Emerging research shows that explaining to patients their pain experience from a biological and physiological perspective of how the nervous system/brain processes pain allows patients to move better, exercise better, think different about pain, push further into pain, etc.*
> LOUW ET AL 2011

Educating your client about the model of chronic pain discussed in Chapter 4 may be one of the most valuable tools you can give them in their journey out of pain. Most of us, whether we are consciously aware of it or not, receive endless negative messages that reinforce misleading and unhelpful notions about pain conditions. We are taught that pain always signifies damage and despair, can lead to years of misery, causes loss of important things in our lives, is out of our control and is frightening. We believe that pain is due to unseen and mysterious structural problems in our bodies including scary looking discs that deteriorate, joints that jam, pelvises that 'put themselves out' at will and fragile spines that let us down when we least expect it. Most of all we learn that pain is out of our control and needs to be solved by a medical expert.

Our limited notions of problem solving about pain usually runs to the extent of seeing the doctor, taking painkillers or opting for surgery. Helping your client to understand that their pain does not indicate tissue damage and that they can gain back control of their life can literally be life changing.

There is compelling evidence that, for chronic musculoskeletal pain disorders, an educational strategy addressing the neurophysiology and neurobiology of pain can have a positive effect on pain, disability, catastrophisation and physical performance (Louw et al 2011).

Studies over the last decade have shown this approach to be effective in low back pain (Moseley 2004, Moseley et al 2004, Puentedura and Louw 2012), chronic spinal pain (Nijs et al 2014), whiplash associated disorder (Van Oosterwijck et al 2011), FM (Van Oosterwijck 2013) and chronic fatigue syndrome (Meeus et al 2010).

Neuroscience-based education differs from other approaches as it focuses on a detailed description of the biology and physiology of the nervous system and the brain's processing of pain and nociceptive input. This differs from biomedical models often used by orthopaedic surgeons and physical therapists, which focus on how damaged tissues, such as bulging discs or worn down joints, are solely responsible for pain. Biomedical models are increasingly being recognised as outdated, having limited efficacy in decreasing pain and disability, and possibly increasing fear in patients, which in turn may increase their pain.

Neuroscience education can be seen as a preventive measure in acute pain (to lessen the probability of the condition transitioning to a chronic situation) and a treatment strategy in chronic pain.

Essential components of the neuroscience message

Educating your clients on the new science of pain does not have to be complicated. There are many fantastic resources that you can use to get your message across. In particular there are a couple of wonderful books by the poster boy of neuroscience education, Lorimer Moseley, called *Explain Pain* (Butler and Moseley 2003) and *Painful Yarns* (Moseley 2007), that can be really useful in explaining the concepts in an easily digestible way. Research has shown that using metaphors and stories is an effective way of increasing understanding (Gallagher 2012). You are going for 'deep' comprehension here rather than superficial knowledge (which does not necessarily change behaviour).

The main points of the neuroscience message are:

- Hurt does not always equal harm, especially in chronic pain situations. Although the pain your client is experiencing is very real it is not necessarily in proportion to any tissue damage.

- Our brains have much more control over the sensation of pain than previously realised. Messages do not just go from 'bottom up' but also 'top down'. In other words, our brains can turn up or down the 'volume' of the pain sensation.

- The nervous system has the ability to increase or decrease its sensitivity (neuroplasticity). Emotions, stress, and our beliefs and behaviour about the pain can cause an increase in pain. Any activities or behaviour that help decrease stress or change negative thought patterns will be helpful in decreasing pain.

- Activity is desirable. If activity hurts this does not mean we are doing ourselves more damage. Building up activity gradually over time is the best approach.

- Pain indicates 'threat' rather than 'damage'. Is there anything your client feels may be a threat to their physical or emotional wellbeing? Is there anything they can do about these factors?

Dos and don'ts of a successful educational approach to chronic pain
Do

- Use stories and metaphors to explain the concepts.

- Work with the client to set achievable goals on returning to desired activities and work.

- Let your client know that there are many things they can do to help their recovery from pain.

- Give your client hope for full recovery from their pain condition.

- Get your client to repeat back to you what they have understood from your explanation so that you can check what they actually heard.

- Use reassuring language that does not add to the tendency to catastrophise. I tend to stay away from scary sounding diagnoses for my clients, as on the whole they are unhelpful. Labels such as arthritis, frozen shoulder, herniated disc and meniscal damage can all conjure up a cascade of catastrophising thoughts in the client's head. If the client is desperate for a label use words like 'simple strain/sprain' that instead carry connotations of natural recovery.

- Reassure clients with acute pain or recent injury that the body is programmed to heal and that the pain will start to feel better in a few days or weeks (depending on the severity of the injury). Let them know there is no reason for the pain to be long lasting. This is true for all injuries including whiplash and herniated discs.

Don't

- Overemphasise the role of structure or anatomy (such as discs or joints) in the causation of pain.

- Use scary language that may cause the client to catastrophise, e.g. diagnoses such as 'arthritis', 'bulging disc', 'crumbling spine' and 'scoliosis'.

- Tell your client the pain is 'in their head'. Be aware this is what they may have heard even if this is not what you said!

- Let your client think they are totally reliant on you, their doctor or any other outside 'expert' to fix their pain.

- Tell your client to stop going to work or to avoid enjoyable activities. Instead work with them on achievable goals using pacing strategies (see below). Encourage them to find the middle ground between avoiding activity and pushing themselves through the pain.

Without a doubt, explaining the new concepts of pain science to your client is an essential part of good practice. However be warned, your clients may not welcome or believe the news that their persistent pain is not a signal of damage. We are all so brainwashed by the prevalent biomechanical model that telling clients their arthritic joint or bulging disc is likely to be only a part of their pain condition is often akin to telling someone the world is flat. Work on your explanations by testing them out on friends and family; back these up in the clinic with visuals or handouts. Match the message to the receiver, e.g. the more scientifically minded client will need the reassurance of research studies.

In contrast, the New Agers might find the idea that their pain is telling them something is more than enough without needing to go into the science.

You will need to find the approach to explanation that best works for your client – as it is vitally important that they understand their pain better in order to be able to take control. Your website can be a valuable tool in this respect as there are some great blogs, videos, talks and research articles explaining these notions. Capture this content on your website and direct your clients to it. In order to make a difference, your client will need a deep understanding of the concepts so that the new information is integrated into their life and beliefs.

Using pacing and gradual exposure

One of the challenges around recovery for clients in pain is determining how to advise them on exercise, movement and the challenge of returning to both necessary and enjoyable activities. All too often clients in pain fall into some level of inactivity due to their pain levels.

Clients' attitudes often fall into the categories of 'boom and bust' (push through the pain then drop with exhaustion) or 'avoidant' (avoiding potentially painful activities altogether).

A more sensible approach involves gradually increasing the level of the activity in question. Movement is important in recovery from chronic pain and it is important your client is encouraged to gradually return to the activities they enjoy.

- Decide with your client which activities they want or need to work on (cycling, walking, tennis, playing with kids, dancing).

- Determine their baseline, i.e. the amount of activity the client can do without pain flaring up. (Might only be 3 minutes cycling on a flat surface but that's a good start.)

- Encourage a planned progression of the chosen activity, e.g. the client does a little more than they did yesterday but not much more (i.e. 4 minutes cycling the next day).

- If the pain flares up return to the previous baseline for a while. **See Figure 11.6**

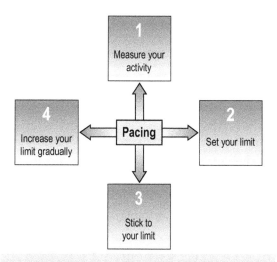

Figure 11.6
Use pacing strategies to gradually help return your client to desired activities

Reducing catastrophisation and unhelpful thought patterns

Chicken Little was in the woods one day when an acorn fell on her head. It scared her so much she trembled all over. She shook so hard, half her feathers fell out.
Chicken Little: Help! Help! The sky is falling! I have to go tell the king!

Catastrophising didn't really work out so well for Chicken Little and neither will it do much good for your clients in pain (you may recall that Chicken Little eventually got eaten by Foxy Loxie along with Henny Penny, Ducky Lucky, Goosey Loosey and Turkey Lurkey who she had also managed to drag into believing her story) (**Figure 11.7**).

Helping your clients to identify and deal with catastrophising thoughts can be an effective self-management tool for chronic pain. The first step to this reassurance is through education and, in many cases, using the approach described above to empower your clients into gaining control over their situation can be extremely helpful in reducing unnecessary fear and catastrophising thoughts.

Unhelpful thought patterns, such as catastrophising, are a major focus of talk interventions, such as CBT, that

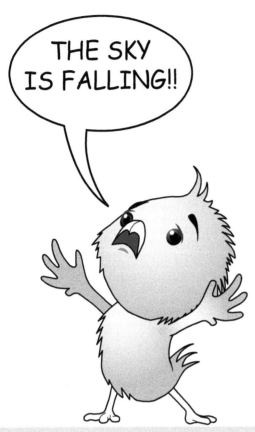

Figure 11.7
Catastrophising didn't work out too well for Chicken Little. Neither will it for your client in pain

have good results for reducing chronic pain. Although some clients may need referral to a CBT therapist, there are also a few simple tools employed by CBT therapists that can be useful self-help skills for clients to learn. The Self-Care Resources (available at uk.singingdragon.com/catalogue/book/9781909141230) can be used as home-work for clients and can help them identify patterns of unhelpful thoughts and behaviours.

Hassles that aren't helping

Another effective self-help strategy is the simple common sense approach adopted by Louis Gifford (2002) where he helps the client identify factors that might be perpetuating their pain condition. He calls these 'hassles that aren't helping'. In the scenario below he describes using this approach with a client in pain following an accident:

Other self-help approaches

There are many other potential self-help approaches that practitioners have found useful in the clinic:

- **Kinesio taping**: this has risen massively in popularity over the last few years, mainly due to the prominent wearing of the brightly coloured tape by high profile athletes at the 2008 Olympics (great product placement by the kinesio taping brand who donated the product to 58 countries). Taping websites feature toned handsome athletes engaged in extreme sporting activities (and the message here is that kinesio taping not only cures your sporting aches and pains but enhances your sex appeal by a factor of 10). I know many practitioners who swear by it as a useful tool in the treatment of pain. The flexible tape can be applied after a session to enhance the results of your work and you can also teach your clients to apply the tape themselves.

  Although anecdotal evidence and some clinical trials suggest that the tape has positive benefits, substantiation by research is somewhat lukewarm. Reviews indicate that kinesio taping may have some benefit for the short-term reduction of pain but there is no support for any

Quite often I have short sessions with patients with ongoing pains called 'hassles that may not be helping'. The word 'hassles' is written in the middle of a piece of paper and the patient is asked to voice all the hassles that relate to their problem – as you jot them down. It's fun, the patients seem to enjoy it and constructive action plans usually evolve out of it.
Once all the 'hassles that are not helping' have been written on the paper I might ask the question – 'Is there anything you think that could be done to lessen these hassles?'
I get another piece of paper and we list the ones that can be worked on. We might get a long list of things. We do one thing at a time and when it gets done it gets ticked off the list, we start with the most annoying and we may just do a little of that until it is eventually done. The patient learns to put a small part of the day aside for 'dealing with hassles'.

We both problem solve the hassles and the patient learns how it can be done. Often the patient feels better because they're getting a sense of control, they're seeing the light at the end of the tunnel, they're able to respond to things in a balanced way and get them done before they become a burden. Some hassles are difficult to deal with. For example, 'the bloke who hit me, who smashed my car up and left me like this, he never said sorry, he didn't even offer to help me ... he's now denying it was his fault!' We can't deal with patients' lives, we all have hassles, but we can take one or two, show how they can be better managed and teach the skills to our patients. But we must be careful not to take over.

LOUIS GIFFORD 2002

effect in the long term. There is also insufficient evidence of other claimed benefits such as improving muscular strength, prevention of sporting injury, or, I'm afraid to say, making you look cool if you are not actually an Olympic athlete (Kalron and Bar-Sela 2013, Montalvo et al 2014, Mostafavifar et al 2012, Williams et al 2012). This is not to say that the benefits reported in individual cases are fantasy – as we know the brain is a powerful modulator of pain so those messages imparted by tape application may well have an effect ('My ankle is now supported', 'My back feels protected', 'My knee is stabilised' and 'Wow, I look hot'). Studies have found kinesio tape to be no more clinically effective than sham tape (Morris et al 2013). Although it may be true that kinesio tape has beneficial effects they are potentially no greater than sticking a big brightly coloured sticking plaster on the area of pain, which frankly could save you a fortune in training courses about how to apply the tape, which has evolved into a highly complex art in itself.

- **Use of hot and cold**: as described in Chapter 6, application of hot or cold can be a useful self-help measure for the client at home. Anything that reduces pain is a good thing and will add to your clients feeling of control over their health.

- **Lotions and potions**: long before the advent of modern medicine, musculoskeletal complaints were treated with herbal remedies. Research supports the use of some topical herbal gels and creams with comfrey cream coming out the clear winner. Clinical trials corroborate that applying comfrey root extract ointment has proven effects in treating low back pain and osteoarthritis (Frost et al 2013). A clinical trial comparing comfrey to a placebo cream in acute low back pain subjects found a whopping decrease in pain of approximately 95.2% in the comfrey group versus 37.8% in the placebo group. The cream also acts quickly with effects felt 1 hour after application (Giannetti et al 2010).

Other popular unguents (posh word for ointment, use it and impress your friends) include capsicum extract and arnica. A review of their use for arthritis found that arnica gel is as good at improving symptoms as a non-steroidal anti-inflammatory drug (NSAID) gel, although it also has a slighter higher rate of adverse effects. Capsicum extract gel had less evidence of efficacy (Cameron and Chrubasik 2013). Our personal favourite is good old tiger balm that seems to be as good as paracetamol at relieving tension headaches (Schattner and Randerson 1996). Smells good too.

It is worth noting that our strong societal belief around rubbing cream into our body to alleviate pain can produce a powerful pain reducing effect by itself. In the comfrey study above, even the placebo cream reduced pain by nearly 40%!

- **Self trigger point treatment**: people love feeling empowered to poke and prod their own sore spots. Teaching your clients how to find and treat their own trigger points can hugely help in pain relief and recovery. **See Figure 11.8**

- **Common sense**: although my mother always accused me of having very little of this, it is a useful faculty to invoke in your clients. With a little time and space for reflection, most of us actually know what we need to do to help ourselves. Less time at work, leaving a stressful job, cycling to work instead of driving, getting out

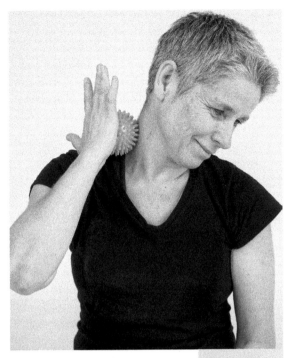

Figure 11.8

of a stressful marriage. Guide your clients to find their own self-care solutions within themselves and they will be much more likely to carry these out than the ones you may have imposed on them.

Teaching self-care strategies

Self-care strategies should be built into an overall t reatment protocol. The client Self-Care Resources (available at uk.singingdragon.com/catalogue/book/9781909141230) are examples of useful self-help exercises. However, you will need to use your skill and judgement to choose the strat-egies that will work most effectively.

In summary, self care for most musculoskeletal pain conditions should cover:

- Education about the neuroscience of pain and the effects of central sensitisation in chronic pain (in a way that helps the client understand).

- Reassurance that hurt does not equal harm.

- Encouragement to carry on with activities of daily living/work or support a graded return to those activities.

- Tips on pacing activities to get the happy balance between 'boom and bust' and 'avoidance'.

- Strategies to reduce catastrophising. These could be as simple as pointing it out, education or the self-help sheets in the resources section. Alternatively the client may need referral to a CBT therapist.

- Support and strategies to help with emotional issues. However, don't slip into the role of counsellor yourself. Remember massage itself can be as effective as a course of psychotherapy. Refer on if your sessions are getting too 'talky'.

- Strategies to encourage enjoyable movement.

- Strategies to decrease central sensitisation, such as meditation, yoga and exercise.

- Remember to make the self-care suggestions fun, enjoyable and easily adapted into daily life. Set achievable goals and reinforce progress.

Some general tips if you are teaching specific exercises such as stretching:

- Explain why the exercises are helpful: understanding will increase compliance.

- Don't overwhelm your clients with exercises. Start with something they can do in a 10–15 minute period, i.e. one mindfulness exercise or three stretches.

- Set achievable goals and monitor progress weekly. Give lots of praise for effort and provide understanding and problem solving if things have not gone to plan.

- Review and change your plan if it is not working.

Tips for stretching or mobilisation exercises:

- Advise your client not to force or push into painful areas. Encourage them to listen and be kind to their body.

- If symptoms are exacerbated then check what they have been doing and how. You may need to reduce the number of repetitions or number of exercises. Exercises should not increase pain.

- Show the exercise clearly to your client as part of the session and watch them do it. Never just hand out a sheet of exercises for them to read themselves.

- If your client is very restricted then doing stretching exercises after a hot bath is a great idea.

- Always get your client to show you the exercises again at the following session to check that they are being performed correctly.

- Teach the client how to breathe and tune into their bodies while stretching.

References

Balasubramaniam M, Telles S, Doraiswamy PM 2012 Yoga on our minds: a systematic review of yoga for neuropsychiatric disorders. Frontiers in Psychiatry 3:117.

Beinart NA et al 2013 Individual and intervention-related factors associated with adherence to home exercise in chronic low back pain: a systematic review. The Spine Journal : Official Journal of the North American Spine Society 13(12):1940–1950.

Bourne C 2012 Co-creating Health : Evaluation of first phase. *Health (San Francisco)*, (April).

Brox JI et al 2008 Systematic review of back schools, brief education, and fear-avoidance training for chronic low back pain. The Spine Journal: Official Journal of the North American Spine Society 8(6):948–958.

Busch AJ et al 2007 Exercise for treating fibromyalgia syndrome. The Cochrane Database of Systematic Reviews 4:p.CD003786.

Busch AJ et al 2011 Exercise therapy for fibromyalgia. Current Pain and Headache Reports 15(5):358–367.

Büssing A et al 2012 Effects of yoga on mental and physical health: a short summary of reviews. Evidence-Based Complementary and Alternative Medicine 2012:165410.

Butler D, Moseley G 2003 Explain Pain, 1st ed. Adelaide: Noigroup Publications.

Cameron M, Chrubasik S 2013 Topical herbal therapies for treating osteoarthritis. The Cochrane Database of Systematic Reviews 5:CD010538.

Cassidy EL et al 2012 Mindfulness, functioning and catastrophizing after multidisciplinary pain management for chronic low back pain. Pain 153(3):644–650.

Cherkin DC et al 2001 Randomized trial comparing traditional Chinese medical acupuncture, therapeutic massage, and self-care education for chronic low back pain. Archives of Internal Medicine 161(8):1081.

Chiesa A, Serretti A 2011 Mindfulness-based interventions for chronic pain: a systematic review of the evidence. Journal of Alternative and Complementary Medicine (New York, NY) 17(1):83–93.

Coughlin AM et al 2000 Multidisciplinary treatment of chronic pain patients: its efficacy in changing patient locus of control. Archives of Physical Medicine and Rehabilitation 81(6):739–740.

Cramer H et al 2012 Mindfulness-based stress reduction for low back pain. A Systematic Review. BMC Complementary and Alternative Medicine 12:162.

Cramer H et al 2013 A systematic review and meta-analysis of yoga for low back pain. The Clinical Journal of Pain 29(5):450–460.

Curtis K, Osadchuk A, Katz J 2011 An eight-week yoga intervention is associated with improvements in pain, psychological functioning and mindfulness, and changes in cortisol levels in women with fibromyalgia. Journal of Pain Research 4:189–201.

Dagfinrud H, Kvien TK, Hagen KB 2008 Physiotherapy interventions for ankylosing spondylitis. Cochrane Database of Systematic Reviews.

De Silva D 2011 No evidence: helping people help themselves. A review of the evidence considering whether it is worthwhile to support self-management. London: The Health Foundation.

Engers A et al 2008 Individual patient education for low back pain. The Cochrane Database of Systematic Reviews 1:CD004057.

Evans S et al 2009 Using the biopsychosocial model to understand the health benefits of yoga. Journal of Complementary and Integrative Medicine 6(6):1, ISSN (online) 1553-3840, doi: 10.2202/1553-3840.1183.

Ferreira ML et al 2010 Can we explain heterogeneity among randomized clinical trials of exercise for chronic back pain? A meta-regression analysis of randomized controlled trials. Physical Therapy 90(10):1383–1403.

Fransen M, Mcconnell S 2009 Exercise for osteoarthritis of the knee. The Cochrane Database of Systematic Reviews 4:CD004376.

Frost R, MacPherson H, O'Meara S 2013 A critical scoping review of external uses of comfrey (Symphytum spp.). Complementary Therapies in Medicine 21(6):724–745.

Furlan AD et al 2002 Massage for low back pain. The Cochrane Database of Systematic Reviews 2:CD001929.

Gallagher L, McAuley J, Moseley GL 2013 A randomized-controlled trial of using a book of metaphors to reconceptualize pain and decrease catastrophizing in people with chronic pain. The Clinical Journal of Pain 29(1):20–25. Available at: http://www.ncbi.nlm.nih.gov/pubmed/22688603 [Accessed 2 March 2015].

Giannetti BM et al 2010 Efficacy and safety of comfrey root extract ointment in the treatment of acute upper or lower back pain: results of a double-blind, randomised, placebo controlled, multicentre trial. British Journal of Sports Medicine 44(9):637–641.

Gifford L 2002 Perspectives on the biopsychosocial model, part 2: the shopping basket approach. In Touch, The Journal of the Organisation of Chartered Physiotherapists in Private Practice 99(Spring Issue):11–22.

Goyal M et al 2014 Meditation programs for psychological stress and well-being: a systematic review and meta-analysis. JAMA Internal Medicine 174(3):357–368.

Green S, Buchbinder R, Hetrick S 2003 Physiotherapy interventions for shoulder pain. The Cochrane Database of Systematic Reviews 2:CD004258.

Haaz S, Bartlett SJ 2011 Yoga for arthritis: a scoping review. Rheumatic Diseases Clinics of North America 37(1):33–46.

Hagen KB et al 2012 Exercise therapy for bone and muscle health: an overview of systematic reviews. BMC Medicine 10:167.

Haines T et al 2009 A Cochrane review of patient education for neck pain. The Spine Journal: Official Journal of the North American Spine Society 9(10):859–871.

Härkäpää K et al 1991 Health locus of control beliefs and psychological distress as predictors for treatment outcome in low-back pain patients: results of a 3-month follow-up of a controlled intervention study. Pain 46(1):35–41.

Hayden JA et al 2005 Meta-analysis: exercise therapy for nonspecific low back pain. Annals of Internal Medicine 142(9):765–75.

Hayden JA, van Tulder MW, Tomlinson G 2005 Systematic review: strategies for using exercise therapy to improve outcomes in chronic low back pain. Annals of Internal Medicine 142(9):776–785.

Henchoz Y, Kai-Lik So A 2008 Exercise and nonspecific low back pain: a literature review. Joint, Bone, Spine: Revue du Rhumatisme 75(5):533–539.

Heymans MW et al 2005 Back schools for nonspecific low back pain: a systematic review within the framework of the Cochrane Collaboration Back Review Group. Spine 30:2153–2163.

Hoeksma HL et al 2004 Comparison of manual therapy and exercise therapy in osteoarthritis of the hip: a randomized clinical trial. Arthritis and Rheumatism 51(5):722–729.

Hoogvliet P et al 2013 Does effectiveness of exercise therapy and mobilisation techniques offer guidance for the treatment of lateral and medial epicondylitis? A systematic review. British Journal of Sports Medicine 47(17):1112–1119.

Howe TE et al 2011 Exercise for preventing and treating osteoporosis in postmenopausal women. The Cochrane Database of Systematic Reviews 7:CD000333.

Hurkmans E et al 2009 Dynamic exercise programs (aerobic capacity and/or muscle strength training) in patients with rheumatoid arthritis. The Cochrane Database of Systematic Reviews 4:CD006853.

Hurley MV, Bearne LM 2008 Non-exercise physical therapies for musculoskeletal conditions. Best Practice & Research. Clinical Rheumatology 22(3):419–433.

Javnbakht M, Hejazi Kenari R, Ghasemi M 2009 Effects of yoga on depression and anxiety of women. Complementary Therapies in Clinical Practice 15(2):102–104.

Jordan JL et al 2010 Interventions to improve adherence to exercise for chronic musculoskeletal pain in adults. The Cochrane Database of Systematic Reviews 1:CD005956.

Kalron A, Bar-Sela S 2013 A systematic review of the effectiveness of Kinesio Taping--fact or fashion? European Journal of Physical and Rehabilitation Medicine 49(5): 699–709.

Kay TM et al 2009 Exercises for mechanical neck disorders. Cochrane Database of Systematic Reviews 4.

Kirkwood G et al 2005 Yoga for anxiety: a systematic review of the research evidence. British Journal of Sports Medicine 39:884–891; discussion 891.

Langhorst J et al 2013 Efficacy and safety of meditative movement therapies in fibromyalgia syndrome: a systematic review and meta-analysis of randomized controlled trials. Rheumatology International 33(1):193–207.

Liddle SD, Gracey JH, Baxter GD 2007 Advice for the management of low back pain: a systematic review of randomised controlled trials. Manual Therapy 12(4):310–327.

Long AF 2009 The potential of complementary and alternative medicine in promoting well-being and critical health literacy: a prospective, observational study of shiatsu. BMC Complementary and Alternative Medicine 9:19.

Louw A et al 2011 The effect of neuroscience education on pain, disability, anxiety, and stress in chronic musculoskeletal pain. Archives of Physical Medicine and Rehabilitation 92(12):2041–56.

McLoughlin MJ, Stegner AJ, Cook DB 2011 The relationship between physical activity and brain responses to pain in fibromyalgia. The Journal of Pain: Official Journal of the American Pain Society 12(6):640–651.

Marinko LN et al 2011 The effectiveness of therapeutic exercise for painful shoulder conditions: a meta-analysis. Journal of Shoulder and Elbow Surgery: Official Journal of the American Shoulder and Elbow Surgeons 20(8):1351–1359.

Matsutani LA, Assumpção A, Marques AP 2012 Stretching and aerobic exercises in the treatment of fibromyalgia: Pilot study [Portuguese]. Fisioterapia em Movimento 25:411–418.

Mayer JM et al 2005 Treating acute low back pain with continuous low-level heat wrap therapy and/or exercise: a randomized controlled trial. The Spine Journal: Official Journal of the North American Spine Society 5(4):395–403.

Meeus M et al 2010 Pain physiology education improves pain beliefs in patients with chronic fatigue syndrome compared with pacing and self-management education: a double-blind randomized controlled trial. Archives of Physical Medicine and Rehabilitation 91(8):1153–1159.

Melloh M et al 2012 Predictors of sickness absence in patients with a new episode of low back pain in primary care. Industrial Health 50(4):288–298.

Michaleff ZA et al 2014 Comprehensive physiotherapy exercise programme or advice for chronic whiplash (PROMISE): a pragmatic randomised controlled trial. Lancet 384(9938):133–141. Available at: http://www.thelancet.com/journals/a/article/PIIS0140-6736%2814%2960457-8/fulltext [Accessed 23 January 2015].

Miller J et al 2010 Manual therapy and exercise for neck pain: a systematic review. Manual Therapy 15(4):334–354.

Miller JS, Litva A, Gabbay M 2009 Motivating patients with shoulder and back pain to self-care: can a videotape of exercise support physiotherapy? Physiotherapy 95(1):29–35.

Montalvo AM, Cara E Le, Myer GD 2014 Effect of kinesiology taping on pain in individuals with musculoskeletal injuries: systematic review and meta-analysis. The Physician and Sports Medicine 42(2):48–57.

Morone NE et al 2008 "I felt like a new person." the effects of mindfulness meditation on older adults with chronic pain: qualitative narrative analysis of diary entries. The Journal of Pain: Official Journal of the American Pain Society 9(9):841–848.

Morris D et al 2013 The clinical effects of Kinesio® Tex taping: a systematic review. Physiotherapy Theory and Practice 29(4):259–270.

Moseley G 2007 Painful Yarns, 1st edn. Canberra, Australia: Dancing Giraffe Press.

Moseley GL 2004 Evidence for a direct relationship between cognitive and physical change during an education intervention in people with chronic low back pain. European Journal of Pain (London, England) 8(1):39–45.

Moseley GL, Nicholas MK, Hodges PW 2004 A randomized controlled trial of intensive neurophysiology education in chronic low back pain. The Clinical Journal of Pain 20(5):324–330.

Mostafavifar M, Wertz J, Borchers J 2012 A systematic review of the effectiveness of kinesio taping for musculoskeletal injury. The Physician and Sports Medicine 40(4):33–40.

Nicholson RA et al 2007 Psychological risk factors in headache. Headache 47(3):413–426.

Nijs J et al 2014 A modern neuroscience approach to chronic spinal pain: Combining pain neuroscience education with cognition-targeted motor control training. Physical Therapy 94:730–738.

noijam 2014 noijam. Available at: http://noijam.com [accessed 19 August 2014].

Ono R et al 2008 Higher internality of health locus of control is associated with the use of complementary and alternative medicine providers among patients seeking care for acute low-back pain. The Clinical Journal of Pain 24(8):725–730.

Pilkington K et al 2005 Yoga for depression: the research evidence. Journal of Affective Disorders 89(1–3):13–24.

Plews-Ogan M et al 2005 A pilot study evaluating mindfulness-based stress reduction and massage for the management of chronic pain. Journal of General Internal Medicine 20:1136–1138.

Posadzki P et al 2011 Is yoga effective for pain? A systematic review of randomized clinical trials. Complementary Therapies in Medicine 19(5):281–287.

Puentedura EJ, Lou A 2012 A neuroscience approach to managing athletes with low back pain. Physical Therapy in Sport: Official Journal of the Association of Chartered Physiotherapists in Sports Medicine 13(3):123–133.

Reiner K, Tibi L, Lipsitz JD 2013 Do mindfulness-based interventions reduce pain intensity? A critical review of the literature. Pain Medicine (Malden, MA) 14(2):230–242.

Rooks DS et al 2007 Group exercise, education, and combination self-management in women with fibromyalgia: A randomized trial. Archives of Internal Medicine 167:2192–2200.

Rosenzweig S et al 2010 Mindfulness-based stress reduction for chronic pain conditions: variation in treatment outcomes and role of home meditation practice. Journal of Psychosomatic Research 68(1):29–36.

Rotter JB 1966 Generalized expectancies for internal versus external control of reinforcement: Psychological Monographs: General & Applied 80(1):1–28.

Rowling J 2007 Harry Potter and the Deathly Hallows. New York: Arthur A. Levine Books.

Schattner P, Randerson D 1996 Tiger Balm as a treatment of tension headache. a clinical trial in general practice. Australian Family Physician 25(2):216, 218, 220 passim.

Schütze R et al 2010 Low mindfulness predicts pain catastrophizing in a fear-avoidance model of chronic pain. Pain 148(1):120–127.

Sengul Y, Kara B, Arda MN 2010.The relationship between health locus of control and quality of life in patients with chronic low back pain. Turkish Neurosurgery 20(2):180–185.

Slade SC, Keating JL 2007 Unloaded movement facilitation exercise compared to no exercise or alternative therapy on outcomes for people with nonspecific chronic low back pain: a systematic review. Journal of Manipulative and Physiological Therapeutics 30(4):301–311.

Slade SC, Molloy E, Keating JL 2009 People with non-specific chronic low back pain who have participated in exercise programs have preferences about exercise: a qualitative study. The Australian Journal of Physiotherapy 55(2):115–121.

Söderlund A 2011 The role of educational and learning approaches in rehabilitation of whiplash-associated disorders in lessening the transition to chronicity. Spine 36(supplement 25):S280–285.

Sohn T, Sohn R 1996 Amma Therapy, 1st edn. Rochester, Vt: Healing Arts Press.

Sullivan AB et al 2012 The role of exercise and types of exercise in the rehabilitation of chronic pain: specific or nonspecific benefits. Current Pain and Headache Reports 16(2):153–161.

Van Middelkoop M et al 2010 Exercise therapy for chronic nonspecific low-back pain. Best Practice & Research Clinical Rheumatology 24(2):193–204.

Van Oosterwijck J 2013 Pain physiology education improves health status and endogenous pain inhibition in fibromyalgia: a double-blind randomized controlled trial. Clinical Journal of Pain 29:873–882.

Van Oosterwijck J et al 2011 Pain neurophysiology education improves cognitions, pain thresholds, and movement performance in people with chronic whiplash: a pilot study. Journal of Rehabilitation Research and Development 48:43–58.

Van Tulder M et al 2000 Exercise therapy for low back pain: a systematic review within the framework of the Cochrane collaboration back review group. Spine 25(21):2784–2796.

Williams S et al 2012 Kinesio taping in treatment and prevention of sports injuries: a meta-analysis of the evidence for its effectiveness. Sports Medicine (Auckland, NZ) 42(2):153–164.

Yogajournal.com 2012 Yoga journal releases 2012 yoga in America market study. Available at: http://www.yogajournal.com/press/yoga_in_america [accessed 19 August 2014].

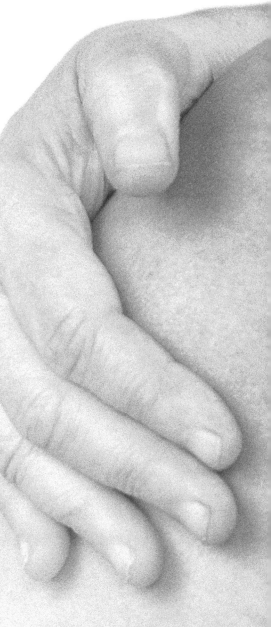

The main act: getting results with common pain conditions using the Jing advanced clinical massage approach

So here is the bit you have been waiting for: a step-by-step guide to the treatment of common musculoskeletal pain conditions for different parts of the body. Each of the chapters will walk you through a detailed protocol including all the elements of the Jing method:

- ***H*** *The use of Hot or cold.*
- ***F*** *The use of Fascial techniques including direct and indirect methods.*
- ***M*** *Treating Muscles with precise trigger point therapy and specifically treating ALL the muscles around an affected joint to release trigger points.*
- ***A*** *Treating relevant Acupressure points.*
- ***S*** *Stretching using techniques such as static, PNF or active isolated stretching.*
- ***T*** *Teaching the client self-help strategies that lie within the massage therapist's scope of practice.*

For the best results in the treatment of pain we recommend combining all the techniques within a treatment session in the way described. Once you become familiar with the method you can feel free to experiment and be creative with the mix.

Remember that your treatment plan for getting clients out of pain is to treat them once a week for up to 6 weeks. Once you see a reduction in pain (usually around week 3) you can lengthen the time between treatments (i.e. once every 2 weeks). When the client is completely pain free a maintenance schedule is recommended, e.g. a once-monthly treatment as part of an overall health care routine.

Low back pain protocol

Introduction

The following protocol, based on the Jing HFMAST approach (see Chapter 1), can be used to good effect with many types of back pain including:

- Non-specific low back pain
- Acute or chronic herniated disc
- Spondylosis
- Spondylolisthesis
- Facet joint irritation syndrome.

Heat application and preparatory work

- **Positioning and draping:** start with your client in a prone position. As always, it is of primary importance that your client is comfortable and as pain free as possible when lying on the table. While prone the client should be supported under the belly with a pillow. It's a good idea to have different sizes of pillow in your treatment room as you may need to experiment with what works best for the client. If your client is uncomfortable when prone you can adapt the protocol to involve the same techniques but with your client side lying. Most importantly DO NOT leave your client too long in the prone position (generally 20–25 minutes is a good rule of thumb but this may be less for people in severe pain). This is a common reason for clients leaving the treatment room in more pain than when they came in.

- **Heat:** prior to working on the affected area, apply moist heat in the form of a heating pad over the low back and buttocks. Heat can also be applied using large hot stones; use two stones on either side of the back and a large one on the sacrum.

- As with all treatments, start by grounding yourself and with introductory still work where you are

simply connecting with your client without feeling the need to 'do'. Have one hand on the sacrum and the other between the shoulder blades. Take time to tune into what you feel, following the rhythm of your client's breath with your hands and allowing your client to connect with your touch. This is the beginning of the relaxation response that is important to healing and you should feel your client's breath slowing down and deepening. **See Figure 12.1**

- **Rocking and mobilisation:** when you feel that your client has started to sink into the experience, you can set in motion a gentle rocking movement of the

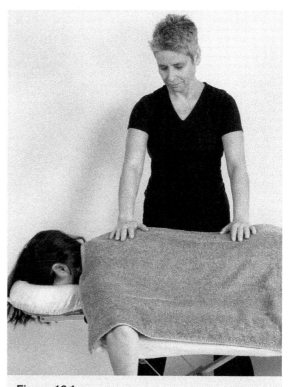

Figure 12.1
Grounding and still work

body. Place both hands on the sacrum and initiate a gentle rock. Find the natural rhythm for your client's body and gradually increase the amplitude of the rock so that it is almost like your client's body is moving by itself with minimal intervention. This should feel like pushing a child on a swing. As you gain momentum you can get into horse stance and use the backs of your forearms to work up and down the sides of the body. Passive mobilisation in this way is a great method for helping your client to let go and is wonderfully healing for sore and damaged soft tissues. **See Figure 12.2**

- **Palming the erector spinae (Bladder channel):** slowly palm down the erector spinae muscle group on the opposite side of the spine to where you are standing. In Chinese medicine terms you are also working the Bladder channel with this technique. Leave the upper hand resting between the shoulder blades and work the other hand slowly down the

back until it rests on the sacrum. You are simply using palmar compression to sink down into the tissues, layer by layer. Then work down with the other hand in the same way before moving to the other side of the table and repeating.

- There are two different ways you can do this stroke:

  - Standing by the side of the table in forward t'ai chi stance, leaning in with your body weight. **See Figure 12.3**

  - Kneeling on the side of the table on all fours, in a 'table top' position, and using your pelvis to lean forward and achieve pressure through the arms. Make sure you keep your arms soft and relaxed; slight shifts of weight in your pelvis will allow you to work deeper in a comfortable way. The more you lean forward, the more pressure you will be able to achieve without pushing. If less pressure is

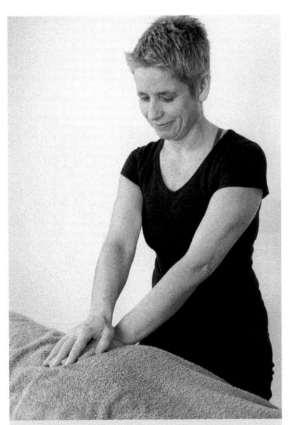

Figure 12.2
Rocking and mobilisation

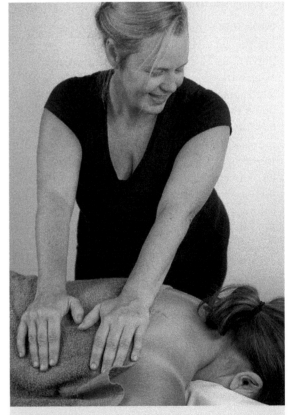

Figure 12.3
Palming the erector spinae (standing)

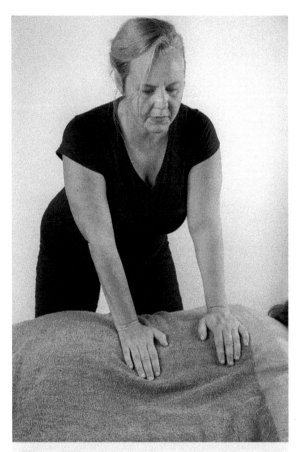

Figure 12.4
Palming the erector spinae (kneeling)

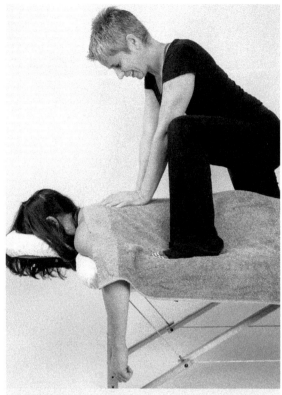

Figure 12.5
Double palming of erector spinae

needed, simply move your pelvis back a bit.
See Figure 12.4

- **Double palming:** you can also work the complete erector spinae muscle group at the same time by using a double palming technique while kneeling on the table in proposal stance (**Figure 12.5**). An alternative is to use soft fists which is a good option if the palming does not feel good for your wrists. **See Figure 12.6, p. 204**

- When reaching the glutes you can use a 'paddy pawing' motion, rocking from one side to the other.

- Remember the dictum 'Assessment is treatment and treatment is assessment.' As you are working, notice areas of tightness and spend longer on these areas, sinking into the tissues to start to release the muscles.

Fascial techniques

- **Next, undrape the back:** remember not to apply oil or lotion at this stage as it will render the following fascial techniques ineffective. Any or all of the following fascial techniques could be used (in any order) with the purpose of freeing areas of fascial adhesions and starting to release trigger points.

- **Direct fascial work with double fists down onto the erector spinae:** stand at the head of the table in forward t'ai chi stance with fists on the back at either side of the spine. Make sure your outside leg is alongside the side of the table so that you can take a small step forward as you work, and don't make the mistake of getting stuck behind the face cradle and having to bend your back. Your fist should be in a soft and loose grip, e.g. imagine you are holding an egg in your hand that you don't want to break. Keep your wrist, elbow and shoulder aligned and use the power of your breath to draw a feeling of

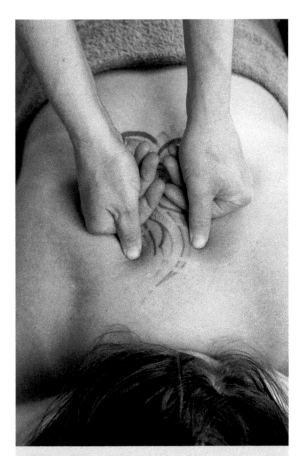

Figure 12.6
Soft fists are an alternative to palms

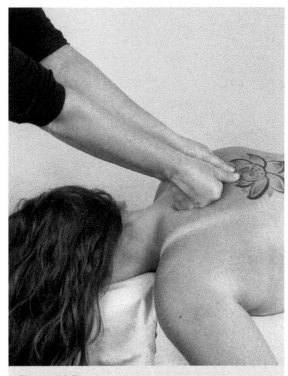

Figure 12.7
Direct fascial work with double fists

energy and qi up from your belly on your in breath. On the out breath visualise this qi shooting up your spine and down your arm like a stream of water flowing through a hosepipe. This visual will help you work 'deeper not harder'.

Use your breath and body weight to gradually sink into your client's tissues; wait until the tissues soften and give way before you SLOWLY start to slide down the back, wait for the tissues to give way in front of you in a wave-like motion. Do not force or try to work too quickly. You are looking for that wonderful gooey sensation of tissue release as you glide through the tissues – like a hot knife slicing through butter. Keep checking back to your body, arms and shoulders to make sure you are not forcing or tensing.

Work down to the sacrum and then repeat two or three times until you feel you have achieved a good release of the tissues. **See Figure 12.7**

- **Fascial finger work over the sacrum:** working the superficial fascia, ligamentous tissue and multifidi muscles located over the sacrum can feel amazing. In t'ai chi stance, stand to one side of the table, facing the sacrum, and work from the midline out to the lateral edge of the bone. Sink down into the tissue with relaxed fingers and oblique pressure to work the whole area with slow, thoughtful strokes. Clients love this one – it just feels great! **See Figure 12.8**

- **Cross hand stretches:** these can be performed on many areas of the low back, for example, with one hand on the sacrum and one over the spine, or over the quadratus lumborum area on both sides. Place your crossed hands adjacent to one another in the area to be released: they should be a few inches apart at this point. Sink down until you have a sense of being on the deep fascial layers that run around and through the muscles. Then put a stretch on this tissue so you have a sense of tension between your two hands – like a piece of material being stretched to a barrier. If you tune until you feel the sense of tissue release described in the fascial chapter (see Chapter 7). This whole process takes around 3–5 minutes so you will need to be patient. Repeat cross hand stretches anywhere as required. **See Figure 12.9**

- **Skin rolling:** this technique can be used on any area of the body to work on the superficial fascia. Here the skin is gently picked up and pulled away from underlying structures. Make sure your thumbs are flat on the body (this helps protect joints from injury) and pick up a 'sausage' of skin and superficial fascia between your thumbs and fingers. Once the skin is pulled away start to slowly push your thumbs forward, lifting the tissues in a smooth continuous motion while the 2nd and 3rd digits feed into this motion causing a rolling effect. The technique can be used over the sacrum and spine. Remember to work slowly allowing time for any restrictions to the release. **See Figure 12.10, p. 206**

- Now you are ready for some broad integration work to relax and prepare the tissues before moving into more specific trigger point work. Apply lubrication such as oil, wax or massage cream at this point. It is better to put this on your hands and forearms first rather than directly on your client. Take care not to apply too much lubrication as this will mean you will be unable to affect the tissues effectively. **See Figure 12.11, p. 206**

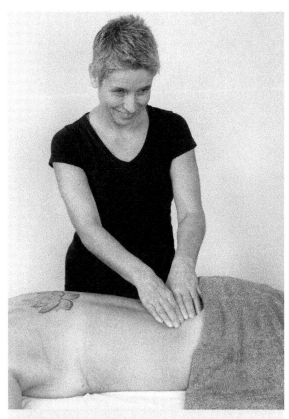

Figure 12.8
Fascial finger work over the sacrum

in with your sense of listening touch, after a while you will start to feel the sensation of the tissue starting to move beneath your hands. Make sure you maintain the stretch and 'follow' the tissues

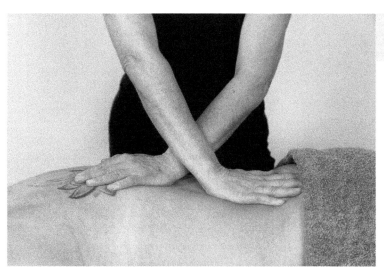

Figure 12.9
Cross hand stretch

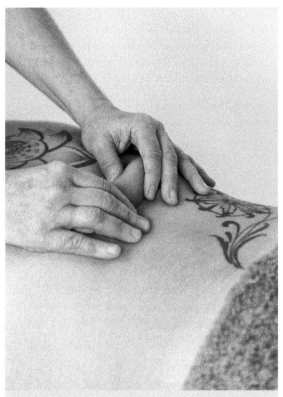

Figure 12.10
Skin rolling over the spine

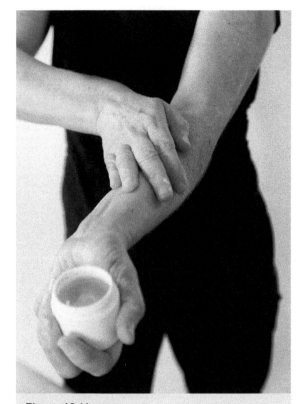

Figure 12.11
Applying lubrication

Muscle techniques and treatment of trigger points

In this section we are treating all the muscles around the joint for trigger points as outlined in Chapter 8.

Broad work to the low back

- **Power effleurage to the low back area:** 'power effleurage' is a term used to describe how effleurage can be a deep and powerful stroke when carried out with optimal body mechanics and a sense of 'listening touch'. Here are a couple of suggested strokes – and again you could use some or all of them.

- **Power effleurage from the head of the table:** in t'ai chi stance, work from the head of the table and glide down either side of the spine using your body weight to work into the erector spinae muscles with your hands. The focus will be on your palms but the whole hand is in contact with the body,

moulding to the contours of the musculature. Glide down to the low back with the stroke, working slowly and deeply, then come back up with a light return stroke and repeat. Breathe out as you work down the body and imagine qi flowing down your arms. **See Figure 12.12**

- **Single forearm massage:** working with the forearms is a great way to save your hands and provides a wonderful sensation for your client. Stand in horse position at the side of the table, knees bent, spine relaxed but straight. Shift your weight onto the leg nearest the client's low back area. Use the soft medial part of your forearm to work into your client's low back, making sure your wrist is floppy and not tense. Shift weight onto your other leg for a light return stroke.

Continue gradually working deeper into the musculature, layer by layer. Cross to the opposite side of the table to work the other side of the low back. **See Figure 12.13**

- **Deep forearm work from the head of the table:** this is a deeper technique, so make sure you start

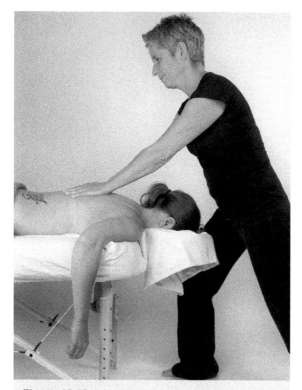

Figure 12.12

Power effleurage from the head of the table

with the other strokes first to soften the area. From the head of table, in t'ai chi stance, start with the ulnar edge of your forearm next to the spine (do NOT use your elbow but make contact using a more broad surface area). Keeping your wrist floppy, lean in and work slowly down the erectors. **See Figure 12.14, p. 208**

- This is also a great time to apply more heat with some dynamic hot stone work. Use any hot stone techniques you know to work into the low back tissues. **See Figure 12.15, p. 208**

- Now you are ready to find and release relevant trigger points: remember the objective in this section is to find and release the key trigger points that are the primary cause of the client's pain pattern. Work with client communication as outlined in the trigger point chapter (read Chapter 8 first if you haven't already done so). Key trigger points should be treated 2–3 times within each session. You will be treating all the muscles around the joint for trigger points.

Treating the erector spinae

- Stand in t'ai chi stance at the head of the table. Starting from the upper back, muscle strip the entire muscle using your thumbs or supported fingers. You are feeling for taut bands and trigger points as you do this work and listening

Figure 12.13

Single forearm massage

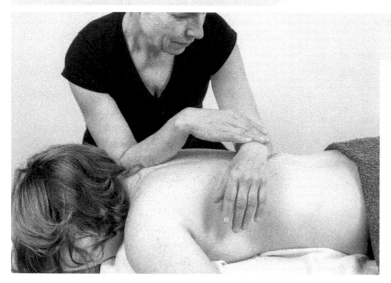

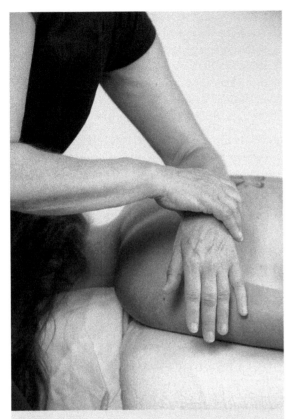

Figure 12.14
Deep forearm work from the head of the table

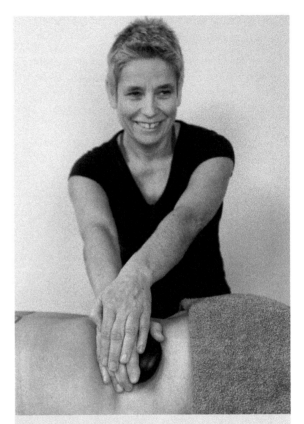

Figure 12.15
Apply more heat with dynamic stone work

to any communication from your client as to whether you have hit a relevant trigger point. Treat any trigger points you find with static pressure for 8–12 seconds until the pain releases (you will need to communicate with your client to assess this). You should go back and treat any key trigger points relevant to the client's pain pattern for 2–3 times per session. Start next to the spine and work from the head to the sacrum in strips (as if methodically 'mowing the lawn'). You will need at least three strips to cover the whole width of the erector spine group. **See Figures 12.16 and 12.17**

- **Power effleurage and integration:** following the specific trigger point work it is great to add some integrating broad work using power effleurage strokes. Be creative and have fun, taking time to dance and enjoy the moving meditation of your work.

- **Fingertip friction to the medial border of erectors and deeper spinal muscles:** this stroke works best with minimal or no lubrication. You may find it helpful to replace the drape and do some palming to absorb excess lubricant before you start.

Stand at the opposite side of the table to where you were working and place your hands side by side so that the fingers are lined up (this technique has earned the nickname in Jing of 'rabbit paws'). Find the spinous processes of the vertebrae and then move slightly laterally so that you slip into the lamina groove of the spine on the opposite side from where you are standing. Sink your fingers down and, starting near the shoulders, move the tissues in a one-directional friction stroke. Take care to not just glide over the surface of the skin; you should be sinking down and affecting the soft tissue found in the

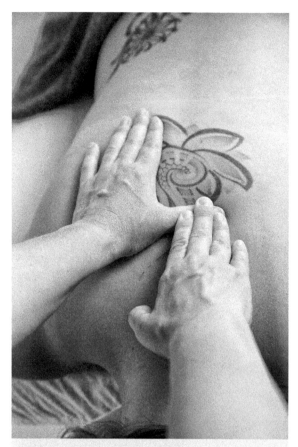

Figure 12.16
Stripping erector spinae for trigger points

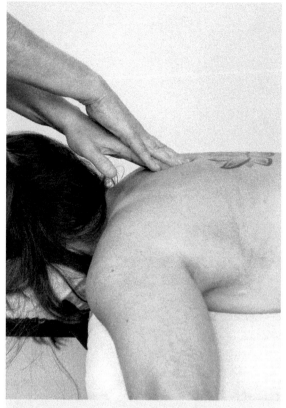

Figure 12.17
Stripping erector spinae for trigger points

lamina groove. Work your way down to the low back. Make sure your friction stroke uses pressure in one direction only, and that the return stroke is light. Do not use pressure in both directions as this can be traumatising to sensitive tissues. If you find tight areas, treat them as trigger points, i.e. wait and hold for a release. **See Figure 12.18, p. 210**

- **Next, carry out fingertip friction to the lateral aspect of the erectors on YOUR SIDE:** place your fingertips on the lateral edge of the erectors and push into the underside of the muscle. Start at the low back area where the muscles are easiest to feel and work up towards the shoulders. The muscles at the top are thinner and it may be more difficult to find the lateral border here.
See Figure 12.19, p. 210

- Repeat at the opposite side of the table so that you have covered both lateral and medial borders of the erectors.

- **Forearm or other power effleurage:** to finish use deep forearm effleurage or other power effleurage strokes, really focussing on opening up the low back and quadratus lumborum region.

Treating the quadratus lumborum (QL)

- There are several steps to treating trigger points in this muscle effectively:

  - **Treat the transverse process attachments of the QL:** to do this your focus needs to be underneath the erector spinae group that lies superficial to this muscle. To treat the transverse process attachments, stand face on at the side of the table and apply pressure at a 45 degree angle between the iliac crest and the 12th rib. Hold static pressure and treat any

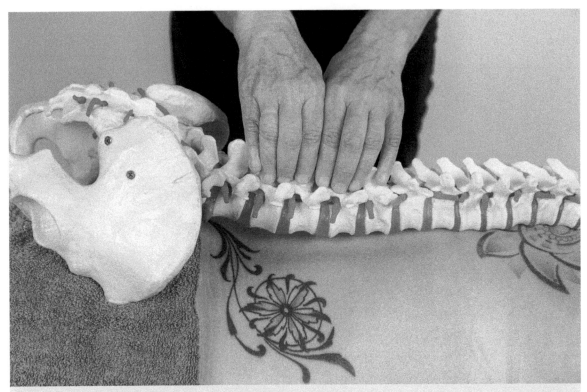

Figure 12.18
Fingertip friction to the medial border of the erectors

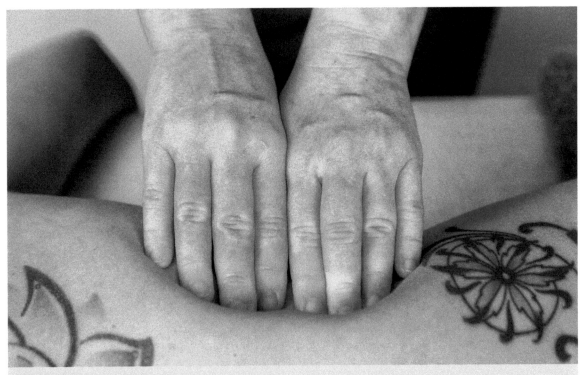

Figure 12.19
Fingertip friction to the lateral border of the erectors

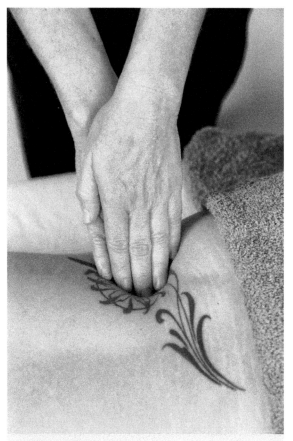

Figure 12.20
Treat the transverse process attachments of QL

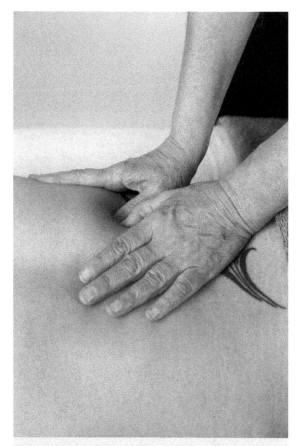

Figure 12.21
Treat the 12th rib attachments of QL

trigger points you find for 8–12 seconds. Explore this small space by orientating your fingers slightly towards the 12th rib or iliac crest. Your focus is underneath the bulk of the erector spinae muscles and towards the midline.

Always use static pressure first. If the muscle is not too tender you can add some slight cross fibre friction, working in one direction only. **See Figure 12.20**

- **Treat the 12th rib attachment:** turn your body so you are in t'ai chi stance and facing the head. Use thumbs to hook underneath and treat the insertion point of the QL on the 12th rib. Use static pressure first, treating any trigger points, then use cross fibre friction if appropriate. **See Figure 12.21**

- **Muscle strip the entire QL:** turn your body so that you are in t'ai chi stance and facing the client's feet. Muscle strip the side of the QL using thumbs or supported fingers, working towards the iliac crest. **See Figure 12.22, p. 212**

- **Treat the inferior attachment point on the iliac crest:** now treat the lower portion of the QL that attaches under the iliac crest. Make sure you push your thumbs under the bone and work from lateral to medial with static pressure and cross fibre friction. **See Figure 12.23, p. 212**

- **Deep effleurage to the QL with the palm of your hand and moving from superior to inferior:** in forward t'ai chi stance work down

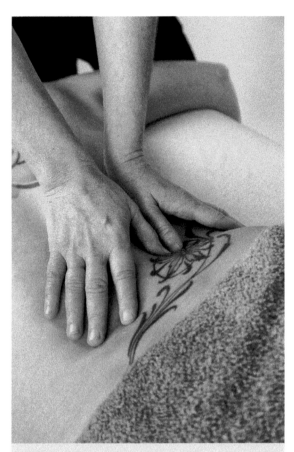

Figure 12.22
Muscle strip the entire QL

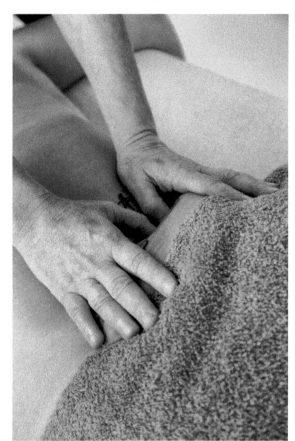

Figure 12.23
Inferior attachment point of QL

the side of the QL with the heel of your hand, gently pushing into the iliac crest at the end to stretch out the muscle.

- **Iliac scissors:** this is a gentle twisting stretch so make sure you always work with client communication. Stand at the side of the table in horse stance. You are working on the opposite side to the QL. Place your upper hand in the low back area between the 12th rib and the iliac crest so that you anchor down the QL. Your lower hand hooks around the iliac crest (hip bone). Take a deep breath and sit back pulling the iliac crest towards you so that you give the low back a gentle twist. Let the hand over the QL slide towards the table with the twist. **See Figure 12.24**

- **Work over the sacrum:** finish the whole sequence with further forearm or palmar effleurage of the entire back and work over the sacral area with the heel of your hand or supported thumbs/fingers.

- **QL stretch:** re-drape the body. This stroke is similar to the iliac scissors except this time you hold the stretch rather than letting the upper hand glide. Use horse stance and the same hand placement as for the iliac scissors technique. Take a deep breath and sit back pulling the iliac crest towards you so you give the low back a gentle twist. Make sure you keep the upper hand anchored down into the QL area. The sensation should feel like a push with one hand and a pull with the other. Work with client communication to find the edge of the stretch

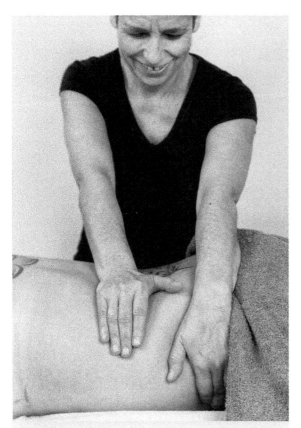

Figure 12.24
Iliac scissors

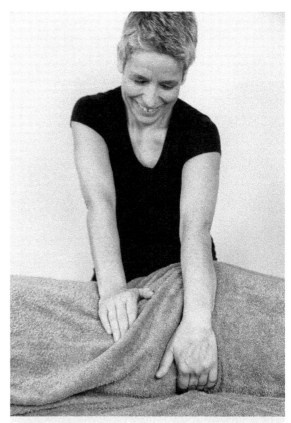

Figure 12.25
QL stretch

sensation and then wait and hold for a release. **See Figure 12.25**

Treating the gluteal muscles and lateral rotators

- **Opening up the gluteal muscles and the lateral rotators:** over the drape, in horse or forward t'ai chi stance, lean the soft part of your forearm into the glutes. Make sure you have a broad contact area with the whole of the forearm, i.e. you are not digging into the tissues with your elbow. Wait and hold in this place for the muscles to release. Your pressure should be straight down towards the table. Repeat so that the whole gluteal area is covered. **See Figure 12.26, p. 214**

- **Deep forearm effleurage to the gluteal area:** undrape the area and use a diagonal drape. Tuck the drape securely under your client's hip

and make sure you are not exposing the gluteal crease. In t'ai chi stance and facing the feet, anchor down the drape with your hand or the inside of your forearm. With the outside arm, work deeply into the area with deep forearm effleurage using the soft medial part of the forearm. **See Figure 12.27, p. 214**

- **Deep stripping with the knuckles:** make a soft fist and, in t'ai chi stance, use the backs of your knuckles to carry out deep stripping of the area, working from the sacrum down to the table **(see Figure 12.28, p. 214)**. A second option is to kneel on the opposite side of the table and strip down with your fist **(see Figure 12.29, p. 215)**. Take care not to trap your client's skin against the table at the end of each stroke.

- **Fingertip friction to the edge of the sacrum:** re-drape the body. Using supported thumbs or

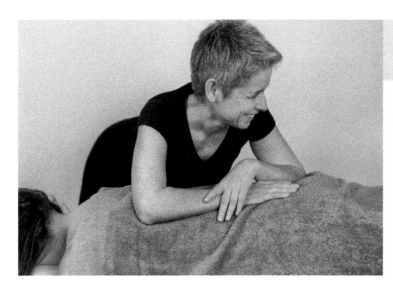

Figure 12.26
Opening up the gluteals and the lateral rotators

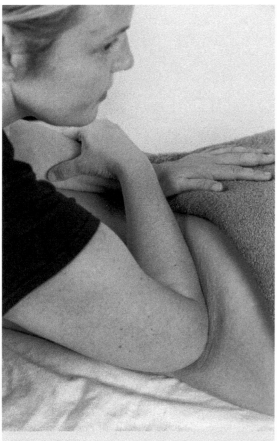

Figure 12.27
Deep forearm effleurage to the gluteals

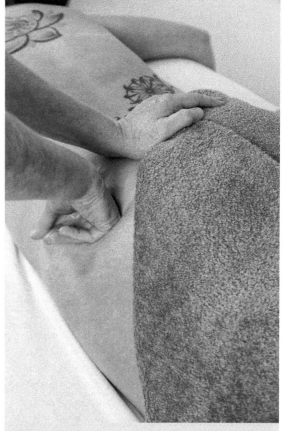

Figure 12.28
Deep stripping with the knuckles from same side

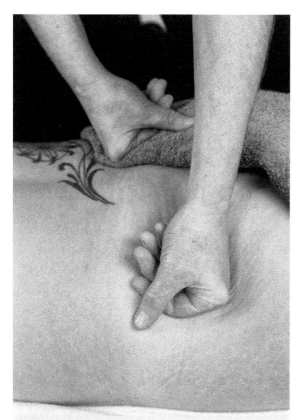

Figure 12.29
Deep stripping with the knuckles from opposite side

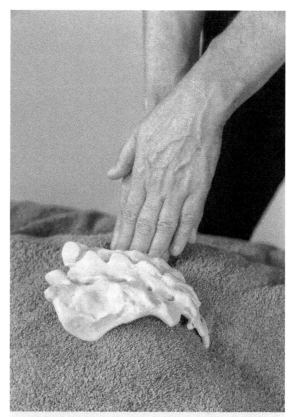

Figure 12.30
Fingertip friction to the edge of the sacrum

fingers, work the edge of the sacrum with cross fibre friction in one direction only. This addresses any trigger points that may be found near the attachments of the gluteus maximus. Cross to the other side of the table to work the opposite side of the sacrum. **See Figure 12.30**

- **Treating trigger points in the gluteal region:** now search for and treat the trigger points over the entire gluteal region. As the glutes are very thick, use a 'listening forearm' to explore the region first. Start about an inch down from the iliac crest, sinking into the glutes with your forearm and identifying any tight areas. When you find these, treat as trigger points and wait for a release. Work outwards and towards the side of the hip, then place your forearm on the next line down and work outwards in a similar manner. Repeat until the entire gluteal region is covered. Make sure you address the inferior aspect near the ischial

tuberosity where trigger points are likely to lurk. **See Figure 12.31, p. 216**

- **For more specific trigger point work:** go back to any tight areas and use a supported thumb or fingers to treat trigger points. You can also do very small friction strokes: apply pressure in one direction only with a light return stroke. Work with the fibres then across the fibres (like a mini 'sign of the cross'). **See Figure 12.32, p. 216**

Treating the piriformis

- **Static friction to the piriformis and lateral rotators:** flex the client's knee so that it is at a right angle and hold gently near the ankle with one hand. Use a t'ai chi stance: the leg nearest to the client's leg should be the one that is back. With your other hand, sink your soft fist into the middle of the gluteal area and drop down with your body weight

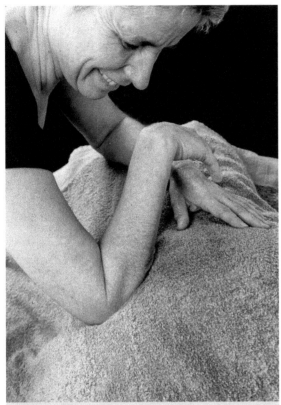

Figure 12.31
Treating trigger points in the gluteals

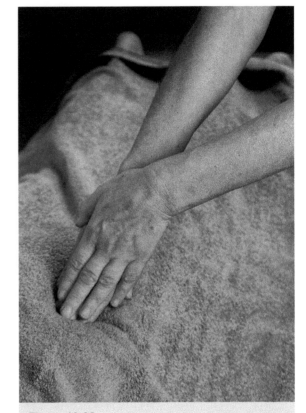

Figure 12.32
More specific trigger point work using supported thumbs

and intent to contact the piriformis and other lateral rotators. Move the client's leg back and forth slightly so that you incorporate internal and external rotation of the femur head.

● **Soft tissue release (STR) of the piriformis:** extend this manoeuver into a STR stretch of the piriformis. Use the heel of your hand or a soft fist into the piriformis area and lock into the muscle while stretching the leg away from the midline (pulling a pint). Hold for 2 seconds then release the stretch and repeat, treating the entire region with this 'lock and stretch' technique. If you need to do more specific work you can use a supported thumb and 'lock and stretch' in the same way. Always do broad work first before specific work.

Practise this stroke in rhythm **(see Figure 12.33):**

• Lock

• Stretch: 1, 2

• Release

• Replace

• Repeat.

● **Treating trigger points in the piriformis:** to treat these trigger points use t'ai chi stance and face the feet. Sink down through the gluteal muscles with supported fingers until you feel a 'speed bump'; this is the piriformis. 'Strum' across the muscle to help release. If you feel trigger points sink down with supported fingers until you feel a release. You can also work with supported thumbs, making sure you keep your hands flat on the body to protect your joints. **See Figure 12.34**

● **Static stretch of the piriformis – 'pulling a pint':** use the same hand positions as for STR (see earlier description). One fist locks down into the

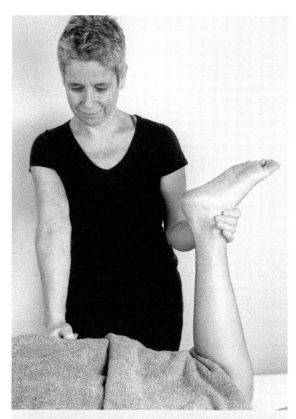

Figure 12.33
STR of the piriformis

piriformis and your other hand holds the leg around the ankle (Figure 12.33). Working with client communication, ask your client to breathe in. On their exhale take the leg toward you as if pulling a pint of beer. Ask your client to tell you when they can feel the stretch – this is very important as it may be more or less than you think. Hold the stretch for between 10 and 30 seconds, encouraging the client to breathe naturally during the stretch. For clients with knee problems, you can use the alternative hand position demonstrated with one hand around the client's thigh. **See Figure 12.35**

● Finish with deep forearm effleurage to the gluteal region or broad release work over the drape.

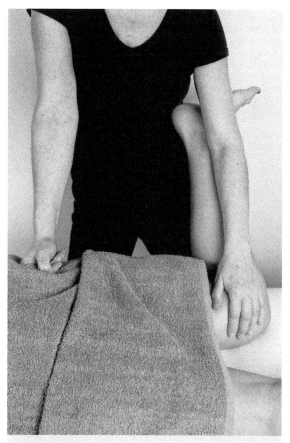

Figure 12.35
Alternative hand position for piriformis stretch

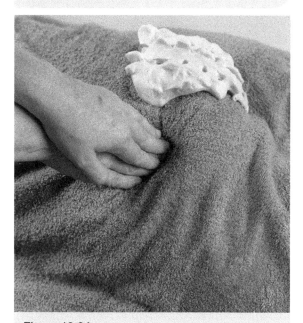

Figure 12.34
Treating trigger points in the piriformis

Treating the gluteus medius, minimus and tensor fasciae latae (TFL)

- Turn your client onto their side so that their hip is uppermost.

- **Palming:** these muscles are all found on the side of the hip. Kneel on the side of the table and lean into the area with your palms, focussing on any tight areas. You can also work the area with a soft forearm while standing in t'ai chi stance. **See Figure 12.36.**

- **Side-lying stretch for hip abductors:** the client lies on their side at the edge of the table; top leg hangs over the side of the table and the bottom leg is bent. The client's hips are stacked vertically, one on top of the other. If the client experiences any low back pain in this position, they can bend forward to round their low back area.

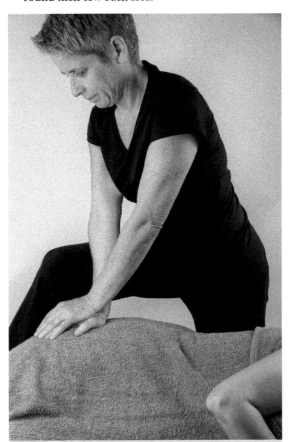

Figure 12.36
Palming gluteus medius, minimus and TFL

Stand behind the client for support and stabilise their hip with one hand. With the other hand press their thigh towards the floor so that their leg hangs off the side of the table. Make sure you work with client communication and their breath as you take them into the stretch. **See Figure 12.37**

Treating the psoas and iliacus

> **CAUTION**
>
> Psoas work is contraindicated during pregnancy

Be very clear to educate your client before you do this work. The abdominal region is a very sensitive area and the importance of this procedure should be explained before the work is done. Be aware that releasing the psoas can be uncomfortable and can also be a site for potential emotional release (as can any muscle in the body).

- Turn your client to be in a supine position.

- Drape the breasts and undrape the abdomen using the draping guidelines in the back to basics chapter (see Chapter 2). The following techniques can also be carried out over the drape if you are clear about where you are on the body.

- **Releasing the iliacus:** the client should flex their knee on the side where you are working. This position shortens and relaxes the iliacus and the psoas so that initial work in this area will not be too intense. With soft fingers, work along the inside rim of the pelvic bowl, waiting for the muscle to soften. Repeat on the other side. **See Figure 12.38, p. 220.**

- **Releasing the psoas:** have your fingers as soft as possible and slowly sink through the superficial tissue. Approaching lateral to the rectus abdominis and at an oblique angle is usually the easiest way of contacting the psoas (if you are not sure where this is get your client to do a small sit up and see the 'six pack' pop up).

> **CAUTION**
>
> If you feel a pulse you are too close to the aorta. Move your fingers slightly laterally. Remember never press on anything that presses back at you!

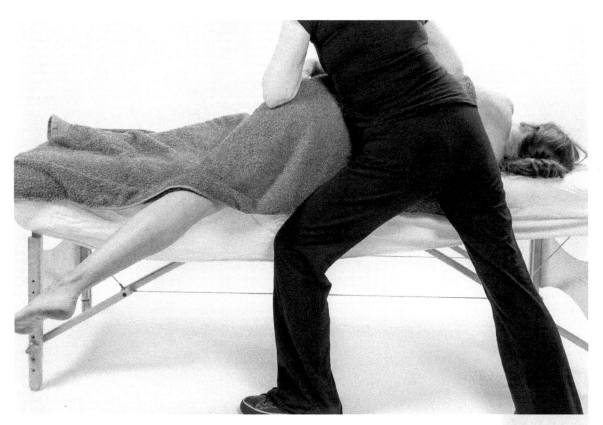

Figure 12.37

Hold static fingertip pressure on the psoas to release the trigger points. Work with the client's breath and be sure to always keep an eye on their face as the psoas is a common site for causing emotional release. **See Figure 12.39, p. 220.**

- **Psoas pin and stretch:** when you have felt some measure of release in the psoas you can finish the technique with a pin and stretch. With the knee still flexed in the triangle position and while keeping your fingertip pressure on the psoas, ask the client to breathe in and then on the exhale to slide their leg along the table until it is straight. Repeat this stroke up to three times to obtain maximum release.

- **Alternative psoas release methods:** although massage students have traditionally been taught to release trigger points in the psoas through palpating directly through the abdomen in this way, there have been recent suggestions in the bodywork community that this may be overly invasive and unnecessary. Here are some alternative methods for releasing the psoas:

- **Cross hand stretch:** the psoas can be released by a cross hand stretch over this area. Have one hand on the upper thigh and the other below the belly button, slightly lateral to the rectus abdominis. Tune into the tissues and follow the release through several barriers. **See Figure 12.40, p.220**

- **Psoas positional release:** place one hand as a listening hand over the psoas area to monitor the tissues. With the other hand, bring the client's hips into flexion and move them around slightly until you notice the place where the tissues start to soften (as felt by the monitoring hand on their belly). Fine-tune the position to find the point of maximal softening. When you have this 'sweet spot', just wait and hold until you feel a full release in the tissues. **See Figure 12.41, p. 221**

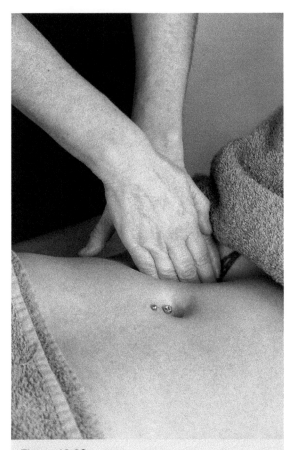

Figure 12.38
Releasing the iliacus

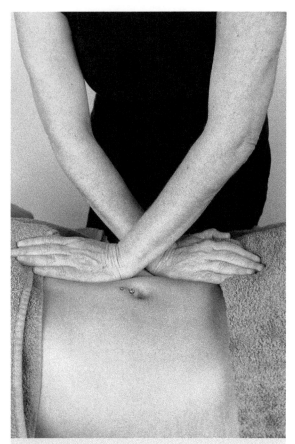

Figure 12.40
Cross hand stretch over psoas

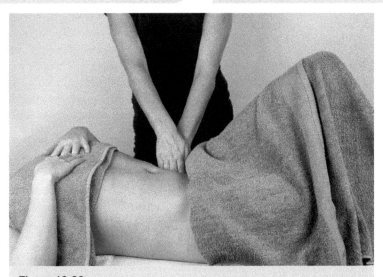

Figure 12.39
Releasing the psoas

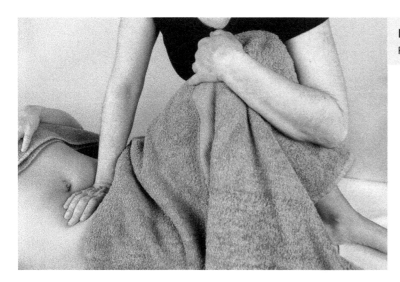

Figure 12.41
Psoas positional release

Acupressure points

Bladder 31–34 (BL 31–34): Upper Bone Hole, Second Bone Hole, Central Bone Hole and Lower Bone Hole

- Use your thumbs to treat local acupressure points BL 31–34 that are located in the sacral foramina (holes in the sacrum). Use static pressure and hold for several seconds. BL 31, 32, 33 and 34 together form the 'Eight Liao' points in Chinese medicine are all useful for local low back and sacrum problems. **See Figure 12.42**

Bladder 36 (BL 36): Support

- This is located in the middle of the transverse gluteal fold approximately where the hamstring insertion is found. This point is used for low back pain and sciatica where the pain runs down the back of the leg. Use supported fingers to apply pressure into the point in a direction towards the client's head. You can also use a soft elbow to work the point. **See Figures 12.43 and 12.44, p. 222**

Bladder 60 (BL 60): Kunlun Mountains

- While the client is supine you can treat acupressure point BL 60, which is found midway between the tip of the lateral malleolus and the Achilles tendon. Manipulate bilaterally with your thumb pressing in towards the midline. **See Figure 12.45, p. 223**

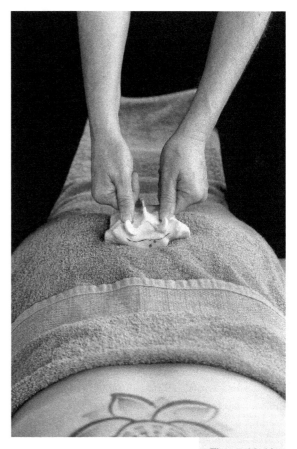

Figure 12.42

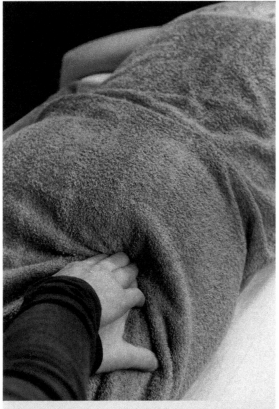

Figure 12.43
Acupressure point: Bladder 36 wtih supported fingers

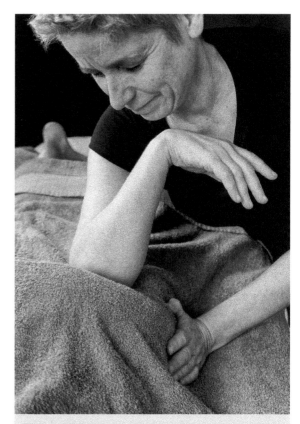

Figure 12.44
Bladder 36 with soft 'listening' elbow

Always finish with still work, holding your client's feet or head, grounding yourself and tuning in. This allows your client to absorb the changes in their body from the session – like saving your work on the computer.

Supine stretches and mobilisations

Gluteal stretch

● Take the corner of the drape and pull it under the thigh so that the client can hold the end of the drape for security. Get into kneeling t'ai chi stance on the table with your outside leg up at right angles and your foot flat on the table. Flex the client's leg at the knee and hip and place it into the fold of your thigh with your outside hand on their knee. Use the inside hand to hold down the other leg and press the client's flexed leg towards their belly by leaning

forward with the pelvis into a lunge. As always work with client communication and breath. **See Figure 12.46, p. 223**

Piriformis stretch

● Experiment with the starting point of the stretch as everyone will feel the muscle stretch in a different position. Flex the client's right hip and knee in a 'triangle position'. Place your client's left foot onto their right thigh in a 'figure-of-four' position. Now get into kneeling t'ai chi stance on the table and place the client's right foot into the fold of your thigh. Take both legs towards their head to stretch the left piriformis. Make sure your client keeps their sacrum on the table. This anchors one end of the piriformis to maximise the stretch. **See Figure 12.47, p. 224**

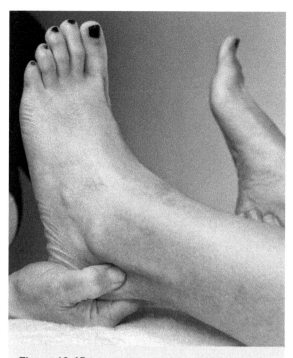

Figure 12.45
Acupressure point: Bladder 60

Mobilisations

- Either kneeling on the table or in standing t'ai chi stance, fold your client's knees to their chest and gently rock their low back with small rocking movements towards and away from their head. Your hands rest lightly on their knees. Use a rate of about one rock per second. If the client has a very sore low back do about 5–10 mobilisations then check in with them about comfort levels before continuing. **See Figure 12.48, p. 224**

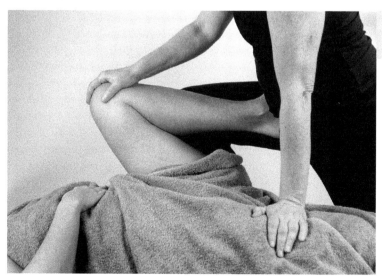

Figure 12.46
Gluteal stretch

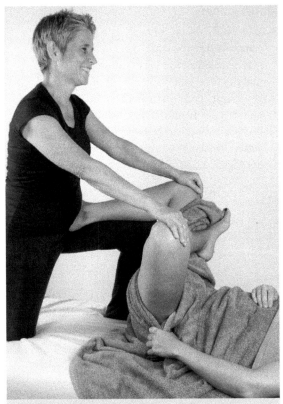

Figure 12.47
Piriformis stretch

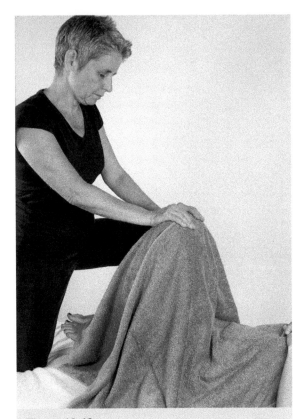

Figure 12.48
Mobilisations for low back

Teaching self-care suggestions for low back pain

Self-care suggestions for low back pain can be found in the Self-Care Resources (available at uk.singingdragon.com/catalogue/book/9781909141230).

Neck and shoulder pain protocol

Introduction

The following protocol can be used to good effect with many types of neck and shoulder pain including:

- Muscular neck and shoulder pain

- Acute and chronic herniated disc

- Headaches

- Temporomandibular joint (TMJ) pain (in conjunction with the techniques outlined in the TMJ chapter (see Chapter 18))

- Carpal tunnel and upper limb disorders (in conjunction with the techniques outlined in the carpal tunnel chapter (see Chapter 15)).

Heat and preparation work over the drape

- Start with your client in a prone position.

- Ensure your client's neck is in a comfortable position in the face cradle (generally slightly flexed downwards) and that their shoulders are relaxed.

- **Application of heat:** start by applying heat to the neck and shoulder area through stone placement or a heating pad.

- **Grounding**: as with all treatments, start by grounding yourself and with some connecting still work. Have one hand on the client's sacrum and the other between their shoulder blades. Take time to tune into what you feel, making a connection with your client.

- **Palming the erectors**: work down the erectors using the palming techniques described in Chapter 12. Use this time to assess areas of tightness and spend longer in these places, sinking into the tissue to start to release the muscles.

- **Paddy pawing the trapezius**: in kneeling t'ai chi stance, palm and compress the upper trapezius

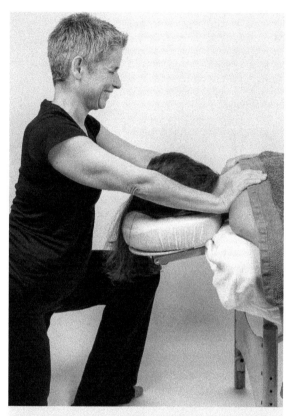

Figure 13.1
Paddy pawing the trapezius

working from the head of the table. Lean into the body using your body weight and an alternate rocking motion. Your arms should be straight to enable the maximum amount of weight transfer without effort, so move back if you are too close to the client's body. **See Figure 13.1**

Fascial techniques

- **Cross hand stretch**: in forward t'ai chi stance, with arms straight but soft, place your hands 3–5 inches apart in the area between the shoulder blades. Adjust your body so you are comfortable and spend

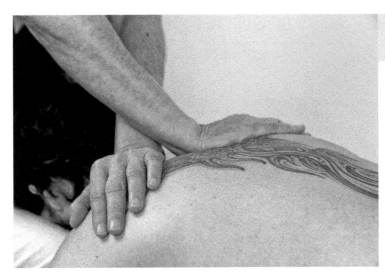

Figure 13.2
Cross hand stretch

time sinking down into the tissues. Once you have connected with the deeper myofascia, put a stretch on the tissues and tune into what is going on underneath your hands. Wait until you feel a release. The cross hand stretch technique can be repeated in different areas. **See Figure 13.2**

- **Direct fascial work with the fist to the trapezius and rhomboids**: in forward t'ai chi stance, sink down into the tissues using a soft fist. Use direct fascial strokes to work slowly through the trapezius and rhomboid area. **See Figures 13.3 and 13.4**

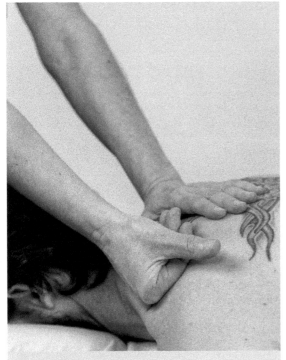

Figure 13.3
Direct fascial work with fist to trapezius

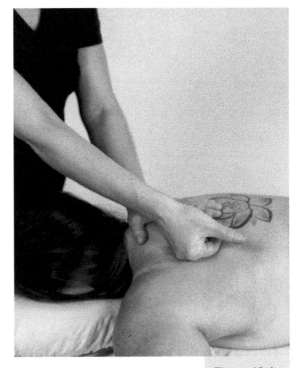

Figure 13.4

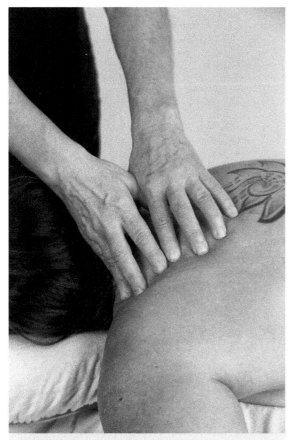

Figure 13.5
Fascial finger work to the upper back

fingers straight but relaxed and soft; your shoulder, elbow and wrist joints are stacked and in a line. Breathe energy up from the earth to your belly then shoot the energy up your spine and down your arms as you sink down into the tissues and slowly start to move through the fascia. You are always looking for the wonderful melting sensation of tissue release and any effort comes from your legs and Hara rather than your arms or hands. **See Figure 13.5**

- **Skin rolling over the back of the neck**. This feels amazing in this area. Stand side-on to the face cradle in forward t'ai chi stance to work the neck. Pick up a 'sausage' of skin and superficial fascia between your thumbs and fingers. Once the skin is pulled away, start to slowly push your thumbs forward, lifting the tissues in a smooth continuous motion while the 2nd and 3rd digits feed into this motion causing a rolling effect. The technique can be used over the neck and upper trapezius. Remember to work slowly giving time for restrictions to release. Pick up and roll the skin from one side of the neck, in a continuous motion, all the way over to the other side. **See Figure 13.6**

Muscular and trigger point techniques

Erector spinae

- **Broad work to the erector spinae group**: releasing this group of muscles is useful for relief from neck and shoulder problems as the erectors connect fascially to the galea aponeurotica that traverses the scalp (superficial back line (Myers 2001)).

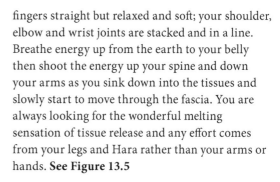

Figure 13.6
Skin rolling over the back of the neck

- **Fascial finger work to the upper back**: the same area can be worked more precisely with deep fascial finger work. Stand in t'ai chi stance and facing the area where you are working. Have your

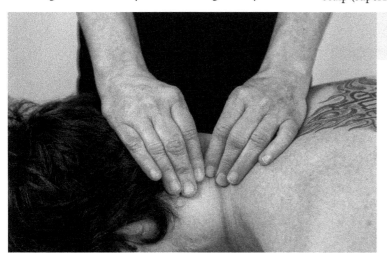

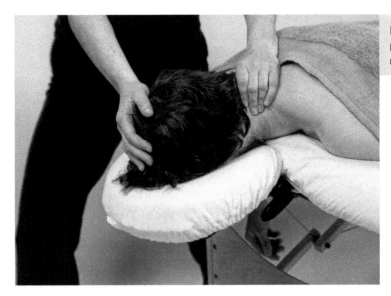

Figure 13.7
Broad work to the posterior cervical muscles

Using techniques from the low back chapter (see Chapter 12), spend some time releasing the erectors using fascial work, power effleurage, trigger point work and specific release to the medial and lateral borders.

Posterior cervical muscles

- **Broad work to the posterior cervical muscles**: in forward t'ai chi stance and facing the head, knead the posterior cervical muscles using pick up petrissage. Grasp the tissue at the back of the neck with a broad grasp: your thumb is at one side and your fingers at the other. Knead the tissues slowly and rhythmically. The hand that is not working rests on the top of your client's head. Move from your Hara so that the stroke is dynamic, with involvement from your whole body. **See Figure 13.7**

- Staying in the same same position, work under the occipital ridge with your thumb. Keep your fingers relaxed and curled around the client's neck. Your thumb presses gently up into the soft tissues under the occipital ridge on your side to compress these small muscles against the bone. Sink in gradually, using static pressure and treating any trigger points you find. Trigger points in the suboccipital muscles located under the skull are a common cause of headache and migraine pain. **See Figure 13.8**

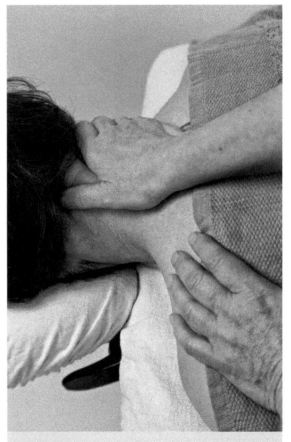

Figure 13.8
Working under the occipital ridge with the thumb

Work from lateral to medial, starting about four fingers width from the midline of the occiput. Once you have treated each point with static pressure you can use cross fibre friction with pressure in one direction only, working slowly and with a listening touch. Make sure you work with client communication as this area can be very tender.

- Staying on the same side of the body, now use your thumb to work down the neck and do more specific work. Sink down with your thumb through the outer layers of musculature until you feel the transverse processes of the cervical spine with their corresponding muscular attachments. These feel like hard tips and are often tender. Treat these points with static pressure, compressing and holding any trigger points. If the points are not too painful you can also follow up with cross fibre friction using very tiny movements.

This work is very specific and requires precision rather than extreme pressure. Your direction of pressure is in towards the midline rather than straight down. **See Figure 13.9**

Upper trapezius

- This precise work to the upper trapezius is best when the muscle is slightly shortened and slackened. This can be achieved by placing the client's arm on the face cradle or on a small stool underneath (or an arm cradle if you are lucky enough to have one on your table). If there is an issue with shoulder mobility, just put a small pillow under the client's shoulder and leave their arm in a neutral position. As always with these techniques, you are searching for and treating trigger points as you go along.

- The upper trapezius deserves some attention, according to Janet Travell, as it is the most frequent site of trigger point activity in the body. We work with the upper trapezius in three different ways:

  - **Compression**: using a pincer technique, grasp the tissue of the upper trapezius between your thumb and forefingers. Start right under the occiput and make sure you have the muscle between your fingers not just skin and fascia.

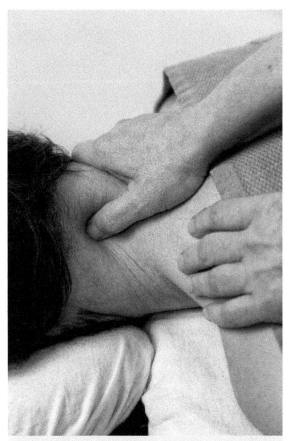

Figure 13.9
Working the cervical transverse process attachments

To achieve this you will need a firm (yet gentle) grip as the muscle has a tendency to slip out from under your fingers. Work down the upper trapezius towards the acromioclavicular (AC) joint; move one thumb width at a time and with static compression, treating any trigger points you find. **See Figure 13.10, see p. 230**

- **Money sign**: go back to the first position under the occiput and, with the same hand position, repeat the compression stroke but this time use a slight back and forth motion to gently roll the tissue between your thumb and forefinger (this is a similar movement to the universal sign language for 'Give me some money!').

- **Uncoiling the trapezius**: the upper trapezius furls over the clavicle like a monk's cowl, and

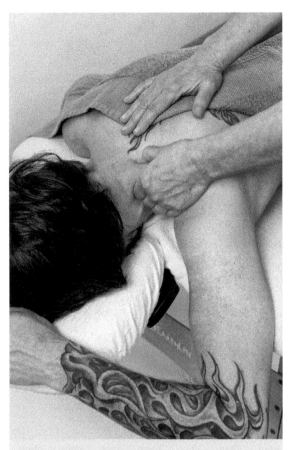

Figure 13.10
Compression and 'money sign' of the upper trapezius

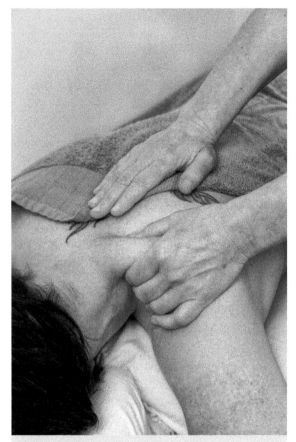

Figure 13.11
Uncoiling the upper trapezius

the commonly found forward head position can result in this tissue feeling tight and restricted. It feels amazing for the client if you roll back this tissue in the opposite direction. Hook your fingertips over the upper trapezius, with your thumb on the posterior tissue and your fingertips gently curled into the space between upper trapezius and clavicle. Use an uncoiling motion as if unrolling a piece of paper to bring the upper trapezius towards you. Repeat a few times. **See Figure 13.11**

Middle trapezius

- **Shearing the middle trapezius**: with the arm still overhead, move your thumbs down an inch or so to work the area of the middle trapezius. Use both hands to 'shear' and move the tissues between thumb and fingers to work the area thoroughly.

Both middle and upper trapezius house many relevant trigger points relating to complaints in the cervical region. **See Figure 13.12**

Attachments on the costal surface of the scapula

The costal surface of the scapula is the anterior surface that is usually positioned against the ribs. By pushing the scapula in a superior direction it is possible to access the costal surface at the superior angle where many a juicy trigger point can be found. There are several muscles that can be accessed on this part of the scapula, including the levator scapula, rhomboid minor and omohyoid.

These attachments can be treated by the following steps:

- Place the client's arm by their side. Never waste the opportunity to provide the client with a

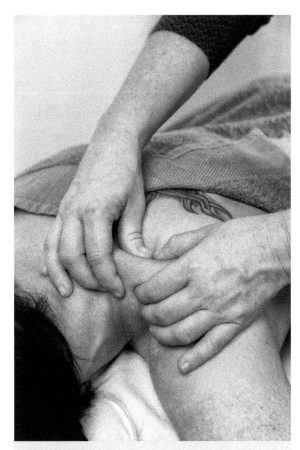

Figure 13.12
Shearing the middle trapezius

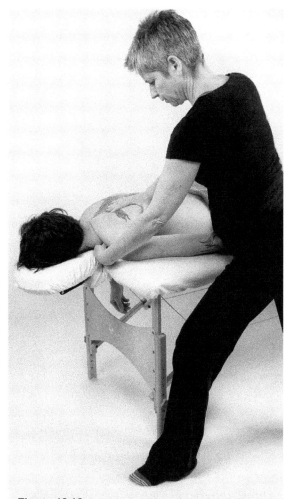

Figure 13.13
Treating the costal surface of the scapula

pleasurable experience by stretching their arm out to the side and then down towards their feet as you move it from one position to another. These little touches help to make your bodywork an elegant dance.

- In forward t'ai chi stance and facing the client's head, push the scapula in a superior direction (towards the head) with your lower hand so that the tip of the scapula is raised slightly above the ribs. **See Figure 13.13**

- Have your other hand positioned with the middle and index fingers in the space between the trapezius and the clavicle and with the back of your hand against the table. Your middle and index fingers should be pointing towards the ceiling. Use one or both of these fingers to press up onto the costal surface of the scapula. If you

are in the right place you should be able to feel bone underneath your fingertips as you press towards the ceiling. Compress the tissue against the bone with static pressure and then use gentle cross fibre friction. Treat any trigger points you find. **See Figure 13.14, p. 232**

- Finish by repositioning the client's arm over the side of the table; again use an elegant and mindful stretch to do this.

- Repeat the above steps on the opposite side, reversing hand and body positions.

- At this point you can now apply oil, wax or lotion.

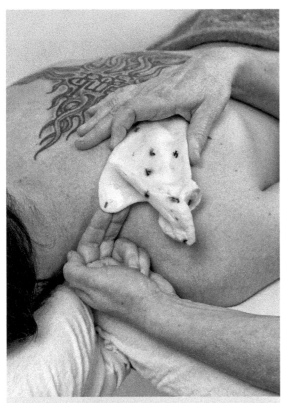

Figure 13.14
Attachments on the costal surface of the scapula

Broad work to the trapezius

- **Broad integration work to the trapezius**: after this very specific trigger point work you can now do some fantastic integrating forearm effleurage to the same region. Applying wax to your arms, kneel at the head of the table in kneeling t'ai chi stance and use the soft anterior part of your forearm to work from the neck out to the AC joint. Keep your wrists floppy and anchor under the occiput with your other hand. As always, the effort of the stroke comes from your Hara and you can use your whole body to lean into the movement. Repeat on the other side.
  See Figure 13.15

- Finish by taking the client's arm into a gentle trapezius stretch, stretching their arm laterally then down towards the feet before replacing their arm on the table.

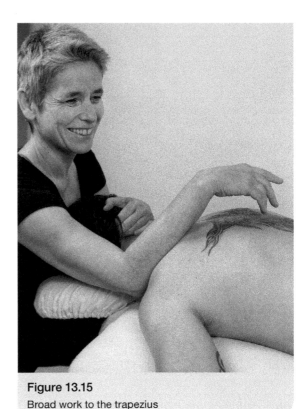

Figure 13.15
Broad work to the trapezius

Rhomboids

- Stand in t'ai chi stance at the opposite corner of the table to the rhomboids you are going to work with (in other words stand at the right corner to work the left rhomboids and vice versa). Muscle strip the rhomboids using supported fingers, thumb over thumb or flat thumb with heel of your hand on top. Treat any trigger points you find. Repeat on the other side. **See Figure 13.16**

Levator scapulae

- Have a clear visual in your mind of where this muscle is located as it can be difficult to isolate by palpation in the cervical area. Standing in t'ai chi stance at the head of the table, strip the levator scapulae from the cervical transverse processes to its attachment at the superior angle of the scapula (where it is much easier to feel). **See Figure 13.17**

- When you reach the superior angle attachment use static pressure and cross fibre friction to work the attachment point. **See Figure 13.18**

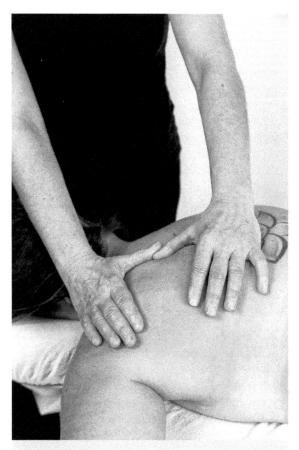

Figure 13.16
Stripping rhomboids

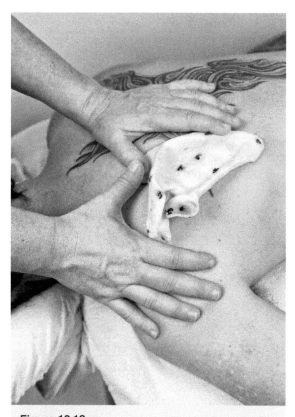

Figure 13.18
Superior angle attachment of the levator scapulae

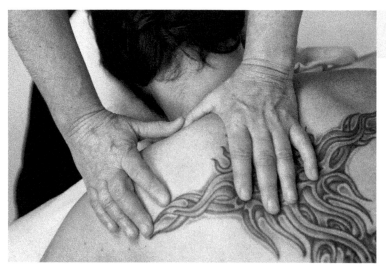

Figure 13.17
Stripping the levator scapulae

Prone pectoral stretch

- While your client is in the prone position you can take the opportunity to give them this great pectoral stretch. Ask your client to place their hands behind their head. Hold their elbows while you get into a low horse stance. Ask your client to take a deep breath in and on the exhale raise their elbows towards the ceiling (with their hands still on back of their head) until they feel the stretch. Hold for 10–30 seconds. Remember both of you need to keep breathing! **See Figure 13.19**

Finishing the prone work

- Finish off the prone work with your own unique combination of strokes to nurture and relax your client and integrate your work. This can include power effleurage, palming or still work. Have fun and be creative!

Side-lying trapezius and scalenes work

- Now turn your client onto their side. For side-lying, your client's legs should be in a figure-of-four position. Bolster under the head and between the legs, making sure the spine is in alignment. It is common for the client to roll forwards or backwards in this position, so make sure their head is aligned with their shoulders and their shoulders are aligned with their hips.

- To work the client's right side they should be lying on their left side with the right side uppermost. Stand at the side of the table in t'ai chi stance facing your client's back. Reach around under their arm with your right hand and hold the front of their shoulder with your fingers curled softly around the top of the shoulder. Make sure your client is resting the weight of their arm on yours and is not holding any tension in the area. If you sense they are not giving you their full weight make a gentle suggestion such as 'Make your arm really heavy for me' and give them positive reinforcement when they do this. This verbal cue works much better than saying 'Relax your arm!' which, paradoxically, usually makes clients tense up. (*Trying* to relax is a bit of a contradiction in terms.)

- With your other (left) hand support the back of their head at the occiput. Use your body weight to lean back into your back leg and give the trapezius a nice full stretch. You can release and repeat this a few times as it feels amazing! **See Figure 13.20**

- Release the stretch but keep your right hand in the same position supporting the client's shoulder. Now use the soft side of your left forearm to give a deep effleurage and stretch to the trapezius and scalenes. Start with the shoulder in a slackened position and lean back as you use your left forearm to work the area. **See Figure 13.21**

- **Now use your fist to strip the trapezius and scalenes**: take the stroke all the way to the occipital ridge. Use your right hand to pull back on the client's shoulder to create space and give a stretch as you work. Make sure your fist is soft as if it were holding an egg rather than ready to start a fight! **See Figure 13.22**

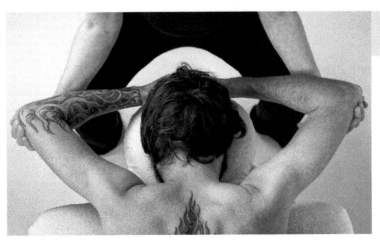

Figure 13.19
Prone pectoral stretch

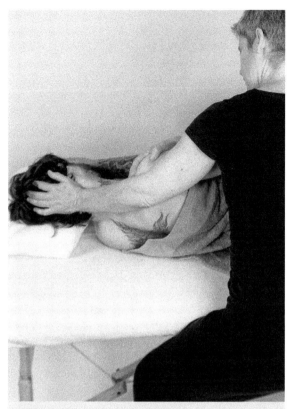

Figure 13.20
Sidelying stretch for trapezius and scalenes

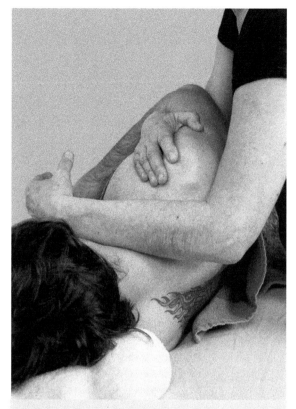

Figure 13.21
Sidelying forearm work

● **Soft tissue release to the trapezius:** now use the hand cradling the shoulder girdle to put the trapezius on a slack by pushing the client's shoulder towards their ear. Use your other hand to lock into a point on the tissue under the occipital ridge. Once you have a lock on the tissue then lean back so that you put the tissue into a stretch. Hold the stretch for 2 seconds then release and find another point and repeat the process. Repeat on several points

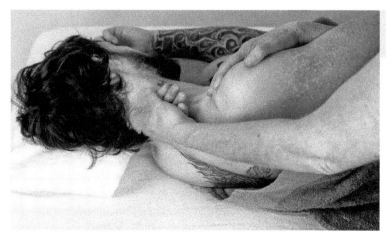

Figure 13.22
Sidelying fist work

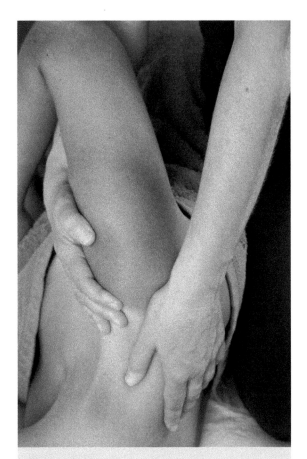

Figure 13.23
STR to trapezius and scalenes

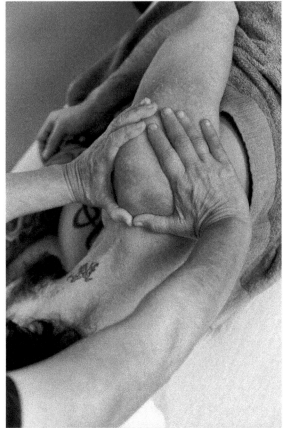

Figure 13.24
'Jing triangle'

along the occipital ridge and then along the trapezius and scalenes.

- Once you have the hang of this you should be able to carry out the process in a flowing rhythm (**see Figure 13.23**):

  - Lock

  - Stretch: 1, 2

  - Release

  - Replace.

- **'Jing triangle'**: stand at the head of the table in t'ai chi stance. Put your hands together to form a triangle with the thumbs and index fingers touching. With this hand position frame the shoulder at the AC joint so that your fingers are resting on the deltoid and your thumbs on the trapezius. This position enables your hands to be

supported as you do this stroke. Use your thumbs to give cross fibre friction to the trapezius, moving the tissue laterally. Work back towards the occiput with each stroke. As you get closer to the occiput switch to using supported fingers instead to do the stroke. **See Figure 13.24**

- **Supported shoulder circumduction**: go back to the shoulder cradle position and put the shoulder through a rotational movement. Complete two or three circular movements, letting the movements come from your legs, feet and Hara, and using your body weight to give a full range of motion (ROM) to the scapula. **See Figure 13.25**

Working the vertebral border of the scapula

- Leave your right hand in the same position of cradling the shoulder and come down into kneeling t'ai chi stance. Place the thumb of your left hand

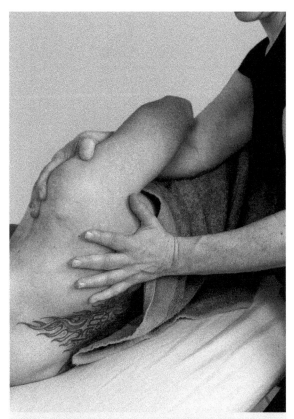

Figure 13.25
Supported shoulder circumduction

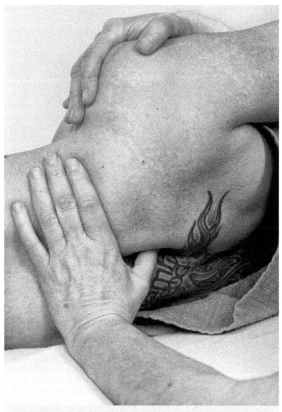

Figure 13.26
Working the vertebral border of the scapula

underneath the medial (vertebral) border of the scapula. Use your front (right) hand to push the scapula towards the back of the body (by leaning back with your body weight) and the thumb of your left hand should disappear slightly under the scapula to enable you to work the soft tissue there without too much effort. Use static compression and work any trigger points you find.

- To protect your thumbs make sure you keep the carpometacarpal (CMC) joint flat against the body. Alternatively, use a supported thumb by making a soft fist; many Jing therapists also love to use a trigger point stone for this technique.
  See Figure 13.26

- Work the client's left side by turning them and repeating the above steps. Then turn your client to be in a supine position.

- **Grounding**: with your client in a supine position, start by holding their head in your hands and tuning into your breath, Hara and sense of your feet against the ground. **See Figure 13.27, p. 238**

Cervical lamina groove

- Sit at the head of the table using a wide seated stance with feet firmly rooted. Your client's head should be at least an inch from the end of the table. Use this time to make sure your client is giving you the full weight of their head. If you feel they are not, encourage them with verbal prompts such as 'Make your head heavy' or 'Let me take the full weight of your head.'

- Using a small amount of lubrication (or none if you wish this stroke to be more of a fascial stroke), place your fingertips at the base of the neck with your fingertips curled upwards and the backs of your hands against the table. Slowly pull back from

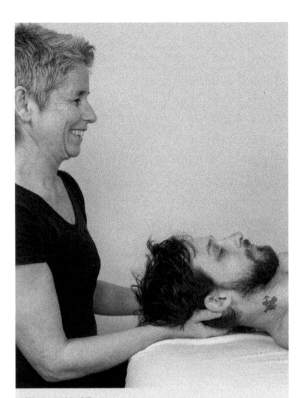

Figure 13.27
Grounding and still work

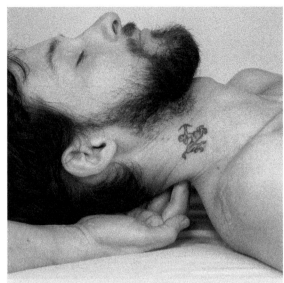

Figure 13.28
Working the cervical lamina groove

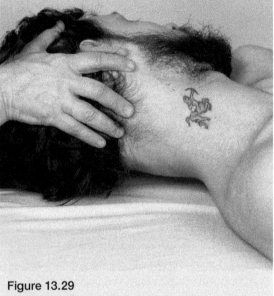

Figure 13.29
Turning the head to expose the scalenes

inferior to superior with fingertips pressing up into the posterior cervical region. Lean your body back as you do this. The key here is to work slowly and precisely.

- As you carry out this stroke, aim for a smooth wave of continuous cervical movement. Tell your client 'Let your head move' if they are holding tension in the neck as you work. This translation and extension movement is the normal and appropriate ROM for these cervical facet joints. **See Figure 13.28**

Scalenes

- Gently traction the head by hooking under the occiput and leaning back. On your client's out breath turn their head to their left side. **See Figure 13.29**

- Muscle strip the right scalenes, using your right hand. First use a soft fist to do broad work to the area and then use your thumb to work in the area between the sternocleidomastoid (SCM) and the trapezius. Treat any trigger points you may find. This is a very important area to work in cases of

referred pain down the arm or carpal tunnel type symptoms. **See Figure 13.30**

- The cervical transverse processes can also be treated from this position. Bring your chair to more of an angle at the corner of the table.

- Using the fingers of your right hand have the fingernails against the lateral border of the SCM

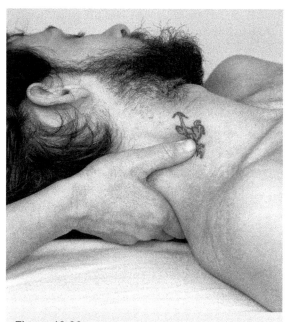

Figure 13.30
Stripping the scalenes

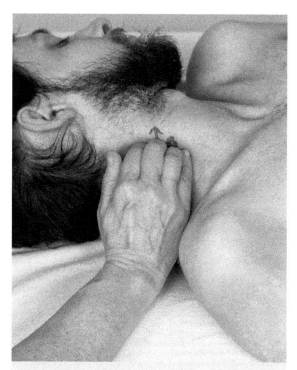

Figure 13.31
Treating anterior cervical transverse processes

and push it slightly superiorly towards the ceiling, so that your finger pads can now contact the tissue normally hidden underneath. If you press gently down towards the table you should be able to feel the anterior surface of the cervical transverse processes where the attachments of the scalenes are located. Use your fingers to apply static pressure. This area can be very tender to treat so take care to communicate with your client and work within their tolerance range. Keep your hand in the same position and apply gentle pressure using one finger at a time – initially your first finger, then the middle finger and then the fourth – so you are able to treat precisely the transverse process attachments. Remember that the nerve bundle of the brachial plexus is in this area so release pressure if the client experiences any shooting or tingling sensations in their neck or down their arms, as this can mean you are on the brachial plexus itself. Use static compression followed by micro cross fibre friction. **See Figure 13.31**

Posterior suboccipitals

Although we have already done some work on the posterior suboccipitals during the client prone position,

this is such an important area that it deserves more attention. By using your sense of listening touch you will be able to palpate and treat each muscle individually. When treating these muscles be very precise and ensure you have located the attachments. Communicate with your client to maintain the correct pressure as most people hold a great deal of tension here and it is the cause of many headache related complaints.

- Gently turn the client's head and move to the side where you are working. To work the client's right side have your chair more towards the corner of the table.

- With your left hand supporting the top of the client's head, use your right thumb to apply pressure deep into the soft tissue at the base of the skull. Work each muscle individually and move medially to laterally between the occiput and C1. Then drop down one thumb width and work between C1 and C2. Use static pressure then cross fibre friction working both with and against the fibres (up and down and side to side – like a miniature 'sign of the cross').

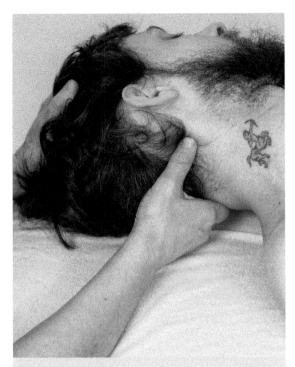

Figure 13.32
Posterior suboccipitals

- Another great way of applying pressure is to use your left hand to move the client's head onto your thumb slightly as you work. **See Figure 13.32**

- Repeat on the other side. Then bring the client's head back to neutral and repeat the translation and extension release.

Sternocleidomastoid (SCM)

The SCM is a key muscle to work for headache complaints, including migraine type pain and jaw issues such as TMJ disorder.

- Move your chair back so that you are sitting at the head of the table. To work the right SCM turn the client's head slightly to the right and bring it a little closer to their shoulder. This puts the SCM on a slack and makes it easier to grasp for trigger point work.

- Rest your right forearm on the table and have your left hand on the head. Use a pincer grasp to gently squeeze and compress the SCM, starting up by the mastoid process. Work slowly as this muscle can be exquisitely tender. As you work down to the clavicular attachment to where the belly gets thinner you can pronate your hand to grasp the muscle. Work with care as the carotid artery is in this region. As ever, don't press on anything that presses back at you! **See Figure 13.33**

- **Working the attachment points**: to work the attachment points on the sternum and clavicle you can hook in with a downward pressure.

Figure 13.33
Pincer grasp on SCM

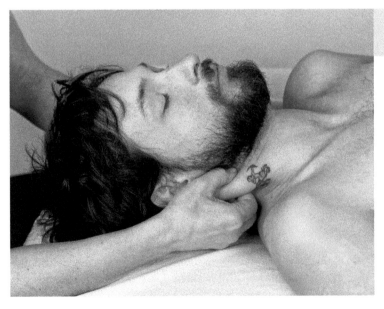

- To finish off use a claw-like hand and rake into the muscle above the point where the sternal and clavicular heads divide. Sweep upward to the occiput (the cranial fascia anchors around the ear). Use static pressure to work the attachment points around the mastoid process.

- Repeat on other side.

Acupressure points in the prone position

The following are three classic acupressure points for treating neck and shoulder pain. The acupressure points can be used at any stage in the prone protocol.

> **CAUTION**
>
> In general, avoid the use of acupressure points in pregnancy as some have a strong descending energy

Gall Bladder 21 (GB 21): Shoulder Well

- **Location**: on the shoulder directly above the nipple and at the highest point of the shoulder. This is a great local point for occipital headache and quickly releases tight trapezius muscles and neck/shoulder pain.

- **Contraindicated**: pregnancy.

- To treat GB 21, in kneeling t'ai chi stance, find the midpoint of the trapezius muscle (more or less

halfway between the place where the neck joins the shoulder and the AC joint). You can work the point bilaterally (both sides at once), so with straight arms sink your thumbs into the tissue (which usually feels hard and tender). Your intention is down towards the feet. Hold the point for 3–5 breaths. Tune into the energy of the point and, as you develop your skills of listening touch, you will be able to feel the energy dissipating and the tissue softening and releasing with your touch. **See Figure 13.34**

Colon 16 (also known as Large Intestine 16): Great Bone

- **Location**: in the depression between the acromion and the scapular spine. A good local point for shoulder pain.

- To find Co 16, move your thumbs laterally along the trapezius towards the AC joint. Just before you reach the actual joint you will feel a small dip or hollow. Press gently into this point with your thumbs; again the direction of your focus is down towards your client's feet. Hold the point for 3–5 breaths. **See Figure 13.35, p. 242**

Gall Bladder 20 (GB 20): Wind Pool

- **Location**: in a depression under the occiput between the upper portion of the SCM muscle and the trapezius. A great point to treat headaches, especially occipital related, and pain in the neck or shoulders.

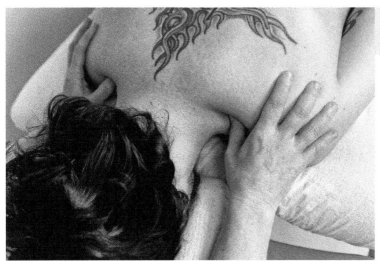

Figure 13.34
Acupressure point GB 21

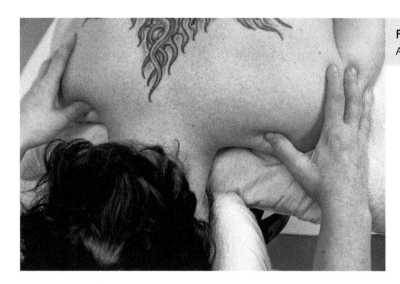

Figure 13.35
Acupressure point Co 16

- To treat GB 20 place your hands over your client's head and hook your third fingers over the skull and into the base of the occiput. You should feel a small hollow between the attachment of the trapezius on the occiput and the SCM on the mastoid process. Lean slightly back so your fingers are pressing up into the point. Hold for 3–5 breaths.
See Figure 13.36

Small Intestine 11 (SI 11): Celestial Gathering

- **Location**: on the scapula in a depression at the centre of the infrascapular fossa, found at the

junction of the upper and middle third between the lower scapular spine and the inferior angle of the scapula. This is a fantastic point for releasing the fascia on the scapula and the whole shoulder girdle. This point is also believed to be helpful for any pain along the Small Intestine meridian that runs along the back of the arm, elbow, face and jaw. To treat SI 11 place a supported thumb in the centre of the scapula where you will usually find a small depression. Hold pressure for 3–5 breaths until you feel a release. **See Figures 13.37 and 13.38**

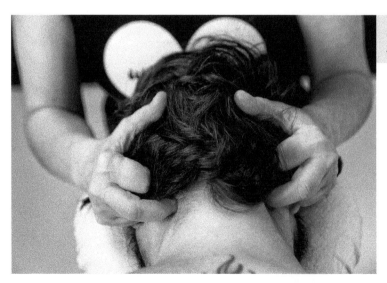

Figure 13.36
Acupressure point GB 20

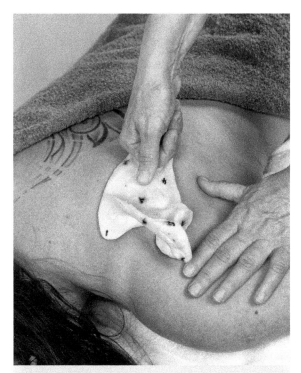

Figure 13.37
Location of acupressure point SI 11

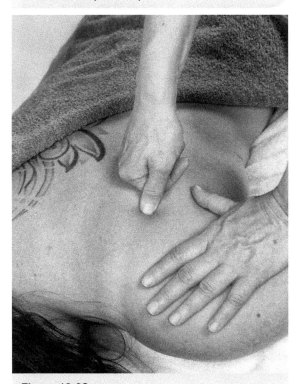

Figure 13.38
Acupressure point SI 11: treatment

Stretches and mobilisations

Manual traction

● Return the head to a neutral position and hook your fingers under the occiput. Gently traction the head back towards you with your fingers in the occiput and while leaning backwards slightly. **See Figure 13.39**

Cervical flexion (neck extensor stretch)

● Hold your client's head with your fingers pointing towards their feet. Lift their head and as you do so swivel your hands so that your fingers are now pointing towards the top of their head, i.e. you should be holding their head like a basketball that you are just about to shoot. The heel of your hands should fit snugly under the client's occiput. Have your elbows on the table and take the client's head

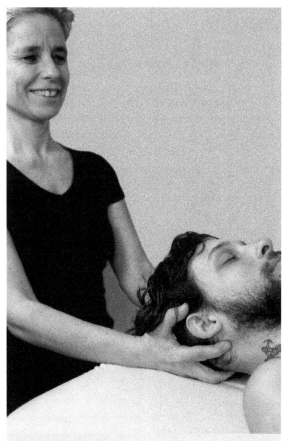

Figure 13.39
Manual traction

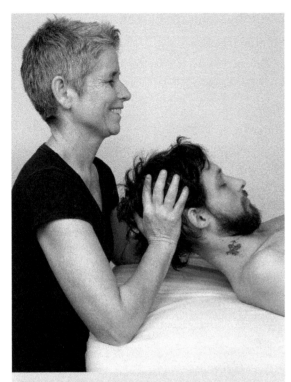

Figure 13.40
Cervical flexion (neck extensor stretch)

towards their chest. You can do this without straining yourself by keeping your elbows on the table and slowly drawing them closer together to increase the stretch. Make sure your client is giving

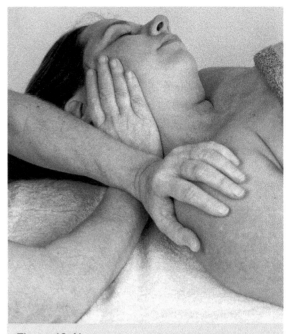

Figure 13.41
Lateral flexion (scalenes stretch)

you the full weight of their head and not doing the movement for you. **See Figure 13.40**

Lateral flexion (scalene stretch)

- Stand or sit at the head of the table. Hold the client's head in your hands. Ask the client to take a deep

Figure 13.42
Cervical mobilisation

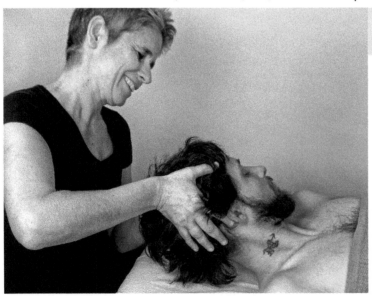

breath and on their out breath bring their ear to their shoulder, keeping their nose pointed to the ceiling. When they have reached the end of their ROM, replace your hands so they are crossed with one hand on the shoulder and one on the side of the head. Get your client to take a breath in and out and take them into a stretch, always working with client communication. Hold for 10–30 seconds. **See Figure 13.41**

Cervical mobilisation

- Carry out a gentle figure-of-eight cervical rotation within the client's comfortable ROM. **See Figure 13.42**

- Finish in your own unique way. **See Figure 13.43**

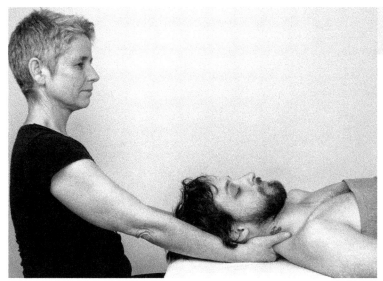

Figure 13.43
Finish in your own unique way

Teaching self-care suggestions

Self-care suggestions can be found in the Self-Care Resources (available at uk.singingdragon.com/catalogue/book/9781909141230).

Reference

Myers T 2001 Anatomy Trains. Edinburgh: Churchill Livingstone.

14

Shoulder girdle pain protocol

Introduction

This protocol can be used to good effect for a number of common musculoskeletal conditions including:

- Frozen shoulder (adhesive capsulitis)
- Rotator cuff injury
- Painful arc syndrome
- Sporting injuries
- Supraspinatus tendinosis.

Heat and preparation work over the drape

- Start with your client in a prone position.
- As we always like to start a treatment with broad work it is good practice to begin with the initial techniques from the low back protocol, such as palming, broad power effleurage and releasing the erectors.
- Depending on the condition you are treating, work on the shoulder girdle will often also incorporate strokes from the neck and shoulder and forearm and wrist protocols.
- Apply hot or cold appropriately at the beginning of the session through a heating pad, stones or other methods.

Fascial work (no oil or wax)

- **Deep fascial work with fists**: start with deep fascial work with fists down the erectors.
- You can also adapt this stroke to work the trapezius and supraspinatus. Stand in t'ai chi stance on the opposite side of the table to where you are working (i.e. stand on the right side of the client to treat their left trapezius/supraspinatus). With your left

hand acting as a still mother hand, use your right hand to sink slowly down into the tissue and work from the medial to the lateral side (start next to the neck and work out towards the acromioclavicular (AC) joint). The trapezius is more superficial, so work this with your initial strokes and then focus your intention deeper to affect the supraspinatus. **See Figure 14.1**

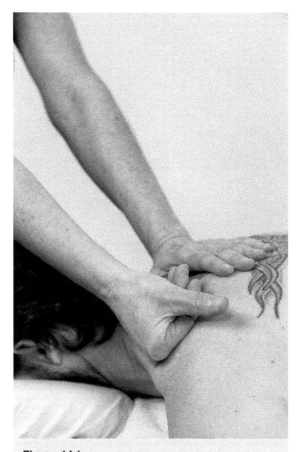

Figure 14.1
Deep fascial work with fists

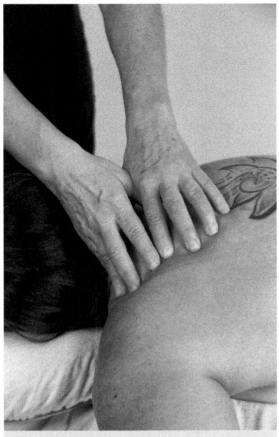

Figure 14.2
Fascial finger work

- **Fascial finger work**: you can also do more specific direct fascial work with the fingers over the rhomboids and infraspinatus area. Have the four fingers of both hands relaxed but with a sense of a springy tensile strength, i.e. there is softness and a slight bend to the joints but they are not floppy. In forward t'ai chi stance with straight arms, line up your fingers and breathe energy up from the earth and through your legs to your belly. Then, with the outbreath, shoot the energy out up your spine, down your arms and out your fingers. Use this energetic sense of intention to slowly work through the tissue with all eight fingers aligned. Remember the effort always comes from the legs and the Hara and not the arms and hands. Keep your shoulders soft and relaxed. Continually check into your body; if you feel yourself tense, straining or using more effort than necessary, simply return your attention to your breath and Hara and feel the power coming from there. **See Figure 14.2**

- **Skin rolling**: this feels great over the scapula, rhomboids and upper back. **See Figure 14.3**

- **Cross hand stretches**: these can also be used around the area, for example:

  - Between the shoulder blades

  - One hand on the back of the scapula, one on the upper arm. **See Figure 14.4**

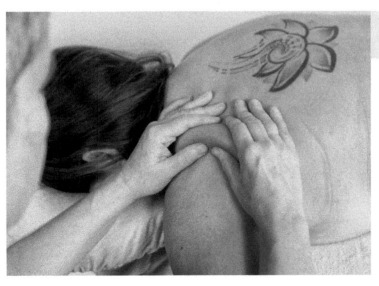

Figure 14.3
Skin rolling over the scapula

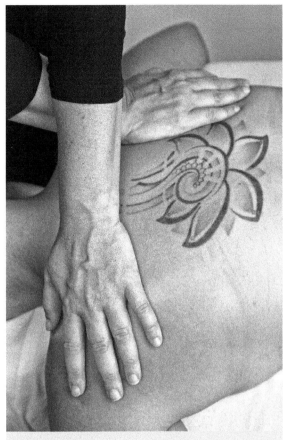

Figure 14.4
Cross hand stretch

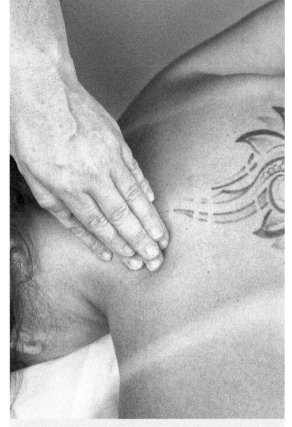

Figure 14.5
Stripping supraspinatus

Muscular and trigger point work

In this section you are treating all the trigger points around the joint according to the treatment principles outlined in Chapter 8.

Supraspinatus

- Stand in t'ai chi stance at the opposite side of table to where you are working. To work the left supraspinatus stand on the client's right side. Using a small amount of wax or oil, muscle strip the supraspinatus from medial to lateral using supported fingers. Work superior to the spine of the scapula and remember that this muscle lies DEEP to the upper trapezius; therefore, focussed deep pressure will be needed. Use your body weight and focus to achieve this and NOT your thumb, hand or arm strength. Treat any trigger points you find. **See Figures 14.5 and 14.6 (p. 250)**

Rhomboids

- From the opposite side of the table, in t'ai chi stance and using supported thumbs or fingers, strip the rhomboids from the spine to the medial border of the scapula. Follow the direction of the muscle fibres and treat any trigger points you find. **See Figure 14.7, p. 250**

Infraspinatus

- Now come to the same side of the table (i.e. the client's left side) to strip the left infraspinatus. Work in the direction of the muscle fibres and then turn your body to work across the fibres. Hold static pressure on trigger points. **See Figures 14.8 and 14.9, p. 251**

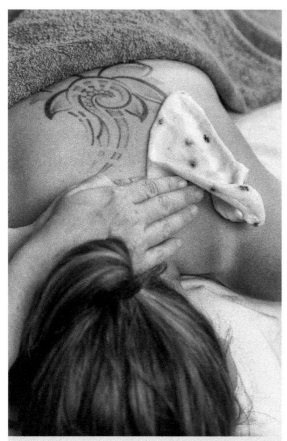

Figure 14.6
Location for stripping the supraspinatus

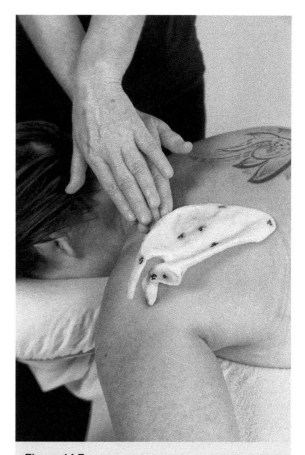

Figure 14.7
Stripping rhomboids

Scapula mobilisation

- **Rotation of the shoulder girdle**: in a low t'ai chi stance, support underneath the anterior surface of the shoulder girdle with your left hand and place your right hand on the posterior scapula. Coming from your whole body, take the shoulder into rotation 3–4 times in each direction.
  See Figure 14.10

- **Scapula sawing**: keeping your lower (left) hand supporting the shoulder, now turn your right hand sideways and slide the ulnar border (i.e. thumb side is towards the ceiling) along the soft tissue at the medial border of the scapula. Use a gliding and sawing motion and follow with the forearm. Work towards the client's head and then back to you. The effort comes from your Hara so

you are moving your whole body as you do this.
See Figure 14.11, p. 252

Deltoids: anterior, middle and posterior fibres

- Take your client's arm to hang over the table by giving it a nice lateral stretch, and then replace it on the table.

- **Posterior fibres of the deltoid**: let your client's arm hang over the side of the table. You are kneeling or seated so you can work all three heads of the deltoid, one at a time, from superior to inferior. Use your right hand to support the arm under the elbow and naturally cup the deltoid with the fingers and thumb of your left hand. Your thumb is now in position to work the posterior and middle deltoid from superior to inferior. Start by the attachment of the deltoid on the spine of the scapula and work

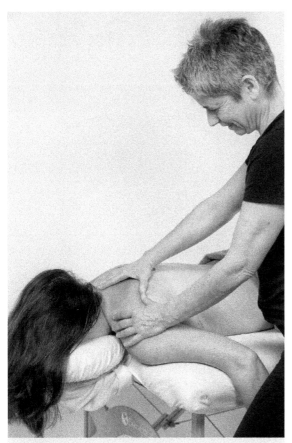

Figure 14.8
Stripping the infraspinatus

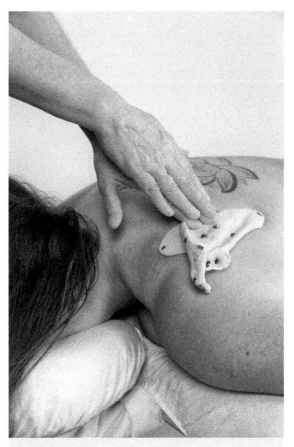

Figure 14.9
Location of the infraspinatus

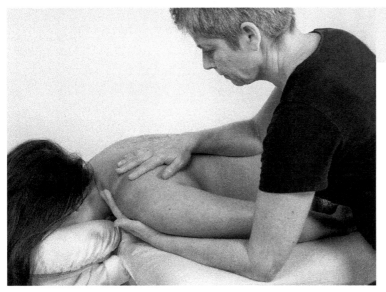

Figure 14.10
Rotation of the shoulder girdle

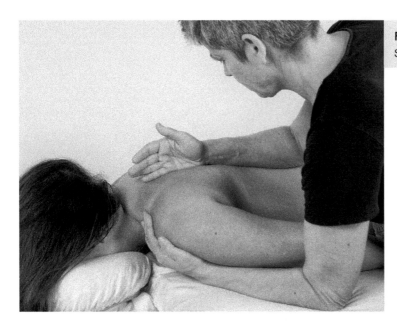

Figure 14.11
Scapula sawing

down the muscle in lines searching for and treating trigger points as you find them. The deltoid spans approximately the top one-third of the humerus, so if you go further down the arm you will be working the triceps (nothing wrong with that but just know where you are). **See Figure 14.12**

- **Anterior fibres of the deltoid**: change the orientation of your body so you are now in kneeling (or sitting) stance and facing towards the feet. From

this position you will be able to cup your hands around the arm to work the anterior fibres of the deltoid with your thumbs. It is more difficult to work the anterior deltoid when the client is in the prone position so we will also return to this area when the client is supine. **See Figure 14.13**

- When you have worked the deltoid belly, friction the tendon attachment found at the inferior end of the muscle, approximately one-third to halfway

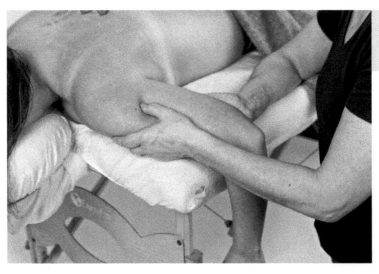

Figure 14.12
Treating posterior and middle heads of the deltoid

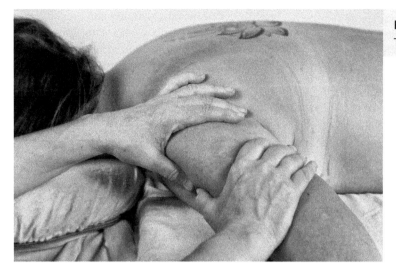

Figure 14.13
Treating the anterior head of the deltoid

down the humerus. Use cross fibre friction with pressure in one direction only and a light return stroke. **See Figure 14.14**

- **Stripping the deltoid**: in t'ai chi stance, muscle strip the entire muscle from distal to proximal (bottom to top). Use supported fingers followed by broad work with a soft fist. **See Figure 14.15**

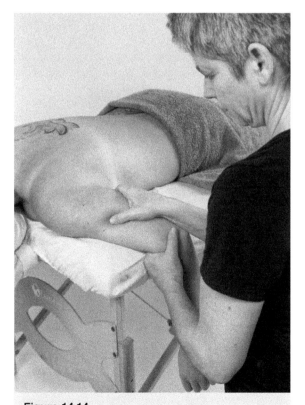

Figure 14.14
Friction to the deltoid tendon

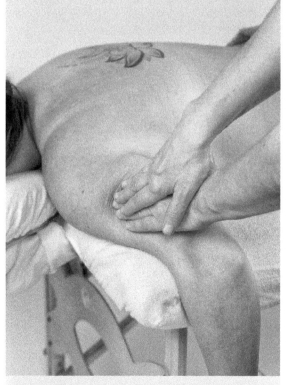

Figure 14.15
Stripping the deltoid

Triceps

- **Broad work to the triceps**: in a seated or kneeling stance, work the triceps broadly with the soft side of your forearm. Hold underneath with your left hand and work the area with your right forearm, leaning into the stroke. Remember to keep your wrists floppy. **See Figure 14.16**

- **Specific stripping to the triceps**: in standing t'ai chi stance and working from distal to proximal (i.e. elbow to shoulder), strip the length of the muscle in clear, methodical strips, with supported fingers. **See Figure 14.17**

Teres major and teres minor

- In kneeling or seated stance with the client's arm still hanging over the side of the table, palpate for the lateral border of the scapula. Start at the inferior end of the lateral border and press into the soft tissue found at the edge. This is teres major. Treat for trigger points with static compression and then friction in one direction only using the thumbs. Gradually work your way along this border in a superior direction (towards the head). As you reach the top third of the border (this is more armpit territory) you will be treating teres minor. **See Figures 14.18 and 14.19**

Supraspinatus, infraspinatus, teres minor and subscapularis (SITS) attachments

- The attachments of the SITS muscles are found on the head of the humerus. Use your fingers to carry out cross fibre friction work to the attachment points (remember pressure is in one direction only). **See Figure 14.20**

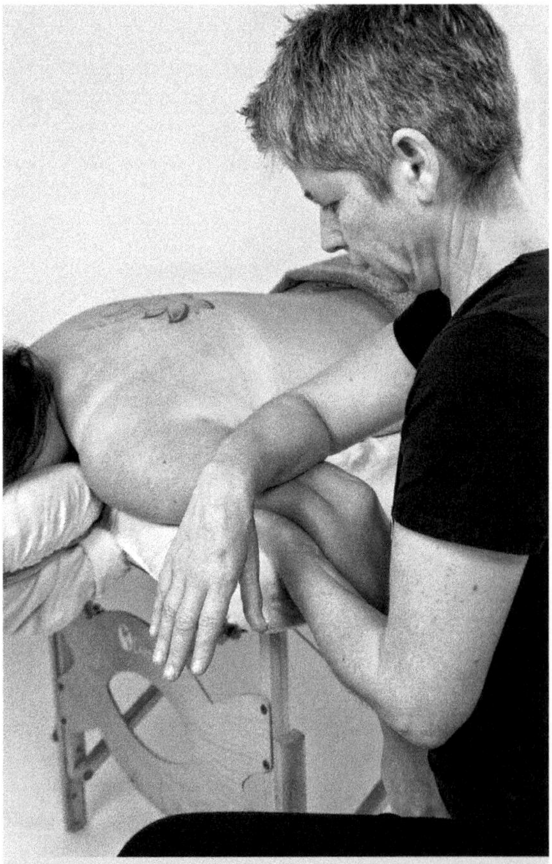

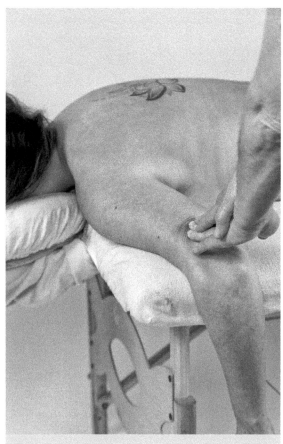

Figure 14.16
Broad work to the triceps

Figure 14.17
Specific stripping to the triceps

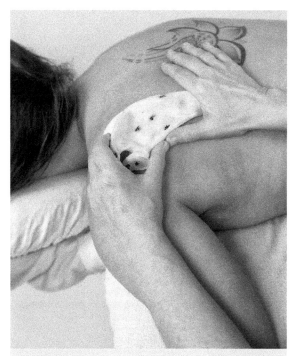

Figure 14.18
Location of the teres major and minor

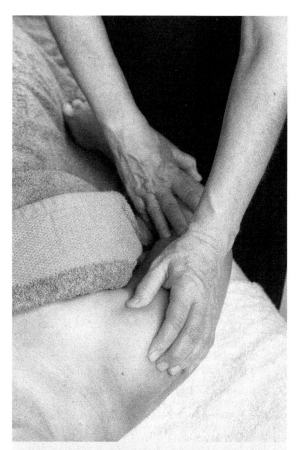

Figure 14.20
Friction to the SITS attachments

Latissimus dorsi stretch

- Stand in a very low t'ai chi stance at the head of the table. For the left latissimus dorsi, use your left hand to grasp your client's arm around the biceps area just superior to the elbow (come around the inside of the elbow to hold the arm). Now pull your client's arm towards you while using your right hand to slide down the latissimus dorsi and slowly stretch the tissue from the armpit to the iliac crest. Hook onto the iliac crest at the end of the stroke and lean back and hold to give a nice full stretch. **See Figure 14.21, p. 256**

- Repeat all the above steps on the opposite side.

Side-lying trapezius work and scapula mobilisation

- Turn your client so that they are in a side-lying position. Your client's legs should be in a

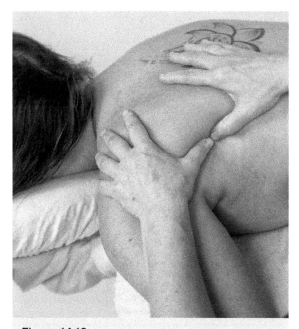

Figure 14.19
Treating teres major and minor

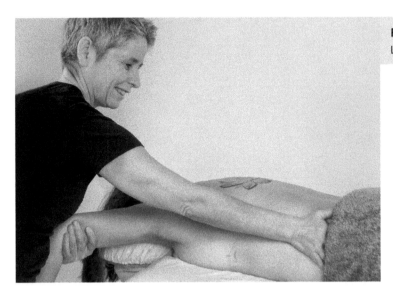

Figure 14.21
Latissimus dorsi stretch

figure-of-four position. Bolster under the head and between the legs, making sure the spine is in alignment. It is common for the client to roll forwards or backwards in this position, so make sure that their head is aligned with their shoulders and their shoulders are aligned with their hips.

- **Side-lying trapezius stretch**: to work the client's right side they should be lying on their left with their right side uppermost. Stand at the side of the table in t'ai chi stance and facing your client's back. Reach around under their arm with your right hand and hold the front of their shoulder with your fingers curled softly around the top of their shoulder. Make sure your client is resting the weight of their arm on yours and is not holding any tension in the area. If you sense they are not giving you their full weight make a gentle suggestion such as 'Make your arm really heavy for me' and give them positive reinforcement when they do this. This verbal cue works much better than saying 'Relax your arm!' which, paradoxically, usually makes clients tense up.

- With your other (left) hand support the back of the head at the occiput. Use your body weight to lean back into your back leg and give the trapezius a nice full stretch. You can release and repeat this a few times as it feels amazing! **See Figure 14.22**

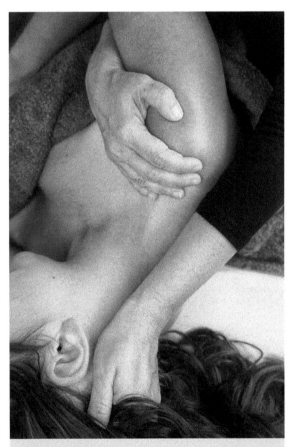

Figure 14.22
Sidelying trapezius stretch

- **Supported shoulder circumduction**: go back to the shoulder cradle position and put the shoulder through a rotational movement. Complete two or three circular movements and let these come from your legs, feet and Hara. Use your body weight to give a full range of motion to the scapula. **See Figure 14.23**

- Leave your right hand in the same position, cradling the shoulder, and come down into a kneeling t'ai chi stance. Place the thumb of your left hand underneath the medial (vertebral) border of the scapula. Use your front (right) hand to push the scapula towards the back of the body (by leaning back with your body weight). The thumb of your left hand should disappear slightly under the scapula to

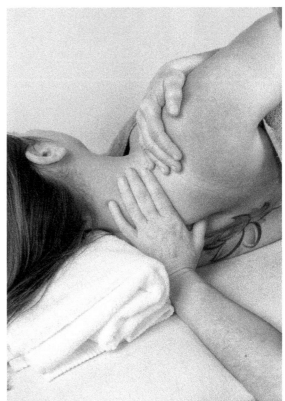

Figure 14.24
Working the vertebral border of the scapula

enable you to work the soft tissue there without too much effort. Use static compression and work any trigger points you find. **See Figure 14.24**

- You can also use a supported thumb (or hot stone) to carry out this technique. **See Figure 14.25, p. 258**

Latissimus dorsi and axillary border of the scapula

- Kneel or stand in front of the client and place their upper arm on your shoulder for support (their right arm goes on your right shoulder). Your right hand is then able to move the shoulder girdle forwards or backwards as needed to put the tissue on more of a slack for ease of access. Using your left hand, use the static compression and money sign techniques to grasp and treat the teres muscles and part of the latissimus dorsi found in this axillary area. For more muscled clients you can also bring your right

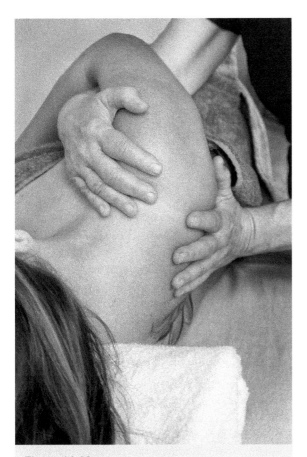

Figure 14.23
Supported shoulder circumduction

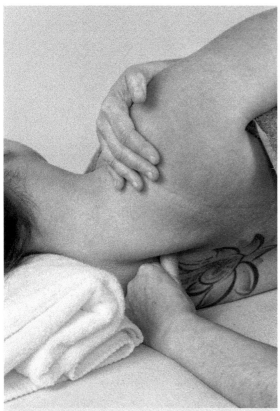

Figure 14.25
Supported thumb technique for working the vertebral border of the scapula

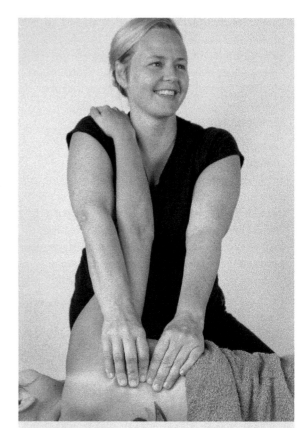

Figure 14.26
Latissimus dorsi and axillary border of the scapula

hand round so that both hands can work the muscle at the same time. **See Figure 14.26**

Subscapularis treated in side-lying position

- You can also treat the subscapularis effectively from the same position as used for the latissimus dorsi and axillary border of the scapula. With your right hand pull the scapula towards you as you use your left thumb to sink down under the latissimus dorsi to contact the anterior surface of the scapula where the subscapularis can be found. This area is incredibly tender so make sure you treat any trigger points you find by static compression, working with client communication on pain levels. **See Figure 14.27**

Serratus anterior

- In the same position, as used for the latissimus dorsi and axillary border of the scapula, you can treat the serratus anterior with supported fingers with cross

fibre friction in one direction only. Serratus anterior is found along the side of the ribcage and is shaped like a bunch of bananas. Portions of this muscle can be accessed in this area by working with the fingers under the flap of the latissimus dorsi. If you place your fingers underneath the latissimus dorsi and pull the shoulder towards you slightly you will find you are able to sink deeper into this area quite easily. **See Figure 14.28**

Latissimus dorsi side-lying stretch

- While your client is lying on their side you can incorporate another great stretch for the latissimus dorsi and lateral fascial line of the body. Gently take the client's arm, above the elbow, in your right hand (make sure you don't have them in a vice-like grip as the skin on the upper arm is quite tender) and with your left hand hook onto the iliac crest. Taking a t'ai chi stance lean back to stretch the side of their body. **See Figure 14.29**

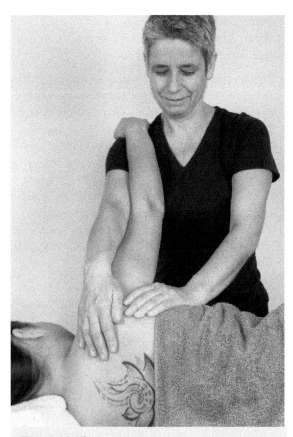

Figure 14.27
Side-lying subscapularis

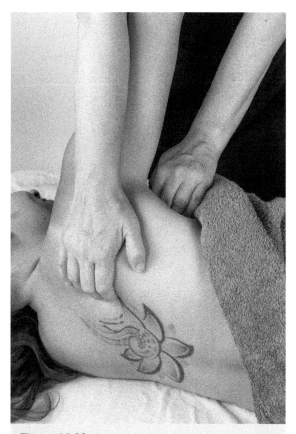

Figure 14.28
Treating serratus anterior

Figure 14.29
Latissimus dorsi side-lying stretch

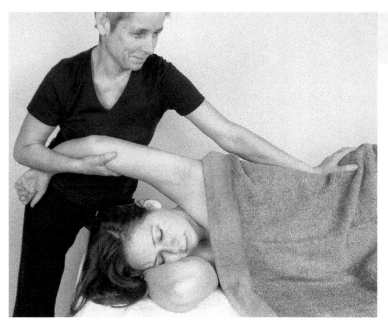

Treating the pectoralis major, subclavius and intercostals

- Turn your client so that they are in a supine position.

- **Sternal attachments of the pectoralis major**: over the towel, work the attachments of the pectoralis major on the sternum (breastbone) with fingertips or thumbs using cross fibre friction. To do this find the sternum and then come off the edge very slightly so that you are on the soft tissue of the pectoralis major. Stand side on to the table in t'ai chi stance and use supported fingers to work with and then against the fibres (back and forth and up and down). Make sure the movements are only small and very precise. You can work the area broadly by using all your fingers lined up side by side. You can also be more specific by using hand

over hand technique and by being very precise about where you are. Work both sides of the sternal attachments. **See Figure 14.30**

- **Subclavius and pectoralis major attachments**: still in t'ai chi stance, swivel your body so you are facing the client's head (keeping eye contact with them). Work the attachments found underneath the clavicle with supported thumb or fingers. This move also works the subclavius muscle that can be very tender. Work with listening touch and keep an eye on your client's face. Sink down through the tissue and up and under the clavicle to fully access the subclavius. Start with static compression and follow with cross fibre friction if the area is not too tender. **See Figures 14.31 and 14.32**

- **Working the pectoralis major and intercostals**: stand in t'ai chi stance on the opposite side to where

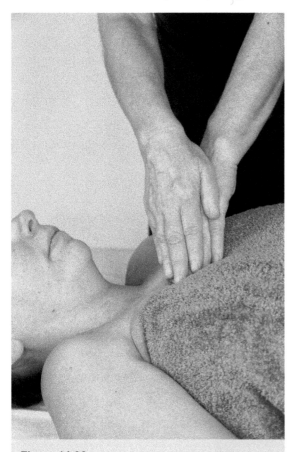

Figure 14.30
Sternal attachments of the pectoralis major

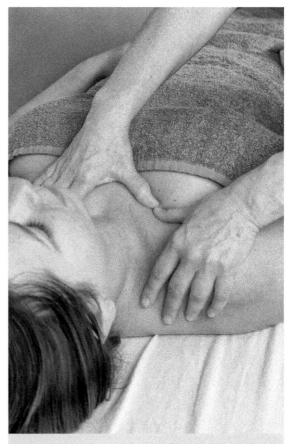

Figure 14.31
Subclavius and pectoralis major attachments

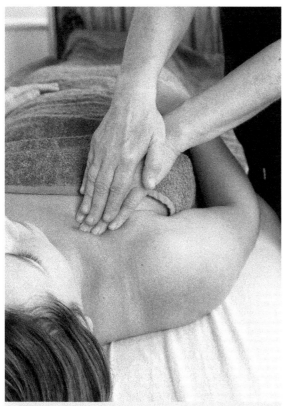

Figure 14.32
Subclavius and pectoralis major attachments

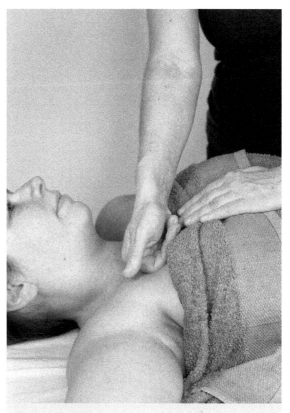

Figure 14.33
Working the belly of the pectoralis major

you are working and use a soft fist to muscle strip the pectorals. You can follow up with more specific work with supported fingers, stripping the pectorals and working in between the ribs to treat the deeper intercostals. **See Figure 14.33**

- **Working the belly of the pectoralis major**: now come to the same side of the table (in this instance the client's right) and support the client's arm by placing it overhead and resting it on your knee on the table. Be careful to work with your client, so you do not bring their arm beyond a comfortable range of motion (e.g. if they have adhesive capsulitis where the range may be severely limited). Grasp the belly of the muscle between your thumbs and fingers of both hands and work the muscle and tendon up to the attachment on the humerus. Use static compression followed by shearing (back and

forth motion between thumb and fingers). **See Figure 14.34, p. 262**

- **Palmar effleurage to the pectoralis major**: swivel your body so that you are now facing the client's head and are in t'ai chi stance. Take the client's arm in your outer hand and use your inner hand to give deep palmar effleurage to the pectorals, working from medial to lateral. You can move the arm into different positions to work different parts of the muscle. Power comes from your belly, legs and Hara; lean into the stroke as you work. **See Figure 14.35, p. 262**

- **Soft tissue release to the pectorals**: in the same position, now anchor down on the pectoral muscle and take the client's arm back into external rotation, holding for a count of 2 seconds. Release your pressure, return the arm to the starting position, and find a slightly different point to lock

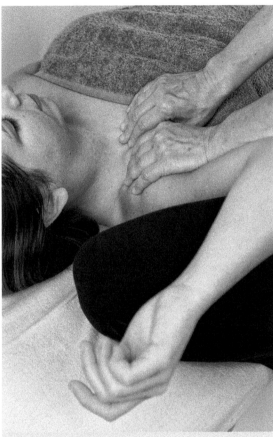

Figure 14.34
Working the belly of the pectoralis major

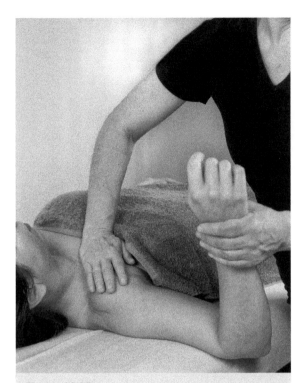

Figure 14.35
Palmar effleurage to the pectoralis major

and repeat the short stretch. Practise this stroke in
a flowing rhythm:

- Lock
- Stretch: 1, 2
- Release
- Replace
- Repeat.

- You can use a broad lock with the palm of your
  hand or a soft fist or a more specific hold with a
  supported thumb. **See Figure 14.36**

Pectoralis minor

You can treat this muscle in two different ways:

1 With your client's arm by their side, stand facing
   the table in t'ai chi stance. Sink down through the

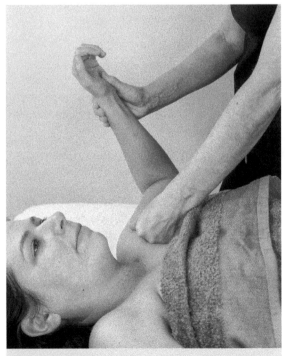

Figure 14.36
STR for the pectoralis major

pectoralis major to contact the pectoralis minor. Get a visual of the muscle in your mind where you see it running on a diagonal from the coracoid process to ribs 3, 4 and 5. Use static pressure or very gentle strumming (slowly rolling back and forth across the muscle with precision and focus) until you gain a release and feel the muscle start to soften. **See Figure 14.37**

2 Kneel at the side of the table and take the client's arm into external rotation. Using soft, relaxed fingers work up and under the pectoralis major; you should be able to feel the ribs against your finger pads and your nails against the pectoralis major. Swim in with your finger pads towards the midline of the body until you feel the 'rope-like' quality of the pectoralis minor. Once you have located the muscle, replace the client's arm on top of your working hand and use your top hand to bring the tissue of the pectoralis major towards you so you can sink in a little deeper. Once you are sure you are on the pectoralis minor, use static pressure to treat trigger points, followed up,

if needed, by very gentle strumming until you gain a release.

> **CAUTION**
>
> Remove your pressure if the client feels any tingling or numbness down their arm, as this indicates you are on the brachial plexus. Reposition your fingers slightly and try the move again

When you have felt the tissue soften, as an added extra to gain a full release, you can stay with your fingers on the muscle and ask your client to take their arm overhead as if swimming the backstroke. If you keep your fingers where they are you should feel an extra lengthening and release at the end of this stretch. **See Figure 14.38**

Integration work to the pectorals

● Finish your work on the pectorals region with some broad work with both fists. Use a 'paddy pawing' motion and work deep into the tissue, shifting

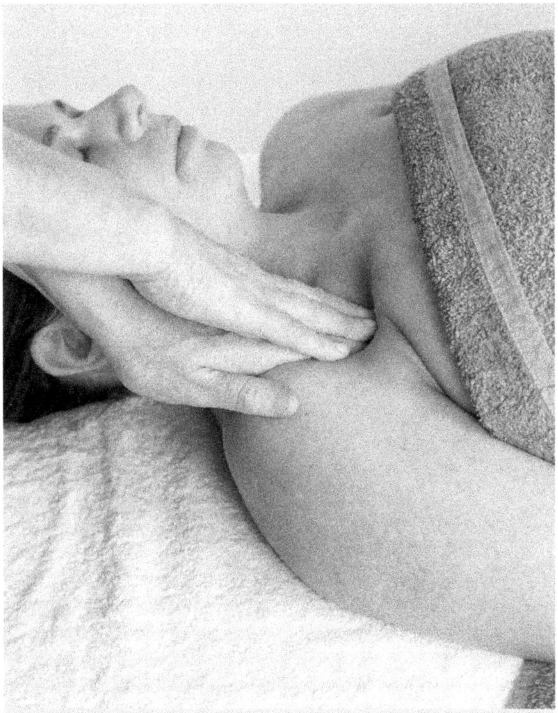

Figure 14.37
Pectoralis minor (1)

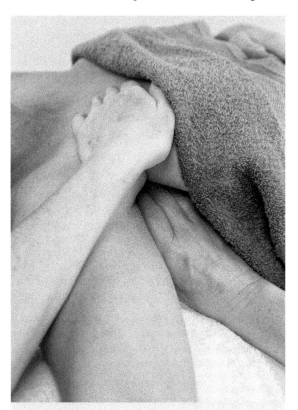

Figure 14.38
Pectoralis minor (2)

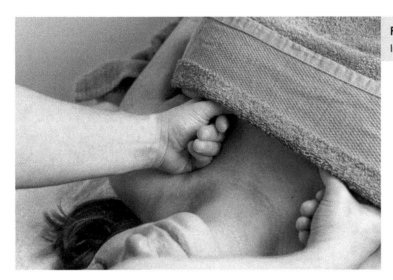

Figure 14.39
Integration work to the pectorals

weight from one side to another. Follow up with some broad short effleurage strokes with your fist, working from medial to lateral. **See Figure 14.39**

Anterior deltoid

- You can treat the anterior deltoid by curling your fingers around the outside of the muscle and using the thumb to work the anterior portion from superior to inferior. **See Figure 14.40**

Subscapularis

The subscapularis is a very important treatment area in shoulder conditions and usually has extremely tender trigger points. So make sure you use your listening touch and client communication.

- With your upper hand hold up the client's arm. With your lower hand slide your fingers into the axillary region between the scapula and the ribs. You should be anterior to the latissimus dorsi (the flap of muscle that constitutes the back of the armpit).

- Swim slowly into this region and, as you curl your soft fingertips downward towards the table, you should feel the bone of the scapula: this is the costal surface that is against the ribs and is where the subscapularis is found. Put the client's arm down with their hand across their body, keeping your own fingertips on the costal surface. Treat the muscle first with static compression and then with gentle cross fibre friction. Work in the direction of the fibres and then across the fibres.

- Note that this muscle is very tender. Keep your eyes on your client's face and make sure they are

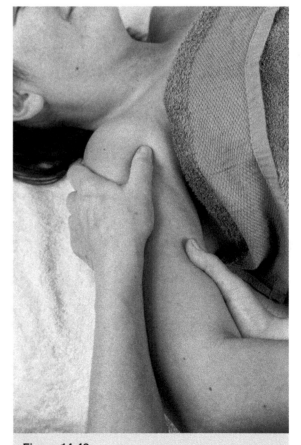

Figure 14.40
Anterior deltoid

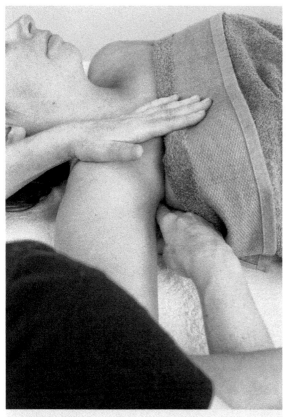

Figure 14.41
Subscapularis

not tensing up against the stroke. Help them to feel in control by getting them to breathe into the area. **See Figure 14.41**

Range of motion

● With your left hand supporting the posterior side of the scapula and your right hand on the anterior side, take the scapulothoracic joint of the shoulder girdle into a full range of motion. Use t'ai chi stance and move your body to achieve a full movement. **See Figure 14.42**

● Now, supporting the arm, take the glenohumeral joint in a range of motion that stays within client tolerance. Work with client communication and your sense of 'listening touch'. If possible, stretch the client's arm overhead and then bring the arm back and across the body for another careful stretch. **See Figure 14.43, p. 266**

Coracobrachialis

● In kneeling t'ai chi stance, displace the overlying biceps towards the lateral side with your outer hand. Use your inside hand to strip the coracobrachialis with your thumb, looking for trigger points. **See Figure 14.44, p. 266**

Biceps

● Using the medial side of your forearm, work the belly of the muscle in broad strips. **See Figure 14.45, p. 266**

● In horse stance do a good old fashioned pick up petrissage to the belly of the muscle. **See Figure 14.46, p. 267**

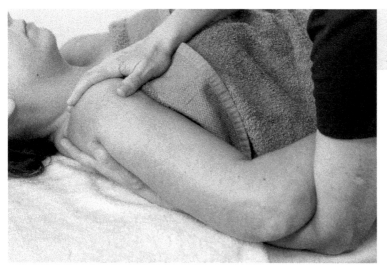

Figure 14.42
Range of motion (scapulothoracic joint)

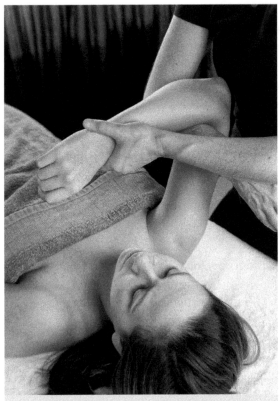

Figure 14.43
Range of motion (glenohumeral joint)

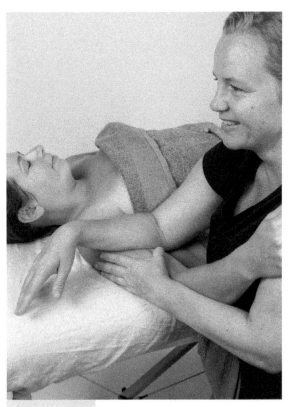

Figure 14.45

Mobilisations

- Take the client's hand and rock, jostle and jiggle the shoulder girdle to give some passive mobilisation. Start with small movements and

Figure 14.44

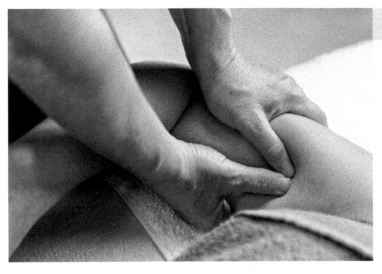

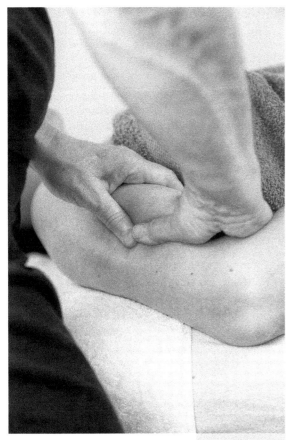

Figure 14.46

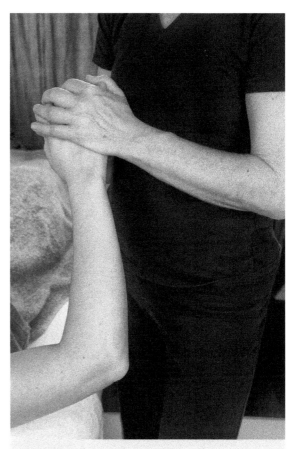

Figure 14.47
Mobilisation

gradually make them bigger. Keep an eye on your client's face as some people find it difficult to 'let go' with these passive movements, particularly if they are in pain. Always work within client tolerance and be sure to get feedback. **See Figure 14.47**

Acupressure points for the prone position

Small Intestine 11 (SI 11): Celestial gathering

- **Location**: on the scapula in a depression at the centre of the infrascapular fossa, found at the junction of the upper and middle third between the lower scapular spine and the inferior angle of the scapula. This is a fantastic point for releasing the fascia on the scapula and the whole shoulder girdle. This point is also believed to be helpful for any pain

along the Small Intestine meridian that runs along the back of the arm, elbow, face and jaw.

- To treat SI 11 place a supported thumb in the centre of the scapula where you will usually find a small depression. Hold pressure for 3–5 breaths until you feel a release. **See Figure 14.48, p. 268**

Stretches

Pectoralis major and triceps stretch

- Client is in a prone position.

- Gently take the client's arm overhead until they are able to feel a stretch. For some people this will be right back on the table while others might need a support from a bolster or your knee. Place your hands on the upper arm and gently press towards the floor for a stretch. **See Figure 14.49, p. 268**

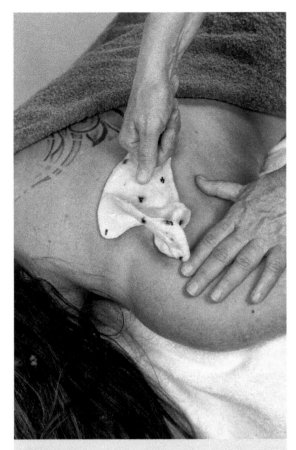

Figure 14.48
Location of acupressure point SI 11

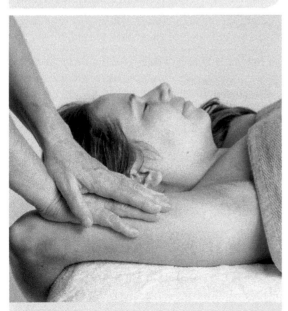

Figure 14.49
Pectoralis major and triceps stretch

Subscapularis stretch

- Client is in a supine position.

- As subscapularis is an internal rotator, taking the shoulder girdle into external rotation will stretch this muscle. Abduct the client's arm and flex the elbow. Working with client breath and communication, anchor down the humerus with your inside hand. Gently take the arm into external rotation (palm towards ceiling) until your client feels a stretch. Keep an eye on your client's face and keep your movements slow. **See Figure 14.50**

Teres minor and infrapsinatus stretch

- Client is in a prone position.

- These muscles are external rotators and can be stretched by taking the arm into internal rotation. With the same hand positions as for the subscapularis stretch, gently take the arm the other way so the shoulder is placed into maximum internal rotation and the palm is facing towards the floor. **See Figure 14.51**

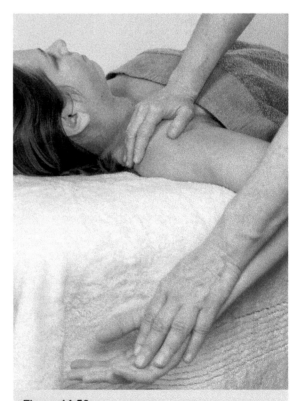

Figure 14.50
Subscapularis stretch

Side-lying 'Devil' pectoral stretch

- A great stretch from Thai massage is the side-lying 'Devil' pectoral stretch. In kneeling t'ai chi stance on the table, traction your client's arm straight up towards you and then gently back towards your body. Make sure you work with client communication and the breath as this stretch can be very strong (hence the name!). **See Figure 14.52**

- Finish in your own unique way.

Teaching self-care suggestions

Self-help suggestions can be found in the Self-Care Resources (available online at uk.singingdragon.com/catalogue/book/9781909141230).

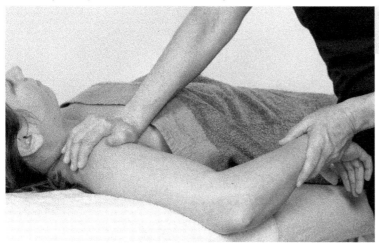

Figure 14.51
Teres minor and infraspinatus stretch

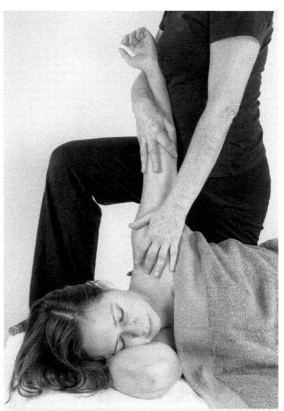

Figure 14.52
Side-lying 'devil' pectoral stretch

Forearm and wrist pain protocol

Introduction

Many forearm, hand and wrist complaints actually originate further 'upstream'. For example, symptoms such as numbness and tingling in the hands and arms (often wrongly misdiagnosed as carpal tunnel syndrome) can originate from entrapment of the brachial plexus by soft tissues, e.g. either the scalenes or the pectoralis minor. Upton and McComas (1973) were the first to suggest the 'double crush' theory proposing that nerve entrapment at the neck means that symptoms are likely to develop further down the arm.

Numbness in the hands and fingers can also be caused by trigger points in several muscles of the neck and shoulder girdle, including suprapsinatus, infraspinatus, subscapularis, serratus posterior, pectoralis minor, triceps and coracobrachialis.

For these reasons, symptoms in the forearm, hands and wrists should also be combined with work from the neck and shoulder and shoulder girdle protocols for the best results.

In our experience, conditions of the hand and wrist can have a large central sensitisation component, especially repetitive strain injury (RSI). If the area is ultra-painful even to light touch you will need to use more fascial work and less trigger point work. In addition, treatments should focus on relaxation and self-care suggestions to reduce emotional and central sensitisation components of the pain.

The following protocol can be used to good effect for conditions including:

- Carpal tunnel syndrome
- Golfer's elbow
- Tennis elbow
- RSI
- De Quervain's tenosynovitis

- Arthritis (both osteoarthritis and rheumatoid arthritis, although modifications to protocols may be needed in acute stages).

Heat and preparatory work over the drape

- For this work your client is in a supine position.

- **Use of hot or cold**: research has shown that, contrary to previous thinking, inflammation is NOT a component of many hand and wrist conditions, such as lateral and medial epicondylitis (tennis and golfer's elbow), so heat can help to release the muscles before fascial and trigger point work. There are various different ways of applying heat to the forearms. If you have a heating pad it can feel great to wrap the whole forearm in this while you do some neck and shoulder work. You can also palm down the forearms with some hot stones.

  Cold can also feel soothing to areas of pain, such as the tendinous insertion points of the flexors and extensors, especially in cases of tennis and golfer's elbow.

Fascial work

A combination of fascial work can be used. Here are some suggested strokes:

- **Cross hand stretches**: this versatile stroke can be applied to many different regions, e.g. over the chest and forearms. **See Figures 15.1 and 15.2, p. 272**

- **Arm pull**: this is a highly effective way of releasing fascial restrictions along the whole fascial chain from hand to neck. Take the client's hand in both of your hands and grasp at the base of the palm whilst spreading the palmar fascia slightly. Place the arm on a slight traction. Now wait until you feel the arm start to move as if voluntarily. Make sure you are not consciously initiating a movement. Once you feel the

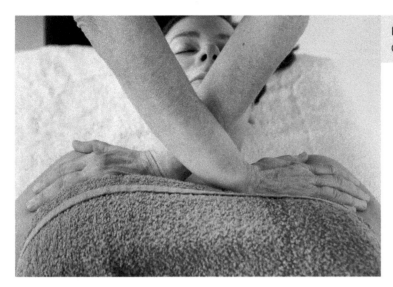

Figure 15.1
Cross hand stretch

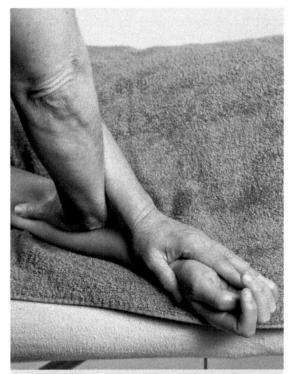

Figure 15.2
Cross hand stretch

response in the tissues then you can follow the movements whilst making sure to keep the arm on a slight stretch. Watch out for still points where the movement ceases as these are places where you need to hold on a stretch until you feel the sensation of tissue release.

If performed with focus and a good listening touch, an arm pull can do the majority of your work for you when treating hand and wrist conditions, so make time to include this stroke. **See Figure 15.3**

Muscular and trigger point work

Scalenes

The scalenes are located between the sternocleidomastoid (SCM) and upper trapezius. The brachial plexus runs between anterior and middle scalenes, so it is common for the nerve to become impinged at this point due to common habits, such as forward head position or shallow breathing which leads to shortened scalenes. As the brachial plexus runs all the way down the arm this can lead to symptoms of numbness and tingling in the hands.

- **Stripping the scalenes**: gently traction the head by hooking under the occiput and leaning back. On your client's out breath turn their head to their left side.

Muscle strip the right scalene muscles, using your right hand. First use a soft fist to do broad work to the area and then use your thumb to work in the area between the SCM and trapezius. Treat any trigger points you may find. This is a very important area to work in cases of referred pain down the arm or carpal tunnel type symptoms. **See Figures 15.4 and 15.5**

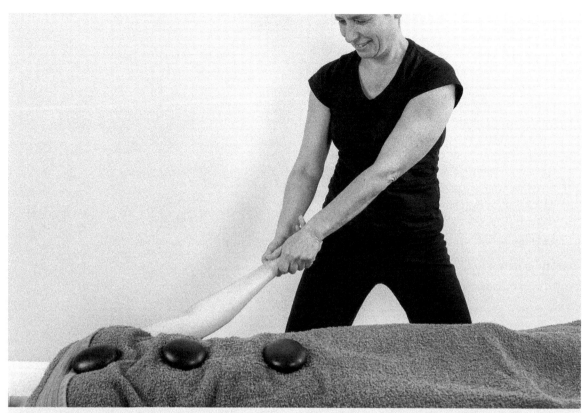

Figure 15.3
Arm pull

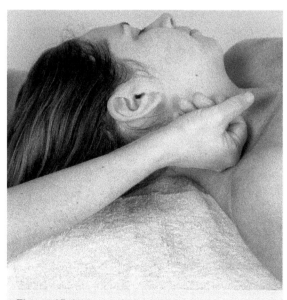

Figure 15.4
Fist work to scalenes

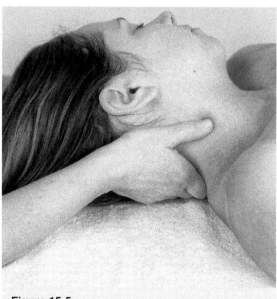

Figure 15.5
Stripping the scalenes

- **Scalene stretch**: stand or sit at the head of the table. Hold the client's head in your hands. Ask the client to take a deep breath and on their out breath bring their left ear to their left shoulder, keeping their nose pointed to the ceiling. When they have reached the end of their range of motion (ROM), replace your hands so they are crossed with one hand on the shoulder and one on the side of the head. Get your client to take a breath in and out and take them into a full stretch, always working with client communication. Hold for 10–30 seconds. Repeat on the other side.
  See Figure 15.6

Pectoralis minor

You can treat this muscle in two different ways:

1 With your client's arm by their side, stand facing the table in t'ai chi stance. Sink down through the pectoralis major to contact the pectoralis minor. Get a visual of the muscle in your mind where you can see it running on a

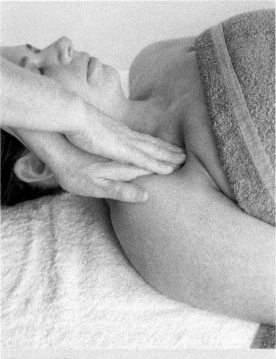

Figure 15.7
Pectoralis minor (1)

diagonal from the coracoid process to ribs 3, 4 and 5. Use static pressure or very gentle strumming (slowly rolling back and forth across the muscle with precision and focus) until you gain a release and feel the muscle start to soften.
See Figure 15.7

2 Kneeling at the side of the table, take the client's arm into external rotation. Using soft relaxed fingers work up and under the pectoralis major. You should be able to feel the ribs against your fingerpads and your nails against the pectoralis major. Swim in with the fingerpads towards the midline of the body until you feel the 'rope like' quality of the pectoralis minor. Once you have located the muscle, replace the client's arm on top of your working hand and use your top hands to bring the tissue of the pectoralis major towards you so you can sink in a little deeper. Once you are sure you are on the pectoralis minor, use static pressure to treat trigger points, followed up if needed by very gentle strumming until you gain a release.

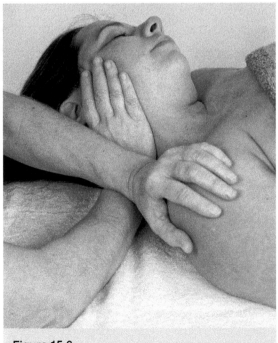

Figure 15.6
Scalenes stretch

CAUTION

Remove your pressure if the client feels any tingling or numbness down their arm, as this indicates you are on the brachial plexus. Reposition your fingers slightly and try the move again

When you have felt the tissue soften, as an added extra to gain a full release, you can stay with your fingers on the muscle and ask your client to take their arm overhead as if swimming the back stroke. If you keep your fingers where they are you should feel an extra lengthening and release at the end of this stretch. **See Figure 15.8**

Forearm extensors

- **Broad work to the extensors**: bolster the forearm if needed – one of those small pillows you purloined on your last aeroplane trip will be perfect for the job. Place your client's hand in the pronated position (palm down towards the table). In t'ai chi stance, muscle strip the entire extensor region from distal to proximal (i.e. wrist to elbow). Use broad strokes first with your fist or forearm followed by specific strokes with supported fingers, searching for and treating trigger points as you go along. **See Figures 15.9 and 15.10 (p. 276).**

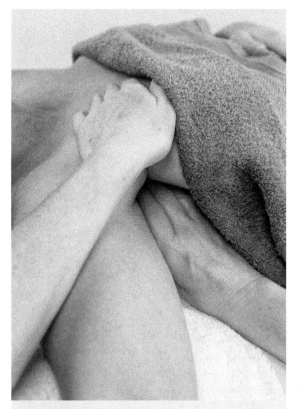

Figure 15.8
Pectoralis minor (2)

- **Friction the common extensor tendon attachment**: the extensor group has a common origin on the lateral epicondyle of the humerus.

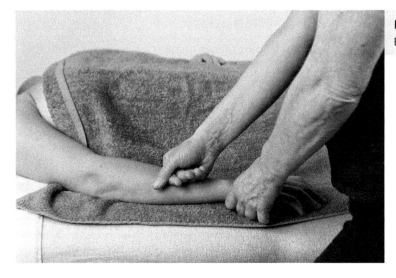

Figure 15.9
Broad work to the extensors

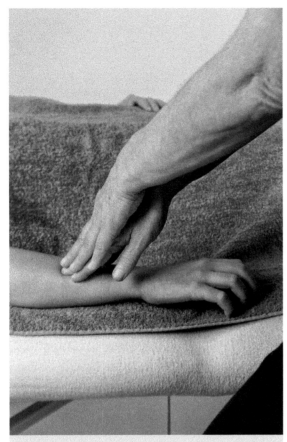

Figure 15.10
Specific work to the extensors

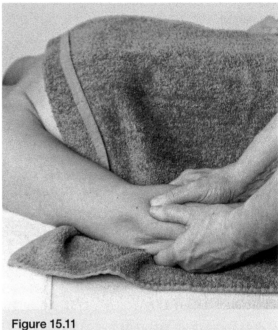

Figure 15.11
Friction common extensor tendon

This is the prominent 'bony bump' found on the lateral side of the forearm. Locate this bony landmark and then come slightly distally onto the soft tissue of the extensor attachments. In cases of tennis elbow this point can be very tender, so work with client communication and do not go beyond your client's tolerance level. Wrap both of your hands around the forearm so that your thumbs are able to carry out cross fibre friction in this area. The movements are very small with transverse pressure in one direction and a light return stroke.
See Figure 15.11

Brachioradialis

This muscle is located on the thumb side of the arm and, surprisingly enough, runs along the radius (anatomy does like to be helpful). Turn the client's arm to a neutral position so that their thumb is facing the ceiling

and carry out the following work to treat this muscle, searching for and treating trigger points with both movements:

- In t'ai chi stance, use a pincer grip to work down the brachioradialis with even inward pressure on both sides of the muscle. Hold the arm at the wrist with the outside hand and work down from elbow to wrist using your inside hand.
  See Figure 15.12

- When you reach the wrist, glide up towards the elbow using the same grip. Use a t'ai chi stance and get your whole body into the stroke so that it is a dynamic movement. **See Figure 15.13**

Supinator

Hiding underneath brachioradialis, the supinator can provide an unexpected contribution to pain conditions. As the radial nerve passes underneath the supinator, entrapment of this nerve can contribute to many different forearm, elbow and hand pathologies. Treat the muscle as follows:

- With the client's hand still in the neutral position, grasp the brachioradialis firmly and displace it towards the client's body using your

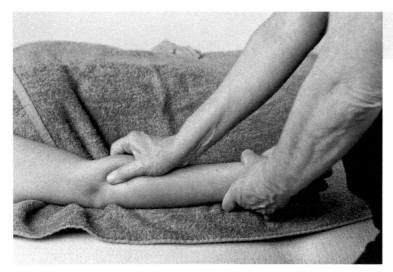

Figure 15.12
Brachioradialis: pincer grip

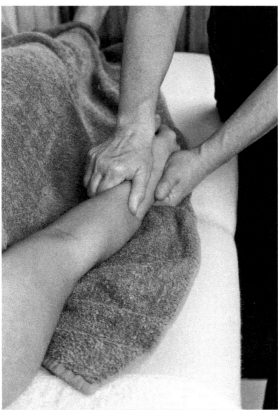

Figure 15.13
Brachioradialis: sliding move

inside hand. If you are working on the client's right arm then use your right hand to do this. Keep the brachioradialis out of the way and with

your other (left) hand, wrap your fingers around the arm and use your thumb to glide up the shaft of the radius. The supinator attaches on the proximal third of the radius, so start a few inches down from the elbow and glide upward with a direct downward pressure right onto the bone. **See Figure 15.14, p. 278**

- Now treat the other side of the supinator. Using your outside (left) hand, displace the brachioradialis away from your client's body. Using your right hand glide up the medial side of the radius with your thumb. **See Figure 15.15, p. 278**

Forearm flexors

- **Broad work to the forearm flexors**: turn the client's hand so that their palm is facing up with their fingers extended. Start at the wrist and muscle strip to the elbow crease. Use broad strokes (with fist or forearm). **See Figure 15.16, p. 278**

- **Specific work to the forearm flexors**: follow the broad work with specific strokes using supported fingers. Work from one side to the other in methodical strips so that you cover the whole area, searching for trigger points as you go. **See Figure 15.17, p. 279**

- **Friction the common flexor tendon attachment**: the wrist flexors have a common tendon attachment point at the medial epicondyle (the bony bump on the medial side of the forearm). In cases of golfer's

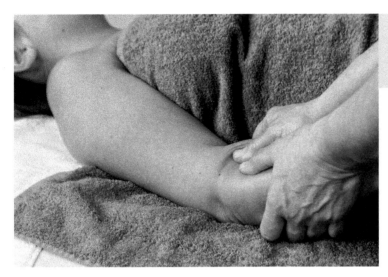

Figure 15.14
Supinator: displace brachioradialis medially and treat lateral side of supinator with left hand

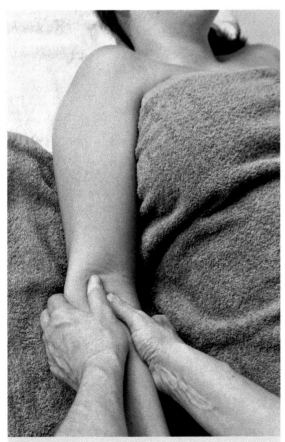

Figure 15.15
Supinator: now displace brachioradialis laterally and treat the medial side of the supinator with the right hand

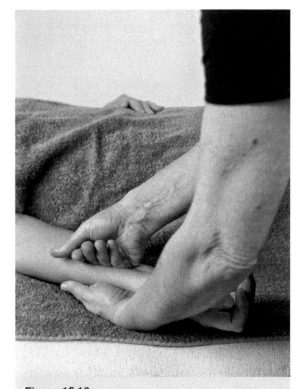

Figure 15.16
Broad work to forearm flexors

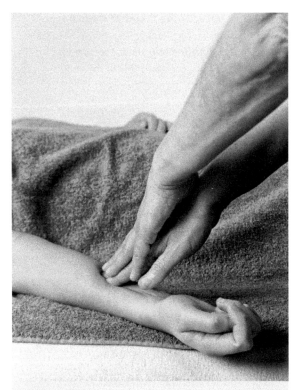

Figure 15.17
Specific work to the forearm flexors

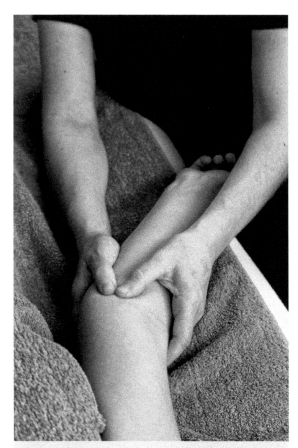

Figure 15.18

Friction common flexor tendon

elbow this point can be very tender, so work with client communication and do not go beyond your client's tolerance level. Wrap both hands around the forearm so that your thumbs are able to carry out cross fibre friction in this area. The movements are very small with transverse pressure in one direction and a light return stroke. **See Figure 15.18**

- **Repeat muscle stripping and friction to the forearm extensors**: this time work deeper both with the muscle stripping and the friction at the lateral epicondyle.

Extensor retinaculum (dorsal carpal ligament)

This is an anatomical term for the strong, fibrous, thickened part of the antebrachial fascia that holds the tendons of the extensor muscles in place. It is located on the back of the forearm, just proximal to the hand.

To treat this area specifically use a minimum of lubrication so the strokes are more fascial in nature.

- **Extensor retinaculum strip and stretch**: one hand holds the client's hand and slowly takes it into flexion. At the same time your other thumb strips deeply with the movement down through the extensor retinaculum. Repeat several times. See Figure 15.19, p. 280

- **Longitudinal friction (the Z stroke)**: wrap both hands around the wrist and have the thumbs horizontal and parallel to each other. Now glide both thumbs simultaneously towards their respective opposite side of the wrist. Repeat several times. See Figure 15.20, p. 280

Dorsal surface of the hand

- **Dorsal surface of the hand (bony side)**: using a very small amount of lubrication and working from

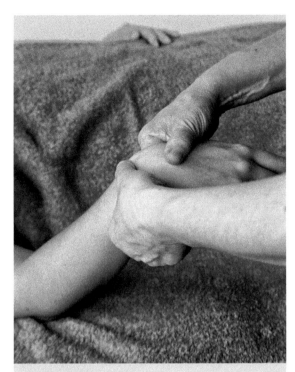

Figure 15.19
Extensor retinaculum strip and stretch

distal to proximal, carry out deep muscle stripping to the muscles located between the metacarpal bones to treat any trigger points. **See Figure 15.21**

- **Webbing between the thumb and forefinger**: this area can be very tender so it is useful to work it specifically. Hold static pressure and use deep thumb work into this fleshy area. **See Figure 15.22**

Brachioradialis and supinator (repeat)

- Repeat the same movements as described under the earlier brachioradialis and supinator sections.

Forearm flexors

- Repeat the same moves as described in the earlier section on forearm flexors. Use deeper pressure to the client's tolerance level.

Palmaris longus

- **Specific muscle stripping to palmaris longus**: the tendon of this muscle merges into the palmar fascia and trigger points in the palmaris longus are thought to lead to Duyputren's contracture (DeLany 2009). Use deeper muscle stripping from palm to elbow on the medial side of the forearm to pay special attention to this muscle. **See Figure 15.23, p. 282**

Flexor retinaculum (transverse carpal ligament)

This is a strong, fibrous band of fascia that arches over the carpal bones at the base of the palm, thus forming

Figure 15.20
Extensor retinaculum: Z stroke

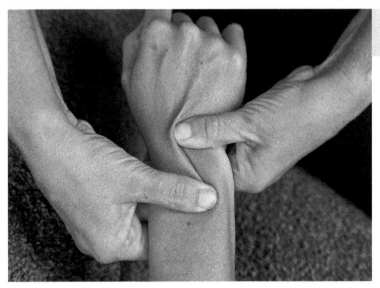

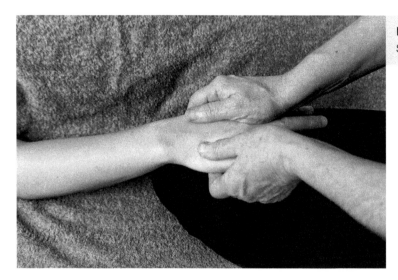

Figure 15.21
Stripping to dorsal surface of the hand

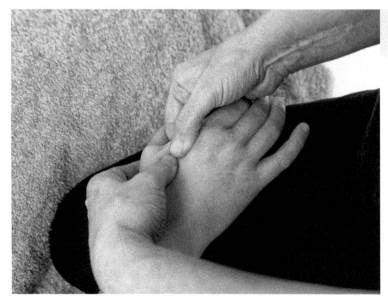

Figure 15.22
Specific work to webbing

the roof of the 'carpal tunnel', the space through which the flexor tendons of the digits and the median nerve pass.

The flexor retinaculm can be treated in exactly the same way as the extensor retinaculum, but remember this structure is anatomically located at the base of the palm rather than at the wrist.

- **Strip and stretch to flexor retinaculum**: working with the client's hand palm up, slowly take their wrist into extension. At the same time your other thumb strips deeply with the movement down through the flexor retinaculum. Repeat several times.
See Figure 15.24, p. 282

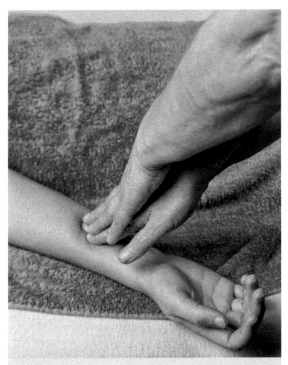

Figure 15.23
Specific stripping to the palmaris longus

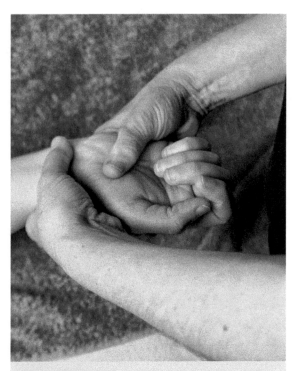

Figure 15.24
Strip and stretch to the flexor retinaculum

- **Longitudinal friction (the Z stroke):** wrap both hands around the palm and have the thumbs horizontal and parallel to each other. Now glide both thumbs simultaneously towards the opposite side. Repeat several times. **See Figure 15.25**

Palmar surface of the hand

The palm of the hand can be split into three different sections for treatment (centre, thenar eminence and hypothenar eminence), which enables you to be thorough and specific in your coverage of this important area. Anyone who works with their hands (including your fellow bodyworkers) will love you for these techniques.

- **Thenar eminence (thumb side):** to treat your client's right hand, take the opportunity to sit on the side of the table and cross one of your legs over the other to make a figure of four so that you have a nice cradle to rest their hand. Use a bolster in your lap if need be.

You can now work the thenar eminence side of your client's palm thoroughly with both

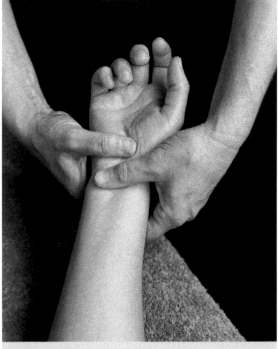

Figure 15.25
Z stroke to the flexor retinaculum

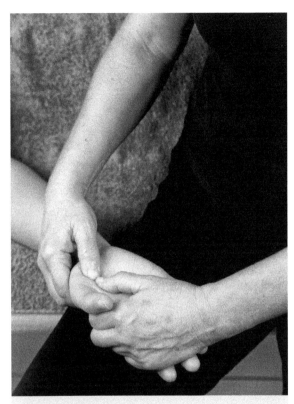

Figure 15.26
Working the thenar eminence

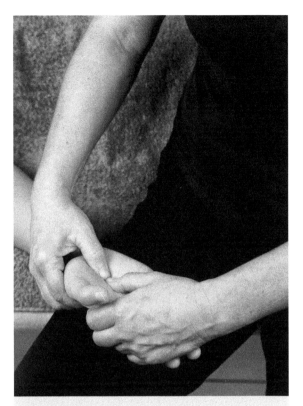

Figure 15.27
Working the centre section of the palm

thumbs. Your fingers are underneath to support the palm. Use static pressure and small cross fibre friction to work the area thoroughly and treat any trigger points you find. **See Figure 15.26**

- **Palmar fascia**: now in the same position use your thumbs to treat the centre section of the palm. **See Figure 15.27**

- **Hypothenar eminence (little finger side):** change your position so that you are now facing the table. With one knee on the table as support, work this area with your thumbs in the same way as described for the palmar fascia. **See Figure 15.28**

- **Work between the metacarpals**: go back to the sitting on the side of the table position and now repeat the palmar work but this time your focus is on working between the metacarpals. Use deep specific friction and stripping strokes. **See Figure 15.29, p. 284**

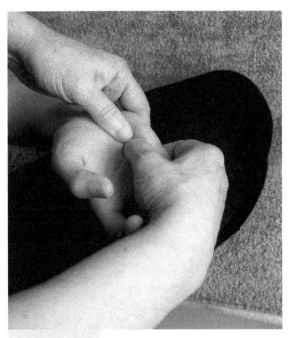

Figure 15.28

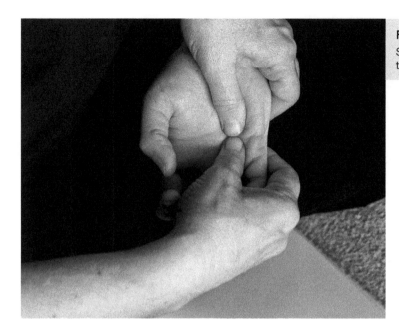

Figure 15.29
Specific work between the metacarpals

- **Decompression of all digits**: still seated on the side of the table, take each joint, one by one, and decompress with slight traction. Each finger has three joints and the thumb has two so take time to treat each of these specifically.

Hold the joint above and below with a firm grasp. Rotate each joint slightly clockwise and anticlockwise and then give the joint a slight traction by pulling it apart (wiggle, wiggle, wiggle, pull – like releasing a stuck drawer). You can use a towel for grip if needed. **See Figures 15.30 and 15.31**

Hand and wrist range of motion

- Now carry out a ROM for the wrist in all directions. Keep the client's upper arm on the table and bend the arm at a 90-degree angle. To treat your client's right arm, hold just below the wrist with your left hand. Interlace the fingers of your client's hand

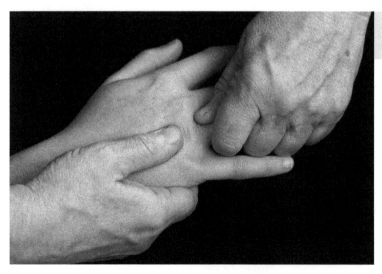

Figure 15.30
Decompression of the digits

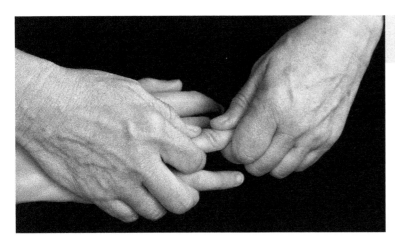

Figure 15.31
Decompression of the digits

with those of your right hand and go through a ROM:

- Extension (take the back of the client's hand towards the table). **See Figure 15.32**

- Flexion (take their palm towards the table). **See Figure 15.33**

- Radial deviation (take their hand sideways towards the thumb side). **See Figure 15.34, p. 286**

- Ulnar deviation (take their hand sideways towards the little finger side). **See Figure 15.35, p. 286**

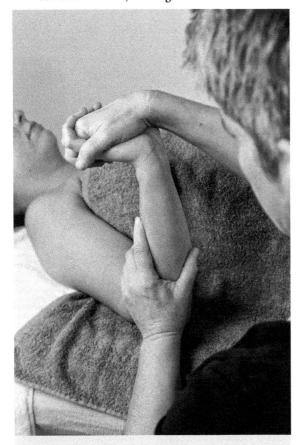

Figure 15.32
Wrist extension

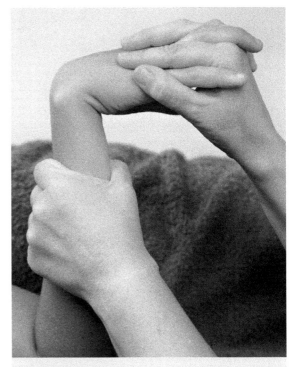

Figure 15.33
Wrist flexion

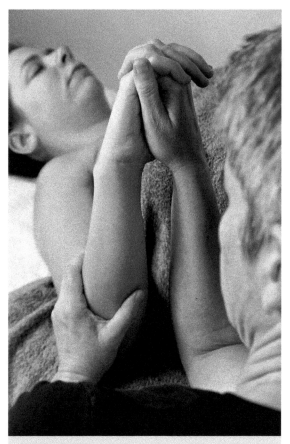

Figure 15.34
Radial deviation

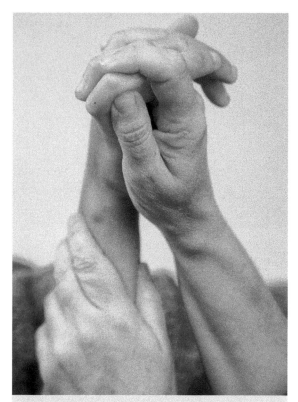

Figure 15.35
Ulnar deviation

- **Hand and wrist traction**: kneel by the side of the table in kneeling t'ai chi stance. Interlock your own fingers with your client's fingers on both sides so that your hands are sandwiching theirs. Bend your own arm and lightly rest it so that it is holding your client's upper arm down onto the table. Your own forearm should now be parallel with your clients and pointing up towards the ceiling. Traction upwards to give a nice release to all the joints in the wrist.

- Continue the traction upwards with your right hand while the other (left) pulls the forearm tissue down in a gliding motion. **See Figure 15.36**

Finishing strokes

- **Finger pull**: this is a traditional massage stroke that feels great. Rub along the sides of the client's fingers with your thumb and forefinger and using a slight rolling motion. At the end squeeze their fingertip

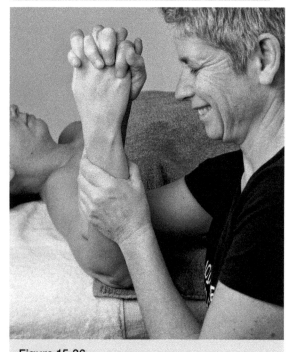

Figure 15.36
Hand and wrist traction

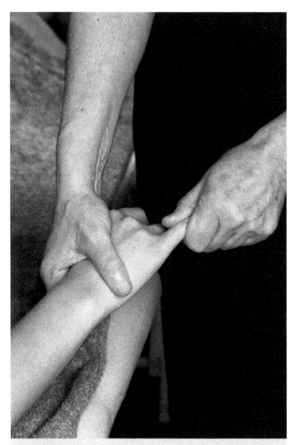

Figure 15.37
Finger pull

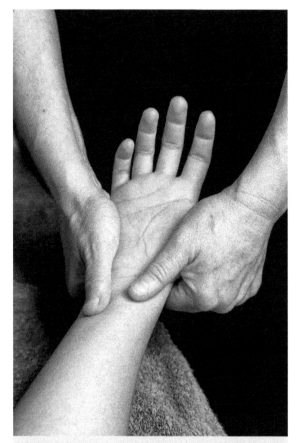

Figure 15.38
Palm press on carpal bones

slightly and snap off quickly. This is thought to energise the meridians which all end in the fingers and toes, from a Chinese medicine point of view. **See Figure 15.37**

- **Palm press on the carpal bones**: grasp the wrist with fingers underneath and palms on top (as if you are breaking a bar of chocolate in half). Use compression then pull your palms apart with a gliding motion. **See Figure 15.38**

Acupressure points

Lung 5 (Lu 5): Cubit Marsh

- **Location**: at the lateral side of the elbow crease, in the depression on the radial side of the biceps brachii tendon. Excellent local point for tennis elbow.

- To find Lu 5, flex the client's elbow slightly to locate the strong biceps tendon. Put your thumb in the small depression on the lateral side of this tendon at the elbow crease. Straighten the client's arm and hold for 3–5 breaths. **See Figure 15.39, p. 288**

Large Intestine 11 (LI 11): Pool at the Bend

- **Location**: at the lateral end of the elbow fold, midway between LU 5 and the lateral epicondyle of the humerus. Another great point for tennis elbow and a powerful point for any problems along the Large Intestine channel, which starts at the index finger and runs along the arm to the face.

- To find LI 11, pronate the client's forearm (palm down to the table). Find the lateral epicondyle (bony bump that sticks out at the distal end of the humerus) and palpate for the small depression

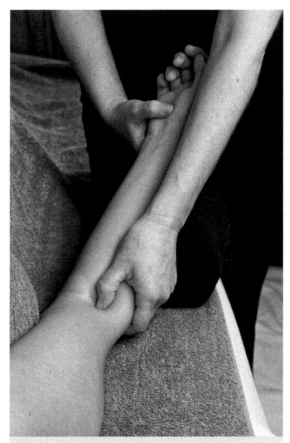

Figure 15.39
Acupressure point: Lung 5

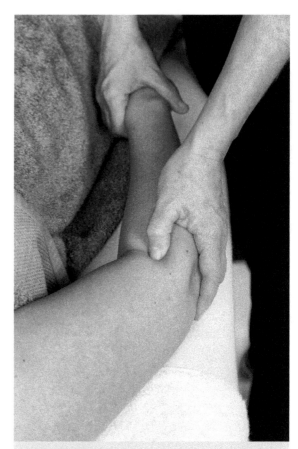

Figure 15.40
Acupressure point Large Intestine 11

between this point and LU 5. Treat the point with your thumb for 3–5 breaths. **See Figure 15.40**

Large Intestine 4 (LI 4): Union Valley

- **Location**: in the webbing between the thumb and forefinger, this point can be found in the centre of the 2nd metacarpal bone on the radial side of the bone. This is a strong point for any problems along the course of the channel. It is useful not just for forearm, hand and wrist problems but is a great point for headaches, toothache or problems in the face.

> **CAUTION**
>
> This point has a strong descending energy and should be avoided in pregnancy, unless you are at the stage of wishing to promote labour!

- To find LI 4, clasp your client's hand as if you are going to shake hands with them. Your thumb should now be lying naturally on the radial side of the first metacarpal. Flex your thumb and press into the bone at this point and you should find a small depression. This is LI 4. Treat the point with static pressure for 3–5 breaths. **See Figure 15.41**

Stretches

Wrist extensors

- Kneel in proposal stance so you are level with the arm you are working. With the client's arm straight and the forearm pronated (palm towards the floor), ask the client to take a breath in. On the out breath, gently take their wrist into flexion to stretch the wrist extensors. Work with client communication so you know when they have felt the stretch. As an added extra you can also curl their fingers over at

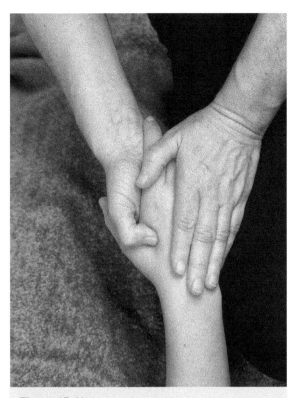

Figure 15.41
Acupressure point LI 4

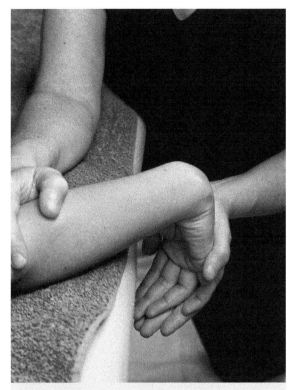

Figure 15.42
Wrist extensor stretch

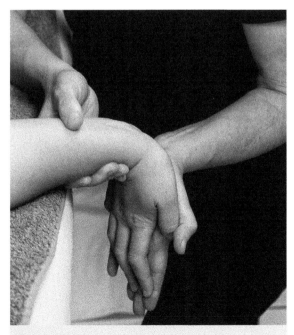

Figure 15.43
Wrist flexor stretch

the end to provide more stretch if appropriate. **See Figure 15.42**

Wrist flexors

- Now supinate the forearm (palm towards ceiling). Working with the breath and client communication, gently take their wrist into extension (with the back of their hand towards the floor). **See Figure 15.43**

Teaching self-care suggestions

These can be found in the Self-Care Resources (available at uk.singingdragon.com/catalogue/book/9781909141230).

References

DeLany J 2009 Spotlight on palmaris longus. Massage Today 9:7. Available at: http://www.massagetoday.com/mpacms/mt/article.php?id=14033 [accessed 8 August 2014].

Upton ARM, McComas AJ 1973 The double crush in nerve entrapment syndromes. Lancet 2:359–362.

16
Hip and pelvis pain protocol

Introduction

The following protocol can be used for more specific work around the pelvic girdle. In conjunction with techniques from the low back pain chapter (see Chapter 12), this protocol is useful to treat conditions such as:

- Sacroiliac (SI) joint pain

- Sciatica

- Sporting injuries such as groin strain

- Osteoarthritis.

Heat and preparation work over the drape

- Start with your client in a prone position.

- **Draping**: due to the nature of the adductor work in the supine sequence of the protocol, it is usually more comfortable for your client to keep their underwear on. Remember to bolster under the belly while your client is prone.

- Apply heat or cold as appropriate.

- **Beginnings**: start with still work. Have one hand on the sacrum and the other on the thoracic area and take time to tune into your client's unique mind–body, breath and vibratory and energetic rhythms.

- **Palming the back of the body**: use the palming techniques described in the low back and leg, knee and foot chapters (see Chapters 12 and 17) to lean in and work the whole of the back of the body with compression. Remember the dictum that 'all assessment is treatment and all treatment is assessment' and use this time to assess the condition of the musculature of the back, pelvis and legs, noting which side feels tighter. This not only gives you important information about where to focus your work but helps your client experience their body as an integrated whole. Tissue tightness around the pelvic girdle will undoubtedly affect and be affected by the

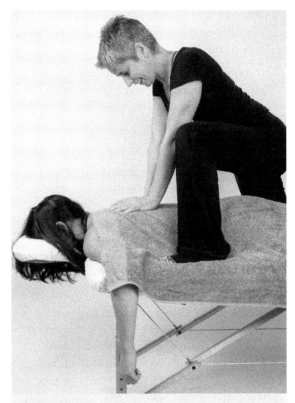

Figure 16.1
Palming the back of the body

myofascial structures above and below, so this step is very important. **See Figure 16.1**

Fascial work

- **Myofascial cross hand stretch to the sacrum and low back**: place one hand on the sacrum and the other lightly over the spine on the low back area. Taking care not to press too hard on the spine, sink into the tissues and separate your hands away from each other to take the tissues into a stretch. Tune into the tissues and follow any twists and turns you perceive whilst keeping the fascia on a stretch. You may find that you are able to tune into a sensation of the sacrum moving slightly from one side to another, eventually coming back to a still place where there is a sense of buoyancy and floating in the tissues. Release the stretch when there is no more effective change. **See Figure 16.2**

- Repeat the cross hand stretches in different areas as needed. For example:

  - On both sides of the back in the quadratus lumborum area (one hand on the iliac crest and one on the low back).

  - Over the gluteal region (for here you will need to sink down deeply both with pressure and your focus and intention).

  - One hand on the gluteal region and the other on the hamstrings.

- **Finger work over the sacrum**: working the superficial fascia over the sacrum feels amazing. Stand in t'ai chi position on the opposite side of the client's body; have your relaxed fingers at an oblique angle to the tissues. Starting at the midline of the sacrum, work the fascia and tissue over the sacrum from medial to lateral. **See Figure 16.3**

- **Modified skin rolling to gluteal area**: a modified form of skin rolling can be used on the gluteal area. It is difficult to use the motion of moving forwards but you can work specific areas by squeezing and rolling the tissue between your fingers and thumbs. Grasp a roll of tissue and lift it away from the body towards the ceiling, then

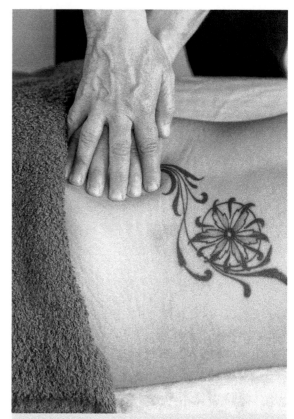

Figure 16.3
Finger work over the sacrum

put the fascia on a stretch between both hands. Those of you familiar with indirect myofascial work will be able to listen in and follow the movement of the tissue until you feel a release.

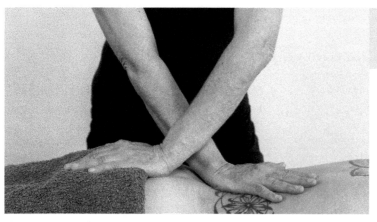

Figure 16.2
Cross hand stretch to sacrum and low back

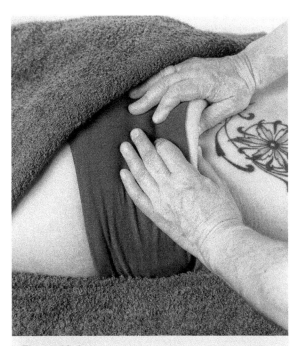

Figure 16.4
Modified skin rolling to the gluteal area

This is like a three-dimensional version of a cross hand stretch. **See Figure 16.4**

Muscular and trigger point work

Broad work to the low back

- Apply lubrication and do some broad work to the low back using power effleurage or forearm effleurage as described in the low back chapter (see Chapter 12).

Release the quadratus lumborum

- Assess both of the quadratus lumborum (QL) muscles for trigger points and tightness and release as described in the low back chapter (Chapter 12). **See Figure 16.5A–D**

- **Broad work to the QL**: finish with some broad work with a soft fist to the QL, really leaning into the tissues to get a nice stretch. **See Figure 16.5E, p. 294**

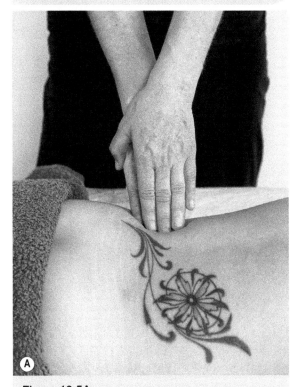

(A)

Figure 16.5A
QL: transverse process attachments

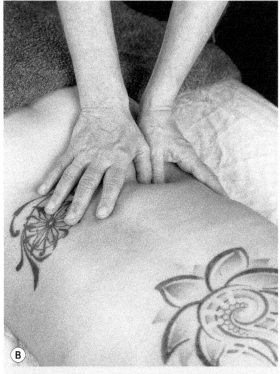

(B)

Figure 16.5B
QL: 12th rib attachment

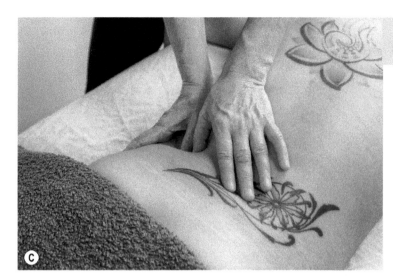

Figure 16.5C
QL: glide down the side

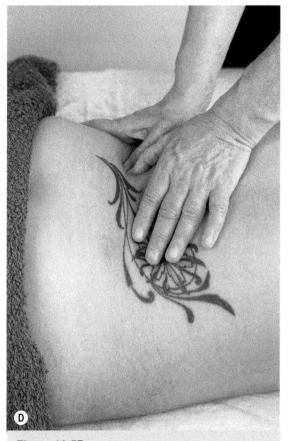

Figure 16.5D
QL: glide down the side

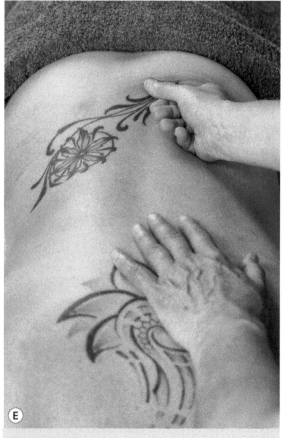

Figure 16.5E
QL: broad work with soft fist

Release the iliolumbar ligament

- Prominent massage author Ben Benjamin states:

Ligament injuries are the most frequently ignored and misunderstood factor in low-back pain. More often than not, chronic pain in the low-back area is caused by tears and subsequent adhesive scar tissue formation in the ligaments. Although the majority of low-back pain actually originates in the sacral ligaments, tears to the ligaments at L1 through L5 and the iliolumbar ligament occur frequently and can be very painful.
Ben Benjamin 2014

- The iliolumbar ligament is located between the transverse processes of L4 and L5 and the posterior iliac crest. It is deep to the thoracolumbar fascia, QL and multifidus. **See Figure 16.6**

- To locate the ligament, first find the posterior superior iliac spine and then slide your supported thumbs in a superior direction. Facing the feet in t'ai chi stance, use cross fibre friction to work the ligament with firm pressure. **See Figure 16.7**

Gluteal area

- **Broad work to the gluteal area**: use a diagonal drape to expose the gluteal area and work over underwear. You can also work over the drape. Start with broad compression work using the forearm, palms or loose fists to open up the area. This also helps to assess which areas need more specific work. For forearm work use horse stance, leaning into the tissues with the soft part of your forearm (don't forget that floppy wrist!). Wait for the tissues to release as the musculature in this region is thick and needs time to respond. Digging and poking or

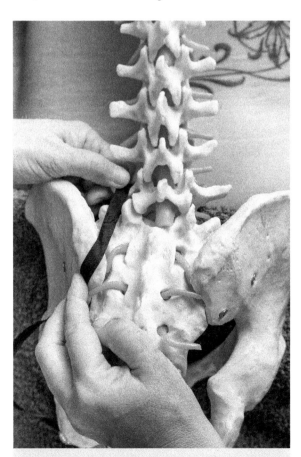

Figure 16.6
Location of the iliolumbar ligament

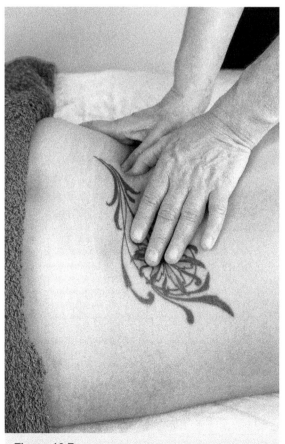

Figure 16.7
Treating the iliolumbar ligament

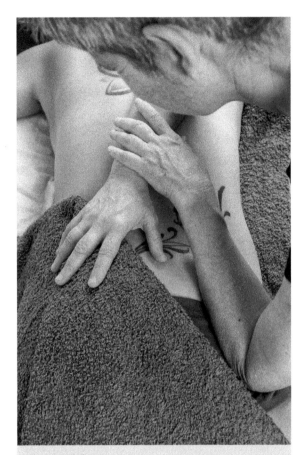

Figure 16.8
Broad work to the gluteal area

working too quickly will only make your work less effective and cause your client unnecessary pain. **See Figure 16.8**

- To work the gluteal area more specifically you can mentally divide the buttock area into thirds:

  - The top third houses the gluteus medius.

  - The middle third is where we find the piriformis.

  - The inferior third is where the obturator internus lives.

Gluteus medius

- This is an important area and the gluteus medius often harbours many trigger points. In horse stance facing the side of the table, first lean in using a broad forearm. To treat your client's right side use your left forearm, the other rests lightly on your

client's back. We joke that this is a bit like leaning on the bar at the end of a long day. Don't be afraid to gradually sink in with your full weight as the gluteal muscles are thick and covered by a layer of adipose tissue, so you have a lot to get through. Slowly bring your broad forearm up into more of an angle so that you can use a 'listening elbow' to sink into the tissue and identify areas of restriction and trigger points. Wait for the tissue to melt and soften. **See Figure 16.9**

Piriformis

- Find the top and bottom of the sacrum and the top of the greater trochanter (the bony bump on the side of the thigh). These three points form a triangle and the piriformis is found right in the centre of this triangle, deep to the gluteus maximus. Hook onto the muscle by sinking down with your elbow

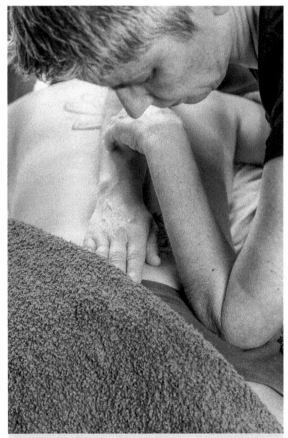

Figure 16.9
Working gluteus medius ('top third' of gluteal region)

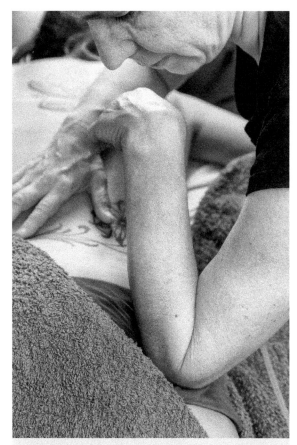

Figure 16.10
Releasing piriformis ('middle third' of gluteal region)

into the tissue. Wait for the melt and release. **See Figure 16.10**

- You may also wish to include techniques from the low back chapter (Chapter 12) to release the piriformis. These are all equally effective.

Obturator internus

- This muscle wraps around and interacts with the pelvic floor. With soft fingers sink into the middle of the gluteal crease so that you locate and contact the ischial tuberosity, which is the bony landmark that you sit on. Keeping in contact with the bone, now use your fingertips to walk through the soft tissue an inch or so superiorly until you contact a slight dip. This area is where the obturator internus turns and comes to the outer body. From here it

moves horizontally to the greater trochanter, running alongside the gemelli muscles.

- Contact the muscle with your fingertips and sink down into the tissues. Now give a slight hook with intention down towards the feet.
- Often waiting and holding with intention and focus will initiate a release in this area, so wait for the softening and relaxation of the tissues. You can enhance this effect, once you have felt the release, by asking the client to lengthen their leg by pushing the sole of their foot down over the end of the table (without pointing as this is just a leg lengthening). **See Figure 16.11A,B, p. 298**

Quadratus femoris

This muscle feels like a small mound or pillow. You can find it just above the gluteal fold and running from the ischial tuberosity to the greater trochanter. Work with supported fingers until you feel a release. **See Figure 16.12, p. 298**

Working the trochanteric notch

- From the head of the table and facing towards the client's feet, find the bony bump of the greater trochanter and then palpate slightly superiorly and posteriorly to find the trochanteric notch. The tendinous attachments of many of the lateral rotators can be usefully accessed here. Use your thumbs to work around the trochanteric notch using static pressure and cross fibre friction (pressure in one direction only). This releases the inferior attachments of the 'deep six' lateral rotator group. **See Figure 16.13, p. 299**

Stretching the deep six lateral rotators

- Use static, proprioceptive neuromuscular facilitation (PNF) or active isolated stretching techniques to stretch the piriformis. Abduct the leg 30 degrees and repeat to stretch the other lateral rotators more specifically. **See Figure 16.14, p. 299**

Sacrotuberous ligament

This broad, solid ligament runs from the ischial tuberosity to the edge of the sacrum. If you palpate into the middle of the gluteal crease you should be able to feel the sacrotuberous ligament as it blends fascially into the insertion point of the hamstrings. If you are having

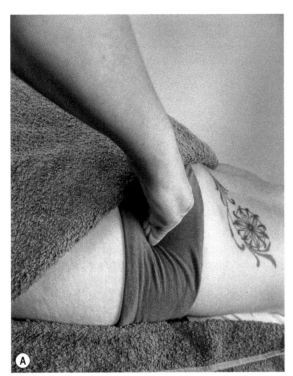

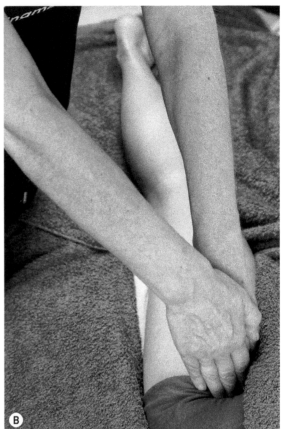

Figure 16.11A,B
Obturator internus

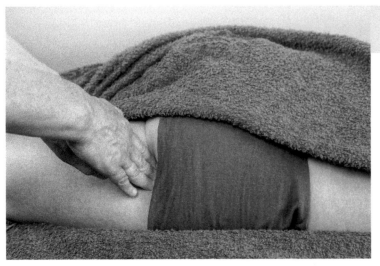

Figure 16.12
Quadratus femoris

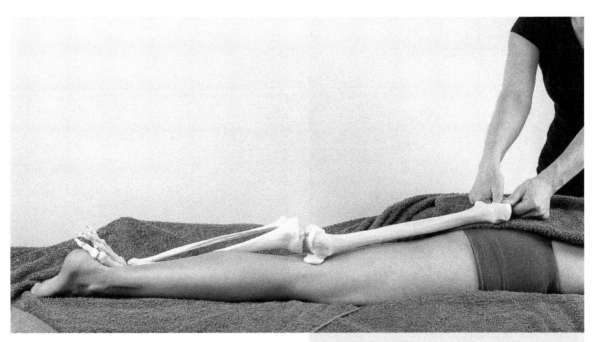

Figure 16.13
Working the trochanteric notch

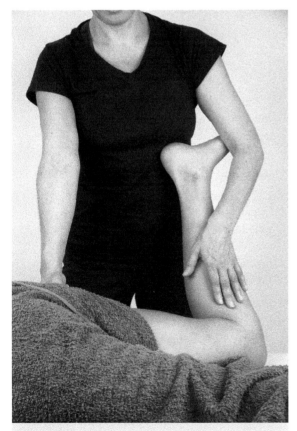

Figure 16.14
Stretching the deep six lateral rotators

difficulty locating the superior hamstring insertion point, ask your client to extend their femur ('Raise your leg towards the ceiling') and you should feel the strong cable pop into your hands.

- To release the fascial attachment of the sacrotuberous ligament as it blends into the hamstrings. Face the client's head in t'ai chi stance. Using your inside forearm sink into the attachment at the ischial tuberosity using a listening elbow. Wait and hold until you feel the sensation of softening and tissue release. **See Figure 16.15, p. 300**

- Then work the ligament with supported fingers or thumbs and using a strumming motion. You will need to work through the thick gluteus maximus belly to contact the ligament. **See Figure 16.16, p. 300**

Release work to the hamstrings

- Use any release techniques from the leg, knee and foot chapter (see Chapter 17) or any other techniques you know to release the hamstrings. **See Figure 16.17, p. 301**

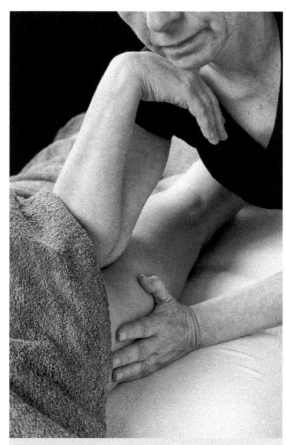

Figure 16.15
Release the sacrotuberous ligament attachment

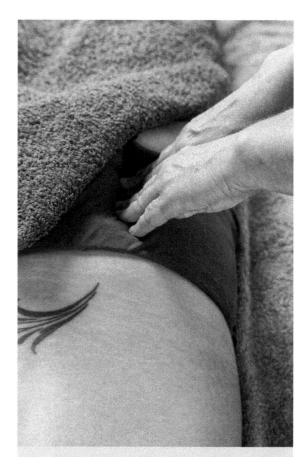

Figure 16.16
Work sacrotuberous ligament with supported thumbs

Working the gluteus medius and tensor fasciae latae (TFL)

- Place your client in a side-lying position with their affected hip uppermost (knees together).

- Kneel with your inside knee on the edge of the table. Your other leg is in contact with the floor. With knuckles or a listening elbow sink down into the tissues and spread the fascia and muscles out from the greater trochanter with fan-like strokes radiating in all directions. **See Figure 16.18**

TFL

- This is the more anterior muscle on the side of the hip. Sink in with the heels of your hands, your fists or a listening elbow. Work with supported thumbs to identify and treat trigger points. **See Figure 16.19**

Gluteus medius and minimus

- You will need a 'listening elbow' to sink down through the tough gluteus medius into the gluteus minimus. Stand in t'ai chi stance and keep your wrist floppy. You can work over the drape if necessary. Treat any trigger points you find. **See Figure 16.20, p. 302**

- **Pin and stretch for gluteus minimus:** abduct the leg to put the muscles on a slack and then sink into the gluteus medius and minimus area with your elbow. The easiest way to lift the leg is to align your forearm with the client's lower leg to provide support. As the leg can be surprisingly heavy once it is abducted, you may wish to support it in this position with your own leg on the table. Get your client to breathe in and out and then lower their leg

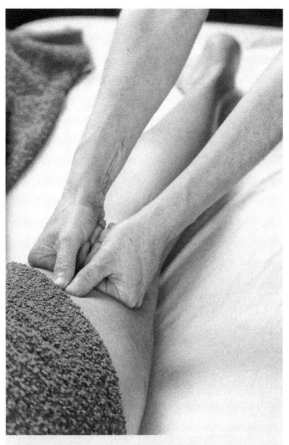

Figure 16.17
Release work to hamstrings

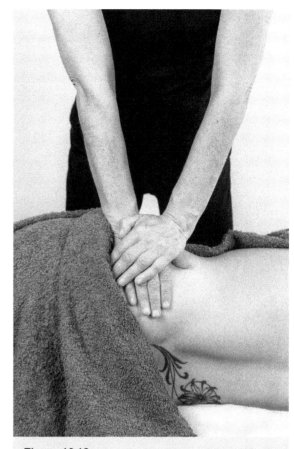

Figure 16.19
Working the TFL

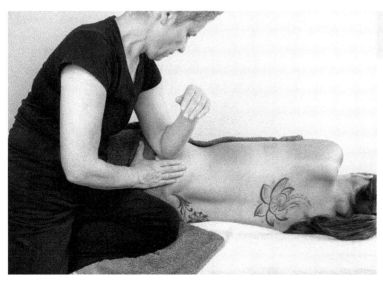

Figure 16.18
Working the gluteus medius and TFL

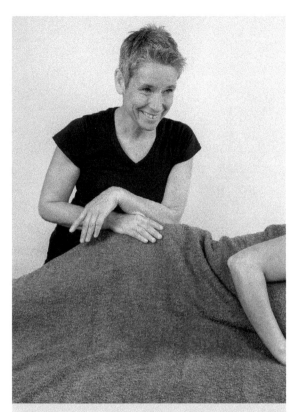

Figure 16.20
Working the gluteus medius and minimus

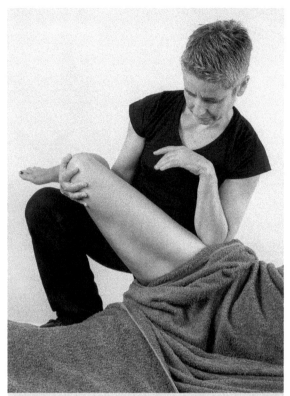

Figure 16.21
Pin and stretch for the gluteus minimus

slowly back to the table to get an effective release. Use caution and work with the client's breath and to their tolerance level as this area can be very tender. **See Figure 16.21**

Iliacus

- **Side-lying iliacus release**: you can release the iliacus from this position by sinking around the rim of the pelvis with soft fingers. Use static pressure and gentle cross fibre friction pressing back towards you to treat and release the muscle and any trigger points. Either work through the drape or do T-draping to expose the iliacus region. **See Figure 16.22**

Internal and external obliques

- **Cleaning the iliac crest**: using a rake-like motion with the pads of your fingers, work the top edge of the iliac crest (like windscreen wipers going in opposite directions). The fingers of both hands start together then move outwards. Treat any trigger

points you find, which are common in the external obliques just above the iliac crest. **See Figure 16.23**

- **Myofascial stretch to the external/internal abdominal obliques and the fascial 'lateral line' of the body**: place one hand on the iliac crest and one on the lateral ribs in a cross hand stretch. Wait and sink into the body for at least 90 seconds and then move the hands in opposite directions to put the fascia on a stretch. Wait and follow any releases. **See Figure 16.24**

- **Cross hand stretch with leg off the table**: to enhance the stretch the leg can also be placed off the side of the table. Make sure the client's body is not twisted and is securely placed on the table. **See Figure 16.25, p. 304**

- **Stripping the external and internal obliques**: in t'ai chi stance, use muscle stripping from the lateral ribs to the iliac crest to address any trigger points in the external and internal obliques. **See Figure 16.26, p. 304**

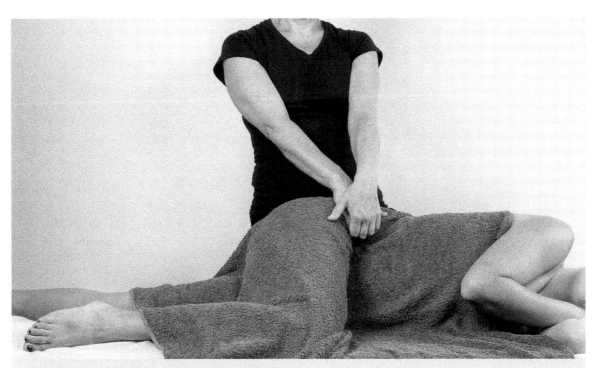

Figure 16.22
Side-lying iliacus release

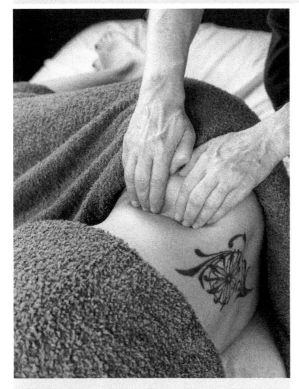

Figure 16.23
Cleaning the iliac crest

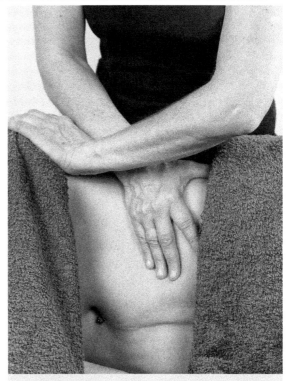

Figure 16.24
Cross hand stretch to external/internal abdominal obliques

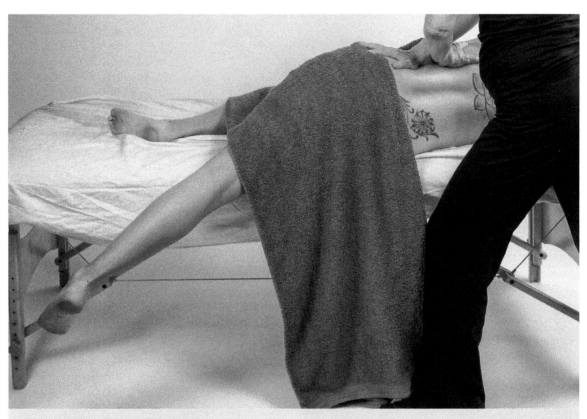

Figure 16.25
Cross hand stretch with the leg off the table

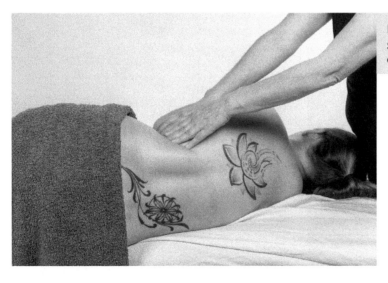

Figure 16.26
Stripping internal and external obliques

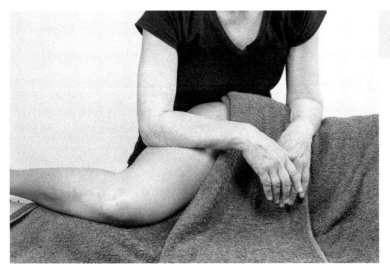

Figure 16.27
Working the IT band

Iliotibial (IT) band

- **Release the IT band**: use your forearms to release the IT band. In horse stance, first use the soft fleshy part of your forearm, moving from the client's hip to their knee. Once the area is warmed up, you can start to use the ulnar edge of your forearm as this gives a deeper stroke. Use caution as this area can be VERY tender. Depending on how you angle your forearm you can work either the more anterior or posterior edges of the muscle. **See Figure 16.27**

Adductors

- Client side-lying with the affected hip towards the table (bottom leg straight).

- **Cleaning the pes anserinus region**: this is the area at the medial knee where the sartorius, semitendinosus and gracilis all converge to form the larger pes anserinus tendon that attaches to the proximal, medial shaft of the tibia. Use the backs of your knuckles or fingers to work this region. **See Figure 16.28**

- **Working the belly of the adductor group**: in t'ai chi stance and facing the inside of the thigh let the palm of your forward hand strip across the belly of the muscle while at the same time the knuckles of your other hand come back towards you. This spreading movement causes the adductors to widen from the midline. **See Figure 16.29, p. 306**

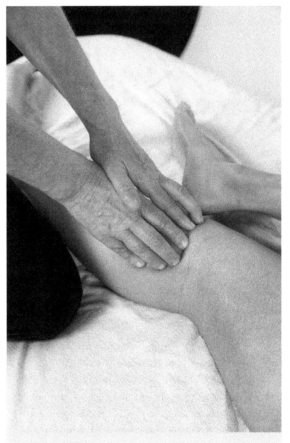

Figure 16.28
Cleaning the pes anserinus region

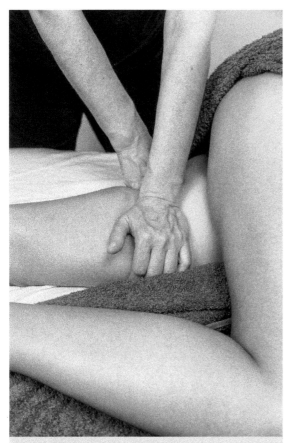

Figure 16.29
Working the belly of the adductor group

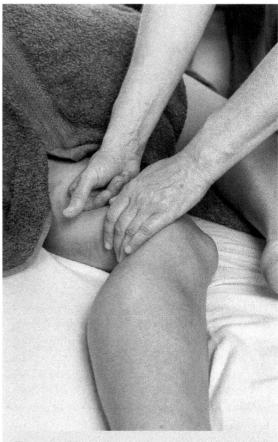

Figure 16.30
Working the belly of the adductors with movement

- **Working the belly of the adductors with movement**: an alternative or addition to this stroke is to stand on the opposite side of the table. Use your fist to strip through the adductors while your other hand passively moves the thigh towards you. See Figure 16.30

- **Treating the proximal adductor magnus attachments on the ischial ramus**: explain to your client why you need to work the adductor attachments and ensure that they feel

psychologically comfortable with this concept. Let them know that you will stop the work immediately if they feel uncomfortable in any way. Keep an eye on their face while you do this work.

- Confidently place your fingers right up to the bone and work the area with cross fibre friction. Use soft fingers and forward t'ai chi stance. See Figure 16.31

Myofascial release (MFR) of the pelvic transverse plane: 'tummy sandwich'

Now turn your client to a supine position to work the fascia of the abdominal region. The majority of the myofascia runs vertically from head to toe but there are places where there are transverse continuities, rather like the hoops of a barrel. One such place is found at the pelvic diaphragm. With your client supine, place one hand under their sacrum and your top hand between the umbilicus and the pubic bone. Make sure the upper

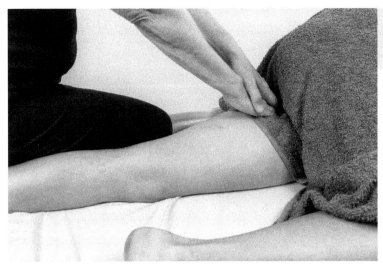

Figure 16.31
Working the adductor magnus attachments on ischial ramus

hand has the little finger side towards the pubic bone to prevent your thumb straying into the groin area inadvertently. Press your hands towards each other very slightly as if you are holding a water filled balloon. Wait for the signs of yielding and tissue release before following the tissue to the next barrier. This whole process could take up to 5 minutes or longer in some cases. **See Figure 16.32**

Psoas and iliacus

- **Cross hand stretch over the psoas and iliacus region**: place one hand just above the iliacus and the other on the upper leg. Sink down and put the fascia on a stretch in opposite directions. Wait and hold for 3–5 minutes until you get a sense of release. **See Figure 16.33, p. 308**

- **Cross hand stretch with the leg off the table**: to enhance a psoas release you can perform the cross hand stretch with the client's leg off the side of the table. Make sure the client does not have low back pain in this position. Also ensure their leg is not overstretched at the groin area which in some cases can be injurious to the skin. **See Figure 16.34, p. 308**

- **Psoas and iliacus release**: release these muscles as per the Low Back Pain Protocol (see Chapter 12).

- **Positional release for the psoas**: place the heel of your hand in the belly of the psoas muscle. Sink down with intent until you contact the muscle. With your other hand move the leg by using the

knee as a fulcrum. If you find areas of tension or trigger points hold and wait for a release. **See Figure 16.35, p. 309**

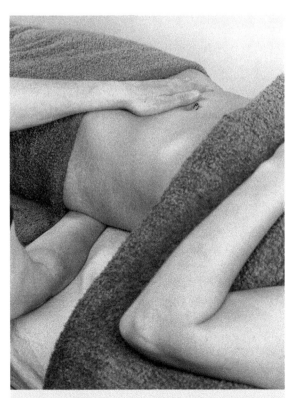

Figure 16.32
Pelvic transverse fascial plane release

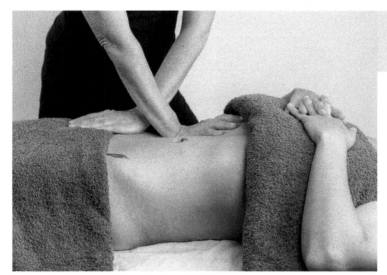

Figure 16.33
Cross hand stretch over the psoas and iliacus

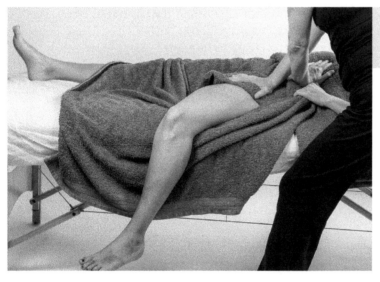

Figure 16.34
Cross hand stretch with the leg off the table

Rectus abdominis

- **Strip the rectus abdominis**: this is the 'six pack' muscle running from the ribs to the pubic bone. In t'ai chi stance, strip the muscle from pubic bone to ribs and treat any trigger points. Always ensure you communicate with your client as to what you are doing, especially at the distal attachments. A useful protection for the client is to ask them to lay their hands horizontally on the pubic bone with their index fingers on the upper edge, so that they feel safe that you will not venture beyond this point.
See Figure 16.36

> **CAUTION**
> With the following techniques, take care not to exert pressure deep into the femoral triangle which contains the femoral blood vessels and nerve. Release your pressure if you feel a pulse directly beneath your fingertips or your client gets a sensation of nerve compression (i.e. tingling, burning, shooting)

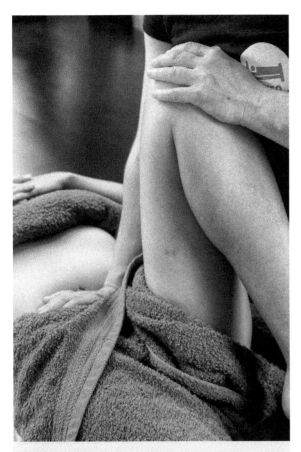

Figure 16.35
Psoas positional release

FEMORAL TRIANGLE

The femoral triangle is considered an endangerment site due to the superficial proximity of certain nerves and blood vessels. The femoral triangle is easily identified, e.g. if your client flexes, abducts and laterally rotates their thigh (in other words puts their leg in a figure-of-four position) you will see a triangular depression in the inner thigh.

The femoral triangle is shaped like a sail and handily the anatomical boundaries can also be remembered using the mnemonic 'SAIL':

- **S** Sartorius's medial border creates the lateral border of the triangle

- **A** Adductor longus forms the medial border of the triangle. The adductor longus is easily identifiable as the most prominent muscle tendon that pops up when the leg is in the figure-of-four position

- **IL** Inguinal Ligament which forms the superior border of the triangle

The floor of the femoral triangle is formed by the pectineus and adductor longus muscles, medially, and iliopsoas muscle, laterally.

(Continued)

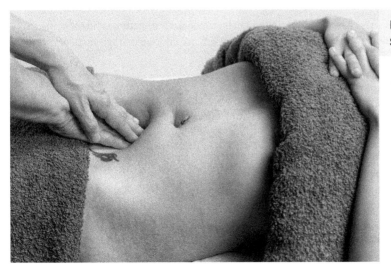

Figure 16.36
Stripping the rectus abdominis

(Continued)

The structures that are contained within the femoral triangle can be remembered by the mnemonic: 'NAVEL'. Running from lateral to medial:

- **N** Femoral Nerve
- **A** Femoral Artery (and several of its branches)
- **V** Femoral Vein
- **E** Empty space
- **L** Deep inguinal Lymph nodes and associated Lymphatic vessels

As the neurovascular bundle is quite superficial, you need to take care while palpating in this area. Release your pressure and reposition if you feel a pulse directly beneath your fingertips or your client gets a sensation of nerve compression (i.e. tingling, burning and shooting sensations)

Pectineus

- **Release the pectineus**: as always, ensure you work with client communication around this sensitive area. Your client is in a supine position with their hip flexed so that their foot is on the table and their leg is in 'triangle' position. Place the flat of your hand on the middle of the medial thigh while supporting your client's leg with your body as you sit on the edge of the table. **See Figure 16.37**

- Locate the prominent tendon of the adductor longus and put your ring finger on the tendon of this muscle. Your middle and index finger should be where the pectineus is found. Slide off this laterally towards the anterior superior iliac spine (ASIS) and into the 'pocket' you find. Slowly sink into the belly of the pectineus. Ask your client to adduct their hip against resistance if you are not sure if you are in the right place.

- Use static pressure and/or gentle cross fibre friction to release trigger points.

- **Range of motion (ROM)**: take the client's hip joint in a complete ROM clockwise and anticlockwise. Use care in cases of osteoarthritis and work with

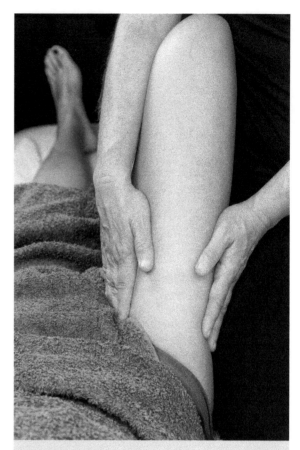

Figure 16.37
Releasing the pectineus

client tolerance. In cases of hip replacement make sure you have checked in your case history which movements are not advisable for your client. **See Figure 16.38**

- **Finish with leg pulls to both legs**: singly and then simultaneously to finally release and balance the pelvis. **See Figure 16.39**

Acupressure points

Gall Bladder 30 (GB 30): Jumping Round

- **Location**: the sacral hiatus is approximately one thumb width from the tip of the coccyx. To find the point draw an imaginary line from the sacral hiatus to the greater trochanter. Divide the line into thirds and GB 30 is two-thirds of the way on this line from hiatus to trochanter.

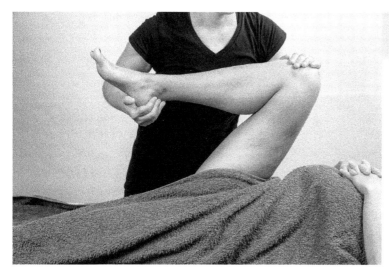

Figure 16.38
Hip ROM

- Use supported fingers to treat the point. **See Figure 16.40**

Gall Bladder 29 (GB 29): Squatting Bone Hole

- **Location**: in a depression at the midpoint between the greater trochanter and the ASIS. A great point for hip pain or sciatica.

- To find the point draw an imaginary line from the greater trochanter to the ASIS (this is the bony

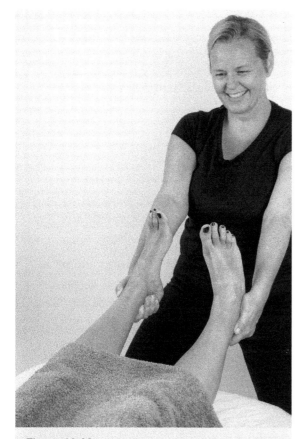

Figure 16.39
Leg pull

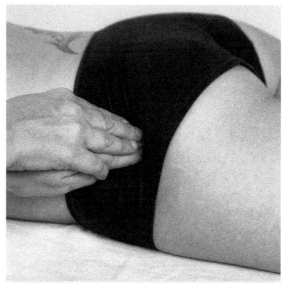

Figure 16.40
Acupressure point Gall Bladder 30

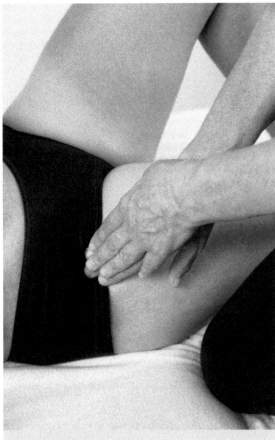

Figure 16.41
Acupressure point Gall Bladder 29

bump at the top of your hip bone). GB 29 is halfway down this line in a palpable depression. Treat with supported fingers, holding the point for 3–5 breaths. **See Figure 16.41**

Stretches

Side-lying stretch for hip abductors

- The client lies on their side at the edge of the table; their top leg hangs over the side of the table and their bottom leg is bent (ensure their knee is clear of the table). Their hips should be stacked vertically on top of one another. If the client experiences any low back pain in this position, they can bend forward to round their low back.

- Stand behind the client using your hip as support to stabilise their hip. Place one hand on the iliac crest

and with the other hand press their thigh, just above the knee, towards floor. **See Figure 16.42**

Side-lying psoas

- Sit on the table with your back to the client so you are supporting their lumbar spine. Flex the client's knee and support the lower leg with one hand on their knee and one hand on their foot.

- Ask the client to breathe in and on the out breath twist your body so you are extending their hip to take the leg back from the table and towards you. This is a good stretch for both rectus femoris and the psoas. Keep an eye on your client's face and work with their breath and communication. **See Figure 16.43**

Supine stretch for the long adductors

- To work on the left leg ask the client to hook their right leg over the side of the table to help anchor the stretch.

- Standing at the left side of the table, take the client's leg in your hands, supporting both above and below the knee. Working with the breath and client communication, start to abduct the leg.

- Now move your body so you are between the table and the client's leg; support the lower leg with your right hand and place your left hand across the medial aspect of the knee. This position prevents stress to the medial collateral ligament.

- Using your body as support, gently take their leg outwards until the client indicates they have felt a stretch. **See Figure 16.44, p. 314**

Supine stretch for the short adductors

- With the client in a supine position. Stand in forward t'ai chi stance and facing the client's feet.

- Ask the client to bend their left knee and place the sole of their left foot against their right leg so they are in a figure-of-four position.

- Position yourself to lightly stabilise the client's right hip against the table with your right hand. Use your other hand or forearm to encourage the bent leg to gently drop towards the table with the breath. If the adductors are very tight you may need to bolster under the thigh. **See Figure 16.45, p. 314**

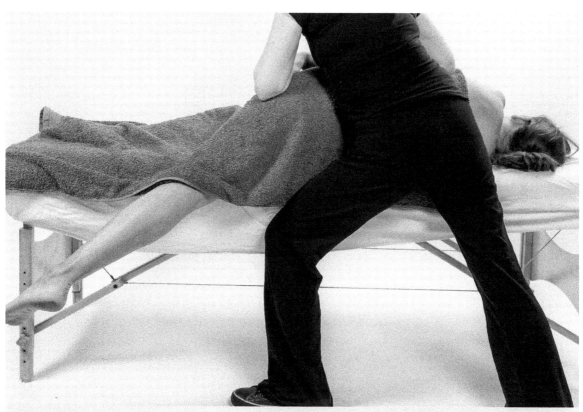

Figure 16.42
Side-lying stretch for hip abductors

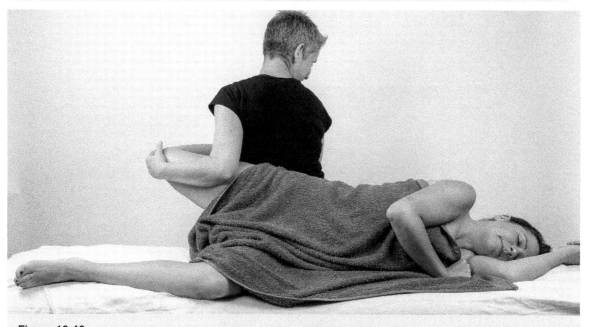

Figure 16.43
Side-lying psoas stretch

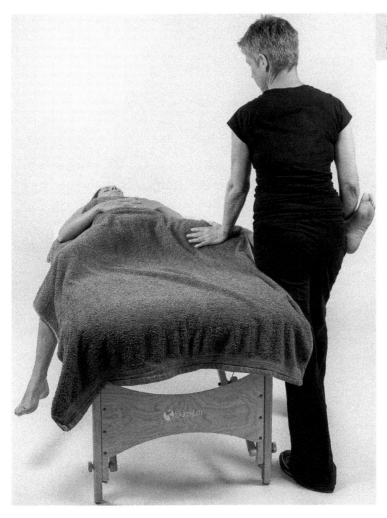

Figure 16.44
Supine long adductor stretch

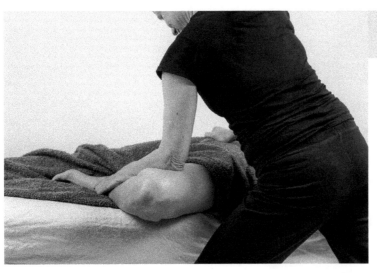

Figure 16.45
Supine short adductor stretch

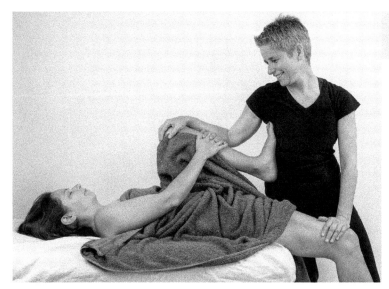

Figure 16.46
Iliopsoas stretch

Iliopsoas stretch

- The client hugs both legs to their chest and positions themselves so their ischial tuberosities are at the end of the table.

- Position yourself so that the foot of the leg that is **not** being treated is against your shoulder or side and you are facing the leg to be stretched.
  See Figure 16.46

- The client lets go of the leg to be stretched. Take hold of their leg and gently lower it towards the floor.

- Gently press the thigh to be treated towards the floor. You will not need any more than a 'suggestion' of pressure as gravity does most of the work for you.

- Ensure that the client's low back is pressed onto the table. This is very important for protecting the low back.

- When both sides are finished have your client bring both knees to their chest. The client then pushes against you with both feet so that they are positioned more fully on the table.

Teaching self-care suggestions

Self-care suggestions can be found in the Self-Care Resources (available online at uk.singingdragon.com/catalogue/book/9781909141230).

Reference

Benjamin B 2014 The mystery of low back pain: Part II. Available from massagetherapy.com: http://www.massagetherapy.com/articles/index.php/article_id/1179/The-Mystery-of-Low-Back-Pain%3A-Part-II. [accessed 6 November 2014].

Leg, knee and foot pain protocol

Introduction

The following protocol can be used in combination with techniques from the hip and pelvis chapter (see Chapter 16) to treat issues in the legs including:

- Strains and sprains
- Patellar tendonitis
- Achilles problems
- Iliotibial (IT) band syndrome
- Shin splints
- Groin strains
- Knee issues (arthritis, chondromalacia patella)
- Osteoarthritis.

Application of heat and preparatory work over the drape

- Start with your client in a prone position.
- **Bolstering:** your client will usually feel most comfortable with a small bolster under their ankles, although you may need to remove this for some of the techniques described below.
- Depending on the client's desired outcome you may need to also include work from the low back and hip and pelvis protocols. The length of time spent on this will depend on your own skill and judgement and the outcome needed by the client.
- **Use of hot or cold:** the nature of your client's complaint will determine your use of hot and cold. Muscle strains are common injuries in the legs, e.g. in adductor longus and hamstrings. Acute injuries may need cold application to help with pain and reduce swelling, whereas pain stemming from trigger points and fascial adhesions will respond better to heat.
- **Preparation work over towel for the legs:** palming down the legs. With one hand on the sacrum, palm

down the leg on the opposite side to where you are standing. Lean in with your body weight using either standing or table shiatsu techniques. The heel of your hand should be centred on the midline of the leg (Bladder channel in Chinese medicine). Cross to the other side of the table to work the other leg.

- Both legs can also be palmed at once using table shiatsu techniques. Get into kneeling stance on the table (make sure you have one knee up – don't straddle!) and lean into the stroke, moving forwards from the pelvis to achieve depth. Your arms should be straight but not locked and with an openness to the joints. Use soft fists on the hamstrings then an open palm when moving onto the calf muscles as these are often more tender. Soften your stroke and use less pressure around the back of the knee. **See Figures 17.1 and 17.2, p. 318**

- When you have palmed the full length of both legs, come to kneeling t'ai chi stance at the foot of the table and sink into the acupressure point Kidney 1 using your thumbs (see acupressure section for details). This point drains excess energy from the upper part of the body, especially the head, and is a wonderful way to start the treatment and ground your client. An alternative is simply to hold the heels. Visualise the energy flowing down from the client's head to their body and then down through your arms and body to the earth. **See Figure 17.3, p. 319**

You can also talk your client through a short visualisation as you do this, e.g. 'On your in breath, draw energy down your spine to your sacrum. On your out breath shoot this energy down your legs and out of your feet into my hands.'

Fascial release

- **Undrape:** ensure client privacy by making the drape tight around the medial part of the leg whilst also making sure you can access the areas

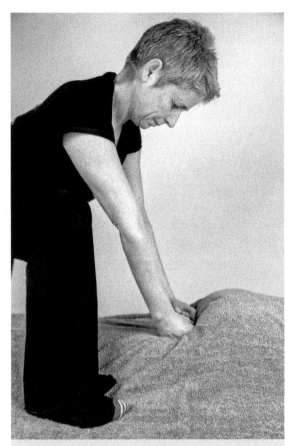

Figure 17.1
Soft fist work on the hamstrings

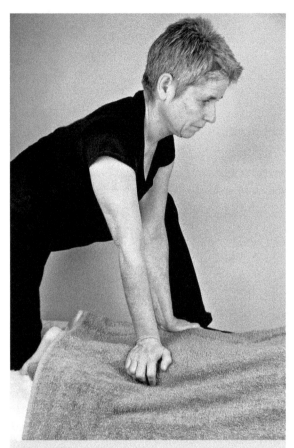

Figure 17.2
Double palming on the gastrocnemius

where you need to work. Follow the draping guidelines in the back to basics chapter (**see Chapter 2**).

- **Cross hand stretches:** these can be used over the whole area. For example:

  - One hand on the glutes and the other on the hamstrings.

  - For knee issues use one hand on the hamstrings and the other on the gastrocnemius.

  - To treat muscle strains begin with cross hand stretches on either side of the area of pain. **See Figures 17.4 and 17.5**

- **Fascial leg pulls:** these are a fantastic tool for both assessment and treatment. As an assessment tool you can use your listening touch to feel your way up the tissues to see where there might be restrictions

(think of pulling a piece of rope that someone has stepped on and trying to figure out where they are).

- To carry out a leg pull, take the weight of the client's leg in your hand. Make sure you have a soft grip. Lean back until you feel the tiniest bit of traction. Wait and hold and follow any movement that is initiated as a result of the stretch. Continue until you feel a softening and a fascial release that will almost feel like the limb is lengthening towards you.

- Wait for several releases, until there is no more movement.

- If at first you do not get a sense of where the limb wants to move, try initiating a very small movement, e.g. giving the leg a little lateral rotation, internal rotation or compression and seeing where it seems to go more easily. It is as if you are saying to the leg 'Do you want to go this way? Yes or no?' **See Figure 17.6, p. 320**

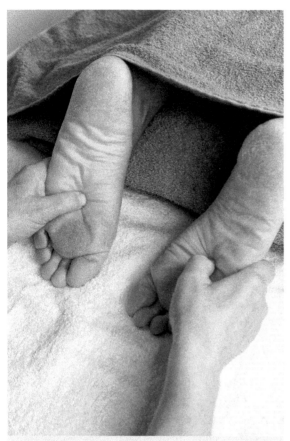

Figure 17.3
Treating acupressure point Kidney 1

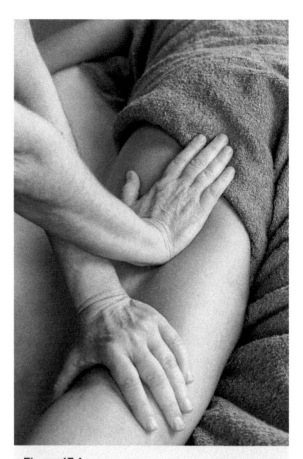

Figure 17.4
Cross hand stretch: hamstrings

Figure 17.5
Cross hand stretch: gastrocnemius

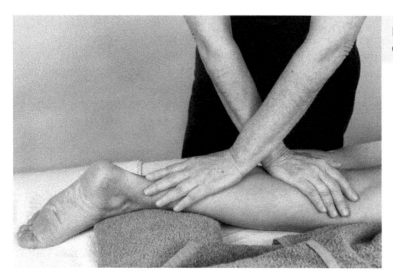

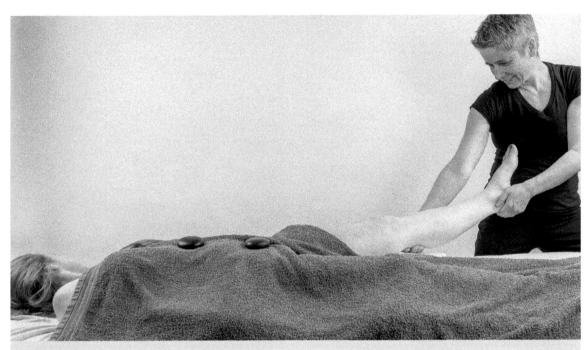

Figure 17.6
Myofascial leg pull

Muscular and trigger point work

Hamstrings

> **CAUTION**
>
> Be aware of the location of the popliteal fossa, i.e. the diamond-shaped area at the posterior knee which is traditionally classified as a massage 'endangerment site'. The superior area of the popliteal fossa is found between the lateral tendon of the biceps femoris and the medial tendons of the semitendinosus, semimembranosus and sartorius muscles. The inferior area consists of the two heads of the gastrocnemius muscle. This area contains the popliteal artery and vein and the tibial and common peroneal nerves, so be careful to work with focus and client communication and don't press too deeply. As Tom Myers famously says 'Don't press on anything that presses back at you!' If you feel a pulse beating under your fingers, move your fingers slightly. If your client gets an unpleasant nerve-type sensation, move your fingers

- **Releasing the common proximal hamstring insertion point:** all three hamstrings insert at the ischial tuberosity. Fascially the hamstrings connect to the sacrotuberous ligament and then onwards to the erector spinae as part of the superficial back line described by Tom Myers. The ischial tuberosity is the bony prominence that is in contact with the chair when you are sitting. In t'ai chi stance facing the client's head find the insertion point by palpating with your fingers halfway along the horizontal gluteal crease. You will feel a strong cable-like structure and if you ask your client to extend their hip ('Take your straight leg a little to the ceiling') you should feel this tendon pop into your fingers. **See Figure 17.7A,B**

  Now place a soft 'listening' elbow at this point (intention is towards the client's head) and sink gradually in and wait for a melting of the tissues. This is also a great acupressure point, Bladder 36, which is treated in exactly the same way. **See Figure 17.8, p. 322**

- **Release hamstring attachments on the tibia and fibula.** To locate the insertion points, ask your client to flex (bend) their knee against resistance (tell them

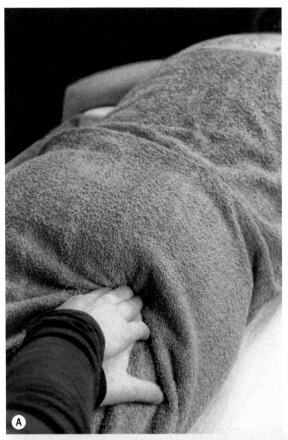

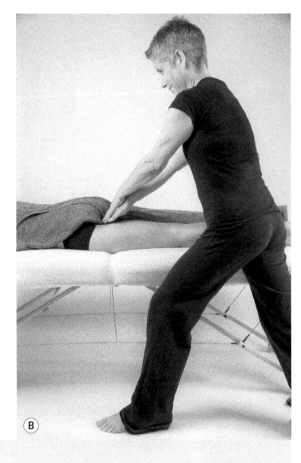

Figure 17.7A,B
Locating the common proximal hamstring attachment

'Bend your knee and try to take your heel to your buttocks'). Resist this action with your hand against their heel and you will see the distal (lower) attachment points of the hamstrings pop up like strong cables. Place the client's leg back on the bolster. **See Figure 17.9, p. 322**

In t'ai chi stance facing the client's head, use static pressure then cross fibre friction (pressure in one direction only) to release these attachments as they insert onto the bones just below the knee. **See Figures 17.10 and 17.11, p. 322**

- **Strip hamstring muscle bellies:** apply a small amount of lubrication. In a low t'ai chi stance, face the client's head and strip the hamstrings using the soft part of your forearm, leaning into the stroke with your body weight. To treat your client's right leg, use your left forearm and your other hand can support your wrist. Make sure you strip all the way

up to the attachment at the ischial tuberosity (you will need to check that the draping allows you to do this while ensuring your client's privacy). You can also include the medial adductor side of the client's leg by angling your forearm more to the medial side. **See Figures 17.12 and 17.13, p. 323**

- The IT band can also be included simultaneously in this stroke. Go into the forearm stroke as before and now hook your right hand over your left wrist so that the flat of your right palm is against the client's IT band. Now as you work the hamstrings with your forearm you are also simultaneously treating the IT band as you glide up the leg. **See Figure 17.14, p. 323**

Remember you are always searching for and treating trigger points, so you will need to work on developing enough sensitivity in your forearms to allow you to detect them accurately. You can also

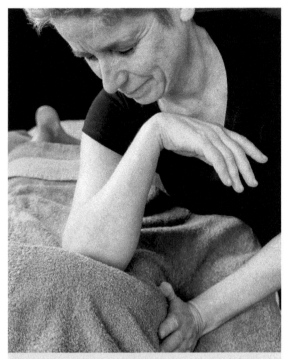

Figure 17.8
Releasing the common hamstring attachment point

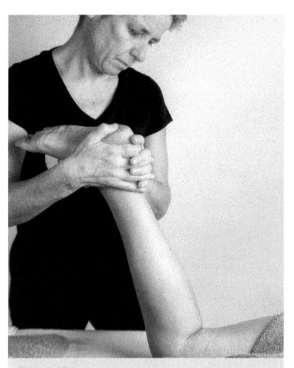

Figure 17.9
Locating the distal hamstring attachment points

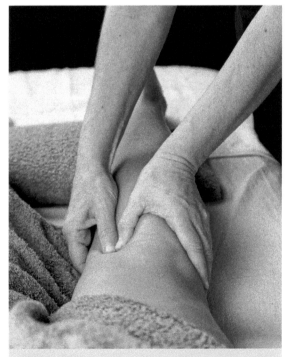

Figure 17.10
Releasing distal hamstring attachments on the tibia

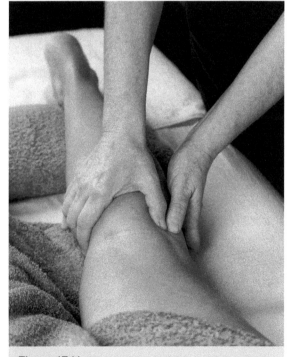

Figure 17.11
Releasing distal hamstring attachments on the fibula

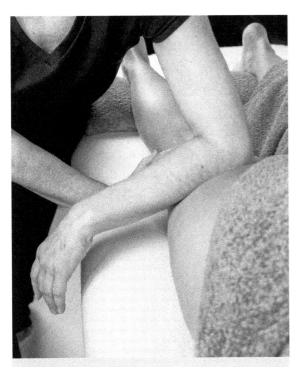

Figure 17.12
Stripping the hamstring muscle bellies

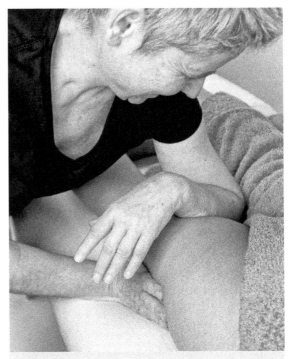

Figure 17.13
Working the medial hamstrings

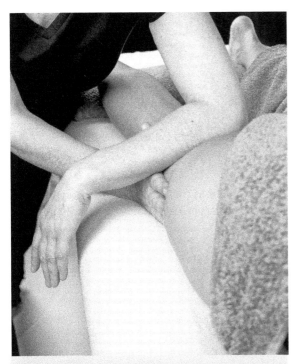

Figure 17.14
Working the IT band and hamstrings simultaneously

follow up the broad forearm work with more specific work with supported fingers if necessary.

- **Soft tissue release (STR) of hamstrings:** flex the client's leg to an angle of 90 degrees. To treat the client's right leg, stand facing the table and with your right hand anchored down on a point on the hamstrings with a broad 'lock', using the heel of your hand or a soft fist. Now take their foot down to the table for a short 2-second stretch. Repeat using different lock points on the hamstrings and getting into a smooth rhythm of lock–stretch–replace–repeat. You can work more specifically using the same technique but using the thumb or fingers – which can be very effective near the hamstring insertion points or to help release stubborn trigger points. **See Figures 17.15 and 17.16, p. 324**

You can also do a short strip of the muscles as you take the leg into the stretch. For this, turn so that you are in t'ai chi stance and facing the client's head. Find a point on their muscle to apply a lock and then do a short stripping movement longitudinally as you take the leg to the table. Repeat on different areas of the hamstrings.

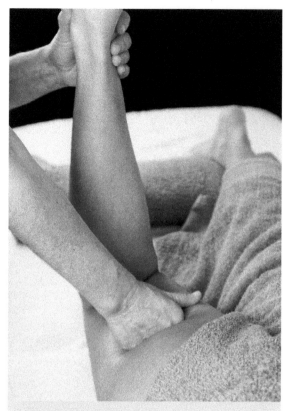

Figure 17.15
STR of hamstrings: the 'lock'

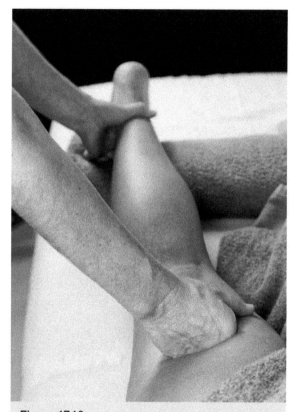

Figure 17.16
STR of hamstrings: the stretch

Popliteus and plantaris

These muscles lie underneath the superficial muscles above and below the knee crease, so take care with your palpation due to the proximity of the delicate nerves and blood vessels in the popliteal fossa.

- Locate the distal attachments of the hamstrings by asking your client to flex their leg against your resistance (as described earlier, see Figure 17.9). Locate the tendon of the biceps femoris on the lateral side of their knee and replace your client's leg either onto the bolster or onto your supporting knee which is resting on the table. The support is necessary as it is important to keep the knee in slight flexion to carry out the technique effectively.

- If treating your client's right leg, wrap your left hand around the medial side of their leg as support and place your right thumb just above the knee crease and lateral to the biceps femoris tendon.

- **To treat the popliteus:** palpate slightly underneath the biceps femoris and right down onto the femoral condyle to locate the soft tissue of the proximal popliteus attachment. Treat with static pressure or one directional cross fibre friction. **See Figure 17.17**

- To treat the plantaris attachment, move superiorly (towards the head) by one thumb width. Use static pressure and one directional cross fibre friction.

- To release the distal attachment of the popliteus, displace the gastrocnemius away from the crease in the knee by dropping with both thumbs between the two heads of the gastrocnemius. Press down into the posterior proximal tibia. There are often some tender trigger points here that are responsible for knee pain. **See Figure 17.18**

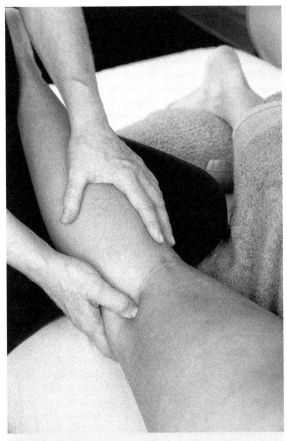

Figure 17.17
Treating popliteus (proximal attachment)

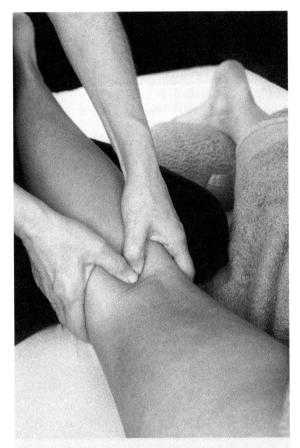

Figure 17.18
Treating popliteus (distal attachment)

Gastrocnemius

Gastrocnemius is the most superficial muscle on the back of the calf.

- **Forearm work to the gastrocnemius:** in t'ai chi stance (or kneeling stance if this is more comfortable) and facing the head of the table, flex your client's knee and place their foot on your inside shoulder. Sandwich their calf between your two forearms and use the soft medial part to glide down through the muscles, working both sides at the same time so you are squeezing the tissue between your arms. You can also work this area more deeply by supinating your forearms so that your palms face the ceiling, which allows you to use the harder ulnar part of your forearm. The calves are usually quite tender so only use this stroke after the other work. **See Figure 17.19, p. 326**

- **Muscle strip the gastrocnemius:** in t'ai chi stance, replace the client's leg on the bolster and, using thumbs or supported fingers, do some stripping work longitudinally through the muscle. Work in strips from the Achilles tendon to the attachments at the knee. Repeat the strips working from medial to lateral or lateral to medial to cover the whole muscle. **See Figure 17.20, p. 326**

- **Windscreen wiper stroke:** in t'ai chi stance and facing your client's head, work their left leg by placing your right hand on the middle of the muscle with your fingers pointing towards their head. Now place your left hand on top and lean into the stroke as you move from lateral to medial so that the bottom hand swivels like a windscreen wiper. This not only feels great but carries out an effective broad cross fibre stripping of the gastrocnemius. **See Figure 17.21 , p. 326**

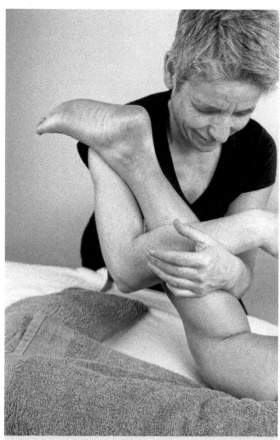

Figure 17.19
Forearm work to the gastrocnemius

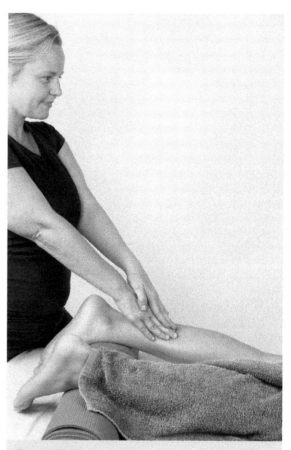

Figure 17.20
Muscle stripping the gastrocnemius

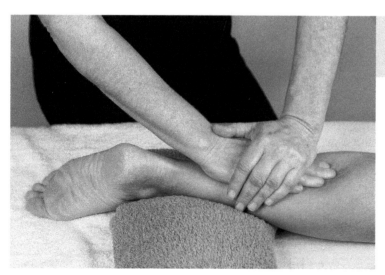

Figure 17.21
Windscreen wiper stroke on the gastrocnemius

Soleus

The soleus is located in the middle muscle layer, deep to the gastrocnemius.

- **Muscle strip the soleus:** stand by the side of the table in t'ai chi stance and put your inside knee on the table. Elevate the client's leg and support it against your diaphragm or sternum; this will enable you to hold their leg in position whilst freeing up both your hands to carry out the stroke. Make sure you are not pressing their foot down into a strong dorsiflexion whilst doing this, as this would put the soleus on a stretch and make the fibres more difficult to treat. Starting near the Achilles tendon, wrap your hands around the lower leg and press in with your thumbs on the muscle groove found either side of the gastrocnemius. Sink deeply towards the middle and you will be on the lateral and medial fibres of the soleus. Glide down the muscle slowly with inward pressure towards the knee. Repeat several times treating any trigger points you find. **See Figure 17.22**

Achilles tendon

- Replace the client's foot back on the bolster. In t'ai chi stance facing their head, work the Achilles tendon specifically with inward pressure using your thumbs on the medial and lateral sides, using a deep stripping motion. **See Figure 17.23**

Deep flexor compartment (the Tom, Dick and Harry muscles)

The deepest muscle layer contains the tibialis posterior, flexor digitorum longus and flexor hallucis longus muscles. A bit of a mouthful! These muscles can

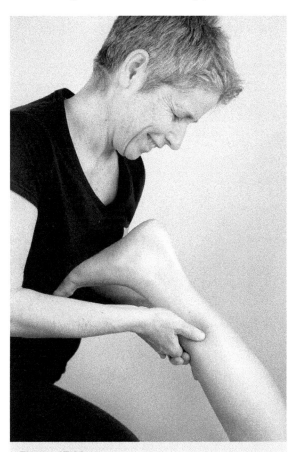

Figure 17.22
Muscle stripping the soleus

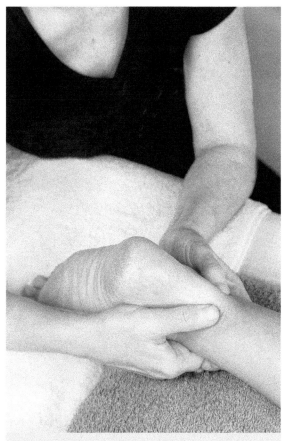

Figure 17.23
Working the Achilles tendon

easily be remembered by the mnemonic: Tom, Dick and Harry. They are a common source of trigger points and can be responsible for many foot and lower leg complaints.

Tibialis posterior and flexor digitorum longus

- To treat client's left leg, place your inside (right) hand in the muscle groove at the edge of the gastrocnemius. Now with your outside (left) hand move the superficial gastrocnemius MEDIALLY which helps your inside thumb sink deeper underneath the muscle. Now use your inside hand to slowly glide up the shaft of the tibia with your thumb whilst at the same time displacing the gastrocnemius medially with your outside hand to cause this muscle to 'fold over' your thumb. You should be able to feel the bone under your thumb as

you press the muscles against the bone. Treat any trigger points you find. Repeat as necessary.
See Figure 17.24

Flexor hallucis longus

- Medially displace the gastrocnemius muscles as before but this time using your inside hand. This now exposes the deep muscles on the lateral side.

- Use the thumb of your outside hand to glide up the shaft of the fibula pressing straight down towards the table. This treats the origins of the soleus and flexor hallucis longus.
See Figure 17.25

Repeat the deep stripping work on both sides simultaneously by elevating the client's leg and supporting their foot with your diaphragm or sternum as before. Using inward pressure with the thumbs glide up the fibula and tibia at the same time (while you are pressing right down onto the bones).

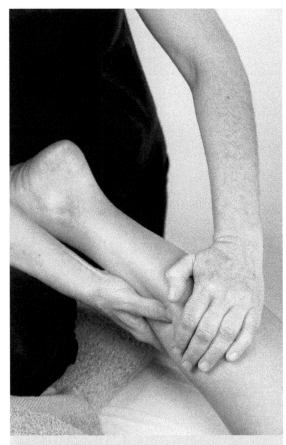

Figure 17.24
Treating tibialis posterior and flexor digitorum longus

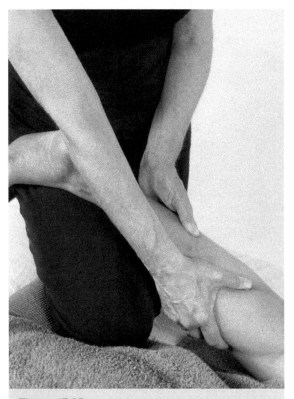

Figure 17.25
Treating the flexor hallucis longus

STR to the Achilles and gastrocnemius

- **STR to the Achilles tendon:** standing side on to the table, put your right knee on the table to support your client's leg at a 90-degree angle. Grasp the Achilles between your thumb and fingers using your left hand. With your right hand press the foot down into dorsiflexion, giving a short stretch of up to 2 seconds while at the same time you pinch and hold the Achilles tendon. Find different points on the Achilles to treat, finding a fluid rhythm of lock, stretch, release and repeat. You can also use a short gliding and stripping stroke down towards the table with the short stretch.

- **STR of the gastrocnemius:** now extend this move into STR of the gastrocnemius. Hold the gastrocnemius with your left thumb on the lateral side and fingers wrapping naturally around the leg. Squeeze the muscle to get a lock and stretch down to the table. Vary your lock position on the muscle and also change the angle of the client's foot slightly each time so you get different types of stretch. You can also use a short gliding motion through the muscle down to the table in addition to just a lock. **See Figure 17.26**

Working the intrinsic musculature of the foot with STR

- Use the same position to work the muscles of the plantar surface of the foot by using the 'lock and stretch' or 'strip and stretch' STR technique. Keep the foot horizontal, find different points on the plantar surface (the sole) with your thumb and take the toes towards the table with your other hand. **See Figure 17.27**

Release the plantar surface of the foot

- Half sit or put your left knee on the table facing the client's feet and hold their left foot underneath with your right hand, resting against your knee. Use the soft medial part of your forearm to work the plantar surface of the foot. Keep your wrist floppy and lean into the stroke. Repeat several times as this feels amazing for your client. At the end of this stroke slowly take your elbow into more of an angle and keep your

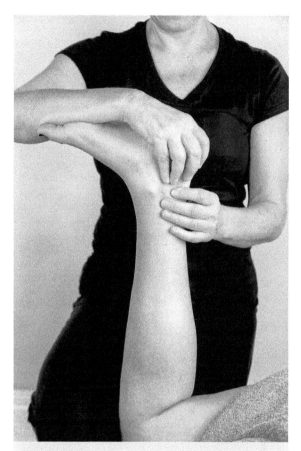

Figure 17.26
STR to the Achilles tendon and gastrocnemius

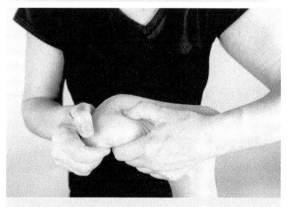

Figure 17.27
STR to the intrinsic musculature of the foot

wrist floppy, use a 'listening elbow' to work deeper into the foot. Sink down slowly using your own breath and bodyweight to do specific point work. **See Figure 17.28, p. 230**

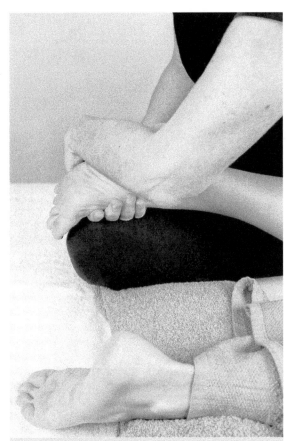

Figure 17.28
Forearm work to the plantar surface of the foot

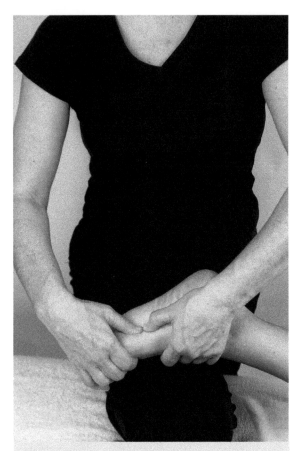

Figure 17.29
Working between the metatarsals

- For more specific work use your thumbs to work in strips from the heel to the pad of the foot.

- When the muscles have softened you can use your thumbs to work the deeper layers of muscles between the metatarsals. Orientate your body so that you are facing the table and put the client's foot on your knee. **See Figure 17.29**

- Facing the head, work around the client's heel specifically with your thumbs or knuckles.

- In the same position finish with soft fist working downwards from heel to toes. **See Figure 17.30**

Ankle decompression

- Now you have released all the soft tissues on the posterior side of the knee, you can apply traction and decompression to the joint. Flex your client's leg to an angle of 90 degrees and place your own

left knee softly on their hamstrings so you are holding their leg down on the table as you work. Wrap your hands around their foot and lift it superiorly towards the ceiling so you are giving traction to the ankle joint. If you are sensitive with your palpation this can become an indirect myofascial stroke, where you listen into the body and follow any twists and turns the tissue might take until you feel the sensation of release. **See Figure 17.31**

- Place your client in a side-lying position with their knees flexed and vertically stacked. Bolster as required.

Tensor fasciae latae (TFL), IT band and vastus lateralis

- The TFL is shaped like a small slice of pie and is found on the side of the hip just posterior to the

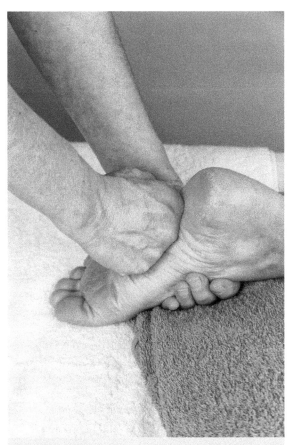

Figure 17.30
Soft fist work to the foot

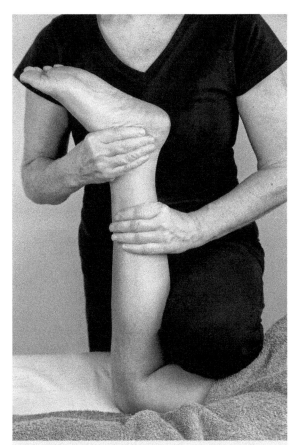

Figure 17.31
Ankle decompression

anterior superior iliac spine (ASIS). Facing your client, in kneeling stance on the side of the table, treat the TFL with compression with the heel of your hand. Have one hand over the other and sink down into the tissues by moving your pelvis forwards slightly. For more specific work use a flat thumb with the heel of the hand over the top to give more weight. Search the whole area for trigger points. **See Figure 17.32, p. 332**

An alternative is to stand at the side of the table in t'ai chi stance and to treat the area with a soft listening elbow. Start by slowly leaning your forearm into the tissues with your elbow joint at an approximate angle of 90 degrees and your wrist floppy. Gradually bring the elbow to more of a pointed angle that enables you to naturally sink deeper into the area without pushing. Remember to keep your wrist floppy and to sink in bit by bit.

If the client feels the pressure is too deep then simply change the angle of the elbow slightly back the other way. **See Figure 17.33, p. 332**

- **Butterfly press on the IT band and vastus lateralis:** stand in t'ai chi stance at the side of the table so that you are in front of your client and facing their IT band. Put the heels of your hands together with your fingers facing outwards and use this position to lean into their body, treating the IT band and vastus lateralis. Work from just below the greater trochanter (bony bump on the side of the hip) to the lateral condyle of the tibia (bony bump on the lateral side of the lower leg just below the knee). **See Figure 17.34, p. 332**

- You can also work this area with broad forearm work. Undrape the area and come behind the client's body in horse stance, resting both forearms

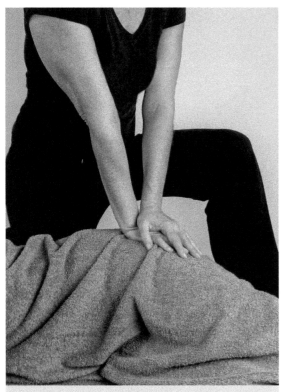

Figure 17.32
Working the TFL with palmar compression

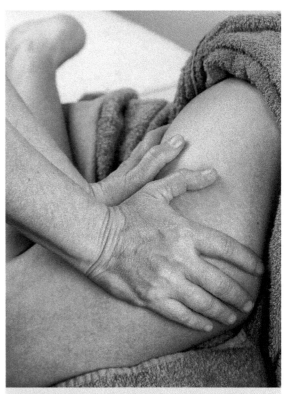

Figure 17.34
Butterfly press on the IT band and vastus lateralis

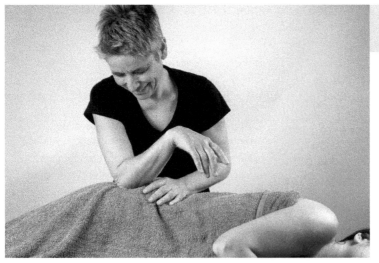

Figure 17.33
Working TFL with a 'listening elbow'

on the hip so that you are leaning in with your bodyweight. If your client is lying on their left side with their right side uppermost, keep your left forearm still while the right forearm slides

SLOWLY down the IT band. If you change the angle of your forearm to angle to front or back you can work the more anterior or posterior side of the tissues as needed. **See Figure 17.35**

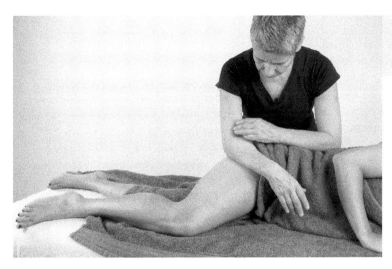

Figure 17.35
Broad forearm work to the IT band and vastus lateralis

- If more specific work is needed, use both of your thumbs or a flat thumb with the heel of your hand over the top for pressure. This can be useful near the insertion points at the side of the knee.

Adductors

> **CAUTION**
>
> Be aware of the delicate structures in the femoral triangle (see Chapter 16)

- **Bolstering:** while still side lying, place the client in a figure-of-four position with a bolster under their bent knee and ankle. The bottom leg is straight so that you can access the medial thigh easily. Make sure the drape is drawn tight at the groin so that your client feels protected but the drape is high enough to expose the area you need to work on, especially the adductor attachments.

- To treat the left adductors your client is in a side-lying position with their right hip uppermost and the inside of the left leg exposed. In t'ai chi stance facing the table, use a soft fist to work across the fibres from medial to lateral.
  See Figure 17.36

- For more specific stripping work, stay in the same position and use supported fingertips to strip the area. Treat any trigger points you find. Work in methodical strips to ensure you have covered the whole area thoroughly.

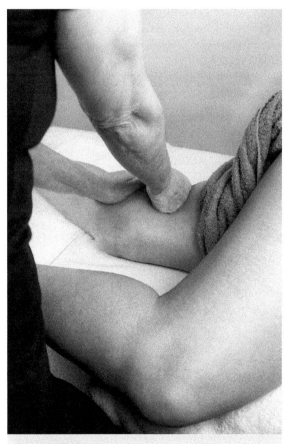

Figure 17.36
Soft fist to adductors

Peroneals

- In the same side-lying position used to treat the left adductors you can treat the peroneals on the upper (right) leg. The peroneals are found on the lateral side of the leg where the seam of the trousers lies. They run along the fibula from just above the lateral malleolus to the fibular head (bony bump just inferior and lateral to the knee). Starting just above the lateral malleolus, glide with direct pressure using your thumbs (or the heel of your hand or soft fist) up the lateral fibula to treat the peroneus longus and brevis. **See Figure 17.37**

Tibialis anterior

- Now move medially to strip the belly of the tibialis anterior with a soft fist, followed by more specific work with supported fingers. If you are unsure of the location of the tibialis anterior, find the sharp ridge of the shin bone and then come laterally. Your fingers will first slip into a groove and then onto the thick muscle of the tibialis anterior. If your client dorsiflexes their foot ('Take your toes towards your head') you should feel the muscle pop onto your fingers.

- Note that the tibialis anterior muscle is quite thick and your pressure will need to be deep in order to have a positive effect. As always when applying deeper pressure make sure you are leaning into the tissues with your bodyweight coming from your Hara, resisting the temptation to push and strain from the upper body. **See Figure 17.38**

- Now come down into kneeling t'ai chi stance and work the intermuscular groove between the tibia and the tibialis anterior by sinking into the groove with your thumbs side-by-side and flat on the body. Use one directional cross fibre friction to sink into the tissues and work from foot to knee.

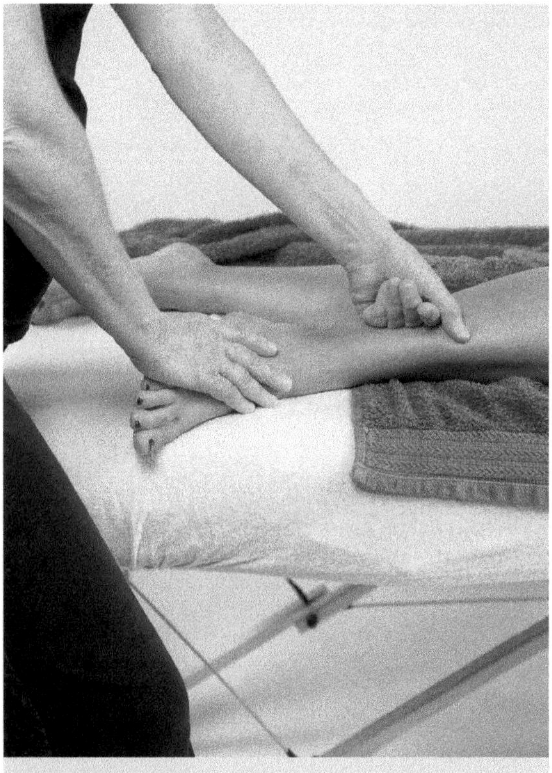

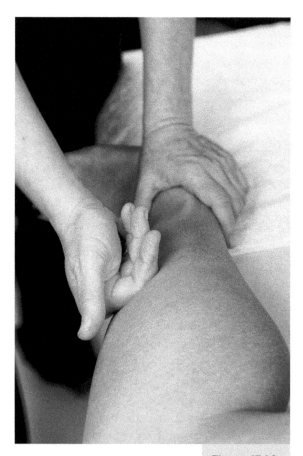

Figure 17.37
Treating the peroneals

Figure 17.38

Extensor hallucis longus and digitorum longus

- Move your thumbs laterally over the tibialis anterior into a second groove found between the lateral edge of the tibialis anterior and the peroneals. Sink medially into the groove using your thumbs (your fingers are wrapped naturally around the client's leg) and work using cross fibre friction. **See Figure 17.39**

> **REMEMBER**
>
> Don't forget the psoas as a possible cause of groin and thigh pain. (Refer to Chapters 12 and 16 for details on how to release the psoas effectively)

Quadriceps muscle group and the patella (knee)

- Turn your client so that they are in a supine position.

- **Cross fibre friction for the patellar tendon and ligament:** in t'ai chi stance facing your client's head, use cross fibre friction above and below the knee to treat the patellar tendon (above the knee) and ligament (below the knee). Wrap both hands around the leg so that your thumbs are free to do the work whilst naturally supporting the leg underneath. **See Figure 17.40**

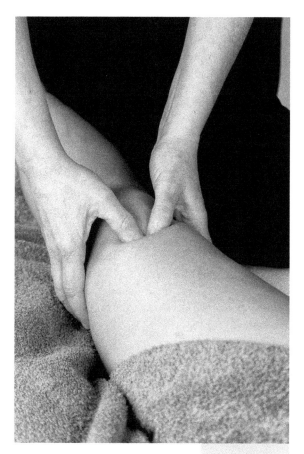

Figure 17.40

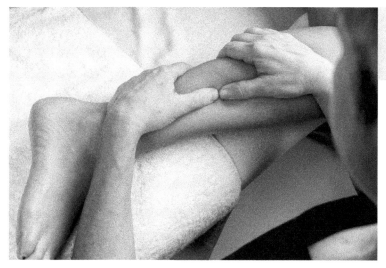

Figure 17.39
Working the groove between the tibialis anterior and the peroneals

- Cross fibre friction on the deep surface of the patella. In kneeling t'ai chi stance, hold the patella between your thumb and fingers, with your fingers around the medial side of the patella and your thumb on the lateral side. Push the patella laterally towards you with your fingers so you are able to reach slightly underneath the edge with your thumbs. With pressure directed towards the ceiling use your thumbs to work the fascia surrounding the posterior surface of the patella using cross fibre friction. Now displace the patella medially (towards the midline of the body) by pushing away from you with your thumbs and press upwards into the under surface of the patella with your fingertips, moving back and forth until you feel a softening and relaxation in the tissue. Look for that biotensegrity sensation of 'floating bone' as described in the fascial chapter (see Chapter 7). **See Figure 17.41**

- **Gentle indirect fascial work around the knee:** there are many occasions where it may be contraindicated to do direct work around the knee, e.g. in cases of acute swelling, bursitis, acute injury or very recent surgery. In these cases we can always use a simple gentle hold above and below the knee. Tune in with focus and intent and visualise the swelling diminishing. If you are accustomed to indirect fascial work you can also tune into the tissues and follow any twists and turns until you feel a release. **See Figure 17.42**

- **Stripping of the quadriceps group:** in t'ai chi stance at the side of the table and facing the client's head, use the heels of your hands or soft fists for broad stripping work. This can also be carried out with a soft forearm (for your client's left leg use your left forearm). Follow the broad work by using supported fingers or thumbs for more specific work. Start at the knee and finish at the ASIS. Work in strips from medial to lateral or

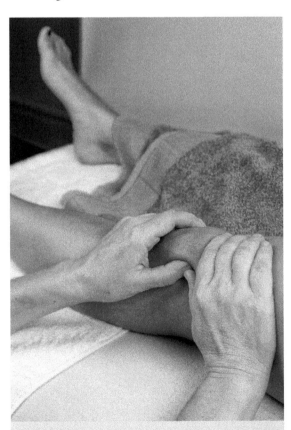

Figure 17.41
Cross fibre friction on the deep surface of the patella

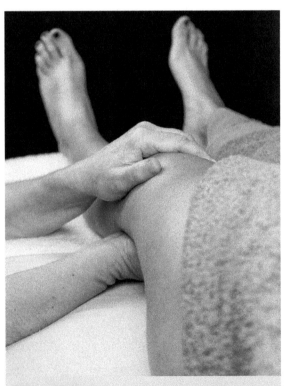

Figure 17.42
Indirect fascial work around the knee

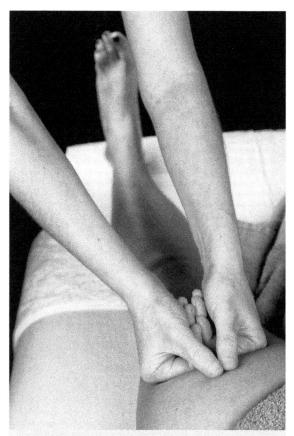

Figure 17.43
Stripping of the quadriceps group

lateral to medial to ensure you cover the full width of the quadriceps group. **See Figure 17.43**

- The vastus intermedius lies deep to the other muscles of the quadriceps group. You may be able to reach the medial and lateral fibres more specifically by displacing the rectus femoris to one side with one hand and using the other hand to strip the muscle; however, in practice this is not always possible on everyone.

- In t'ai chi stance facing the head, use direct pressure with supported fingers directly downwards towards the table to treat the superior attachment of the rectus femoris at the anterior inferior iliac spine (AIIS). Locate the tendon by first finding the ASIS (this is the easily palpable bony bump on the front of the hip) then slide down a thumbs width to find the AIIS. Coming off this bony landmark is a prominent tendon and if you ask your client to flex their hip ('Take your knee to the ceiling') you should feel it pop up strongly. Use static pressure on the tendon to treat any trigger points.

Adductors

- **Compression of the adductor attachments:** the proximal attachments of many of the adductor group muscles lie on the pubic ramus. It may often be necessary to treat these attachments to achieve a positive clinical outcome. There are a number of ways that this area can be treated in a professional manner that ensures client comfort and privacy. The way you choose will depend on your knowledge of the client, the clinical outcome desired and your own comfort levels.

- **Option A:** ensure correct and detailed draping of the inner thigh area. Clients will probably be more comfortable with underwear on. Explain what you are doing to the client and why you need to do it. Use thumbs or fingertips to press into attachment points searching for trigger points and compressing each adductor attachment when you find it. The client can also lay their hand along the pubic crest, just above where you are working, as a protective barrier. This work can be done with the client in a supine position or with their leg in an outwards figure-of-four position (a bolster may be needed). **See Figure 17.44, p. 338**

- **Option B:** explain why these attachment points need to be treated. Demonstrate how the client can self treat these muscles for trigger points.

- Finish with stripping of the adductor group using broad then specific pressure.

Mobilisation of the hip joint

- Stand in t'ai chi stance facing the client's head. To mobilise the client's right hip joint, flex their hip and knee and put your left hand on their knee and your right hand on the sole of their foot. Now take their hip joint through a complete ROM, starting with smaller circular movements that gradually get bigger. It helps to move your own body from your Hara as you do this to ensure a full ROM. **See Figure 17.45, p. 338**

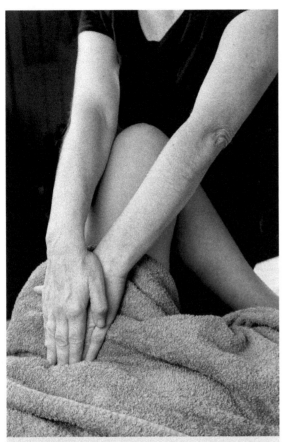

Figure 17.44
Compression of adductor attachments over drape

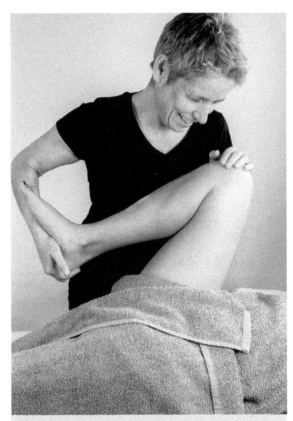

Figure 17.45
Mobilisation of the hip joint

STR of the tibialis anterior

- **Lock and stretch STR:** stand facing the side of the table. The tibialis anterior is found on the lateral side of the shin bone. Lock into the muscle with the thumb of your upper hand (the one nearest the client's head) and, with the other hand, take their foot to table (in other words into plantar flexion). Hold the stretch for 2 seconds. Release and repeat using different points on the muscle.

- **Strip and stretch STR:** as an addition or alternative, stand at the base of the table. To treat the client's left leg place your right soft fist on the tibialis anterior. With your other hand take their foot into plantar flexion as you simultaneously do a short stripping motion through the muscle. Find a different place, replace and repeat. **See Figure 17.46**

Dorsal surface of the foot

- **Fascial release of the ankle retinaculum:** standing at the end of the table in t'ai chi stance, sink into the tissue on the top of the foot with a soft fist. Start with your client's foot in dorsiflexion (toes to their head) and then use your outside hand to slowly take their foot into plantar flexion as you glide through the tissues (toes towards the table). **See Figure 17.47**

Once you have done some broad work you can also work the area with your fingers. For this, start with both hands wrapped around your client's foot with your thumbs underneath and fingers on top (dorsal side). Again start in dorsiflexion and ask your client to carry out active movement into plantar flexion as you move through the tissues.

- Now with a small amount of lubrication, use your thumbs to strip the dorsal side of the foot. **See Figure 17.48, p. 340**

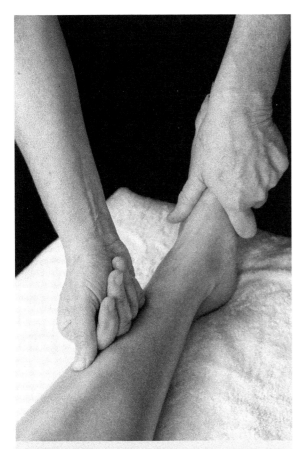

Figure 17.46
Strip and stretch STR of the tibialis anterior

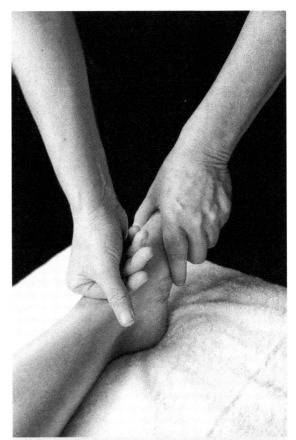

Figure 17.47
Fascial release of the ankle retinaculum

- **STR 'lock and stretch' or 'strip and stretch' for the dorsal side of the foot.** Lock into different points on the dorsal side of the foot and take the client's toes towards the table for a short stretch. **See Figure 17.49, p. 340**

- **Decompression of the toe joints and mobilisation of the foot:** rotate each toe and apply traction to EVERY joint just as you did with the fingers in the carpal tunnel chapter (see Chapter 15). **See Figure 17.50, p. 340**

- Rotate the foot with a twisting motion. **See Figure 17.51, p. 341**

- **Flex and extend the toes:** come to the side of the table in kneeling t'ai chi stance and, with interlocked fingers, sandwich the client's toes between the palms of your hands. Take their toes into several movements of flexion and extension.

- Mobilise the ankle in both clockwise and anti-clockwise directions. In t'ai chi stance at the base of the table, hold the client's foot underneath their heel with one hand and with your other hand at the top of their foot near the toes. Take the foot into a full ROM, using the whole of your body to lean into the stroke so that the movement is coming from your Hara. **See Figure 17.52, p. 341**

Acupressure points

Kidney 3 (Ki 3): Great Ravine

- **Location:** in the depression midway between the tip of the medial malleolus and the Achilles tendon. An excellent local point for heel and ankle pain; also very effective for low back pain.

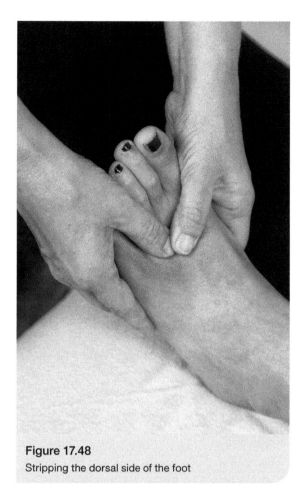

Figure 17.48
Stripping the dorsal side of the foot

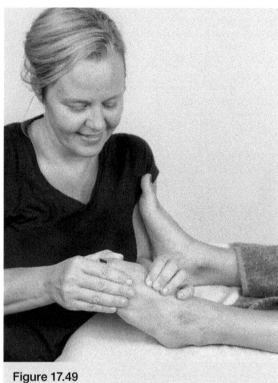

Figure 17.49
STR for dorsal side of the foot

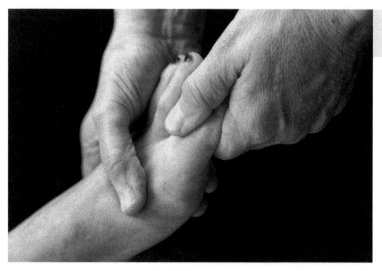

Figure 17.50
Decompression of toe joints

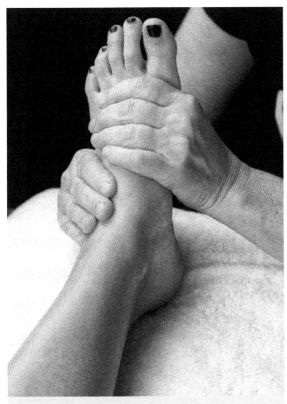

Figure 17.51
Rotating the foot with a twisting motion

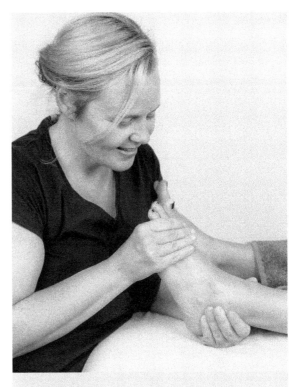

Figure 17.52
Flex and extend the toes

- This point can be manipulated bilaterally. From the base of the table press with your thumbs into the small depression between the Achilles and the medial malleolus. **See Figure 17.53**

Spleen 6 (Sp 6): Three Yin Junction

- **Location:** 3 tsun directly above the tip of the medial malleolus in the depression on the tibia. This point is where the three meridians of Kidney, Liver and Spleen intersect and is useful to tonify the body.

- This point can be manipulated bilaterally. Measure three thumb widths (the same as four fingers) up from the medial malleolus. Press with your thumbs into the small depression you will find in the tibia and hold for 3–5 breaths. **See Figure 17.54, p. 342**

Kidney 1 (Ki 1): Gushing Spring

- **Location:** on the centre line of the sole of the foot, one-third of the distance from the base of the toes to the heel. This is an excellent general calming point.

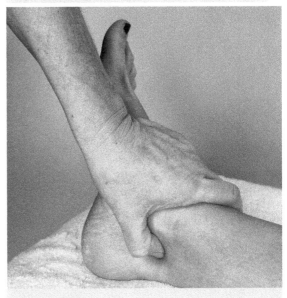

Figure 17.53
Acupressure point Kidney 3

- This point can be manipulated bilaterally with the thumbs, holding for 3–5 breaths. **See Figure 17.55, p. 342**

Stretches

The following stretches can either be incorporated as part of the treatment or at the end of the session.

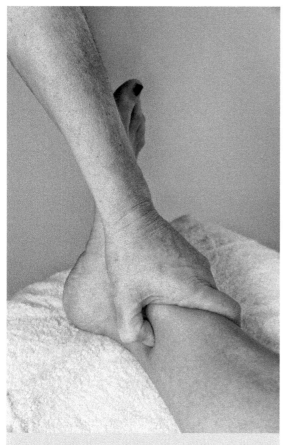

Figure 17.54
Acupressure point Spleen 6

Quadriceps

- The client is in a prone position. In t'ai chi stance facing the feet, place your inner hand on the client's sacrum and traction towards their feet. Use your outside hand to flex the client's leg at the knee. Working with breath and communication take their heel to their buttock to stretch the quadriceps group. **See Figure 17.56**

Bent knee hamstrings stretch

- The client is in a supine position. You are in t'ai chi stance at the side of the table or in proposal stance on the table.

- Flex the client's leg at the hip and support the back of their thigh.

- Now use your inside hand to gently straighten their leg as far as flexibility allows. Put your hand on your client's heel so you are pushing the leg up towards the ceiling. Work with the breath and client communication. **See Figure 17.57**

Straight leg hamstrings stretch

- The client is in a supine position. They may bend their other knee and place their foot flat on table if this is more comfortable.

- Use kneeling t'ai chi stance on the table.

- Put the client's straight leg on your shoulder. Gently bring their straight leg into a stretch using your chest or shoulder as support so that you don't have to hold the heavy leg. Encourage the client to keep their knee straight.

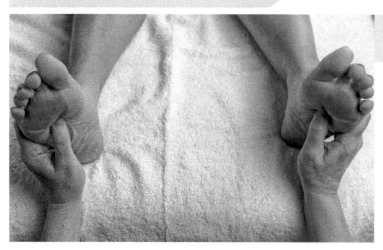

Figure 17.55
Acupressure point Kidney 1

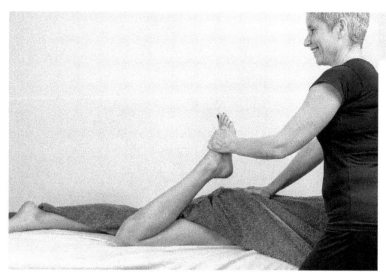

Figure 17.56
Quadriceps group

Keep an eye on their other leg. If it comes off the table during the stretch (indicating tight psoas on that side) you can anchor it down with your free hand or your knee. **See Figure 17.58**

Gastrocnemius stretch

- The client is in a supine position. Stand in t'ai chi stance. To stretch the gastrocnemius hold the client's heel in your hand with your forearm

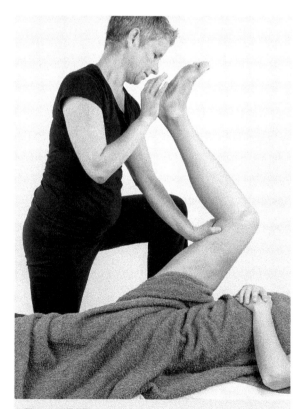

Figure 17.57
Bent knee hamstrings stretch

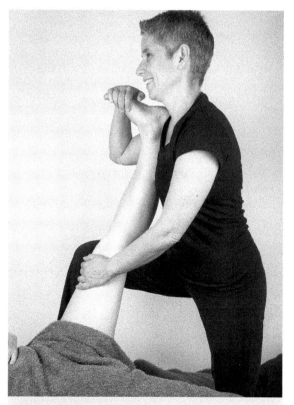

Figure 17.58
Straight leg hamstrings stretch

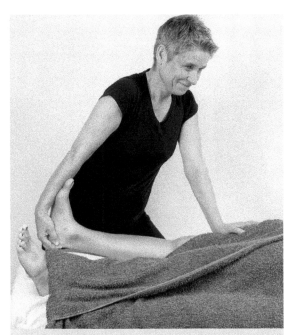

Figure 17.59
Gastrocnemius stretch

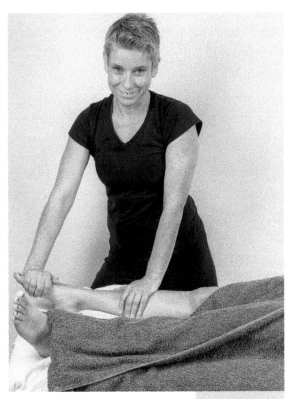

Figure 17.60

placed along the sole of their foot. Take their foot into a strong dorsiflexion to stretch the gastrocnemius. Place your other hand on their thigh to keep the knee straight. **See Figure 17.59**

Tibialis anterior

- The client is in a supine position. Stand face on to the side of the table and take the client's foot to the table while anchoring on the shin with your other hand. **See Figure 17.60**

- To stretch both legs simultaneously, stand at the end of the table and press both of the client's feet to the table.

- Finish with still work.

Teaching self-care suggestions

These can be found in the Self-Care Resources (available online at uk.singingdragon.com/catalogue/book/9781909141230).

Temporomandibular joint pain protocol

Introduction

The techniques in this chapter stem directly from clinical experience as outlined in the quote:

> *During my 15 years experience as a dental nurse I had watched so many people suffer with TMJ and its associated symptoms (including toothache, migraine, visual disturbances and ear disorders) while the usual orthodox treatment protocols seemed to be ineffective at best, or painful and potentially damaging at worst.*
>
> *Then almost 14 years ago after training in massage, and with the support of my dental surgeon and a willing group of TMJ patients I developed a massage and trigger point protocol that saw sufferers move out of pain and misery, and back into enjoying their lives. Many clients were reporting a reduction in symptoms from their first treatment and every one of them were either completely resolved if not dramatically improved within 4–6 treatments. That protocol became the basis for the techniques outlined in this chapter which has now been taught to hundreds of therapists around the UK and Europe, who are freeing people from the misery of TMJ.*
>
> *Trigger Point Therapy is changing people's lives. It is that simple and that powerful.*
>
> TRACEY KIERNAN, EX-DENTAL NURSE AND JING MASSAGE THERAPIST AND TEACHER

The techniques in this chapter have been used to great effect for a variety of common jaw disorders including:

- Temporomandibular joint (TMJ) disorder
- Bruxism (extreme teeth grinding)
- Migraines
- Headaches
- Unexplained face and jaw pain.

For maximum effect, the techniques can also be combined with those from the neck and shoulder protocol (see Chapter 13).

Heat and preparatory work over the drape

- The client is in a prone position. Start with heat application over the neck and shoulder area.

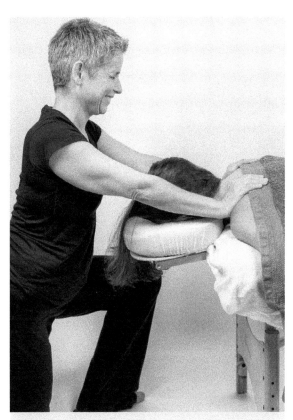

Figure 18.1
Paddy pawing of the trapezius

- Begin with a few minutes of still work over the towel. One hand rests between the scapula and the other on the sacrum.

- Palm and compress the upper trapezius from the head of the table. Use an alternate rocking motion using your body weight to lean into the tissues – like a cat doing 'paddy pawing'. **See Figure 18.1, p. 345**

Muscular and trigger point work

Posterior cervicals

- In forward t'ai chi stance facing the head, knead the posterior cervical muscles using pick up petrissage. Grasp the tissue at the back of the client's neck with a broad grasp: your thumb is one side and your fingers the other. Knead the tissues slowly and rhythmically. The hand that is not working rests on the top of the client's head. Move from your Hara so that your stroke is dynamic, with involvement from your whole body. **See Figure 18.2**

Suboccipitals

In the same position, work under the occipital ridge with the same side thumb (see description for posterior cervicals). Use static pressure first then cross fibre friction with the pressure in one direction only. Treat any trigger points you find. Trigger points in the sub-occipital muscles located under the skull are a common cause of headache and migraine pain. **See Figure 18.3**

Upper trapezius

- Undrape the upper back. Apply wax or oil at this point.

- In kneeling stance, use a soft fist or forearm effleurage to open up the upper trapezius. Support the head at the occiput with one hand and lean in with your bodyweight at the end of the stroke to give a slight stretch to the trapezius. **See Figure 18.4**

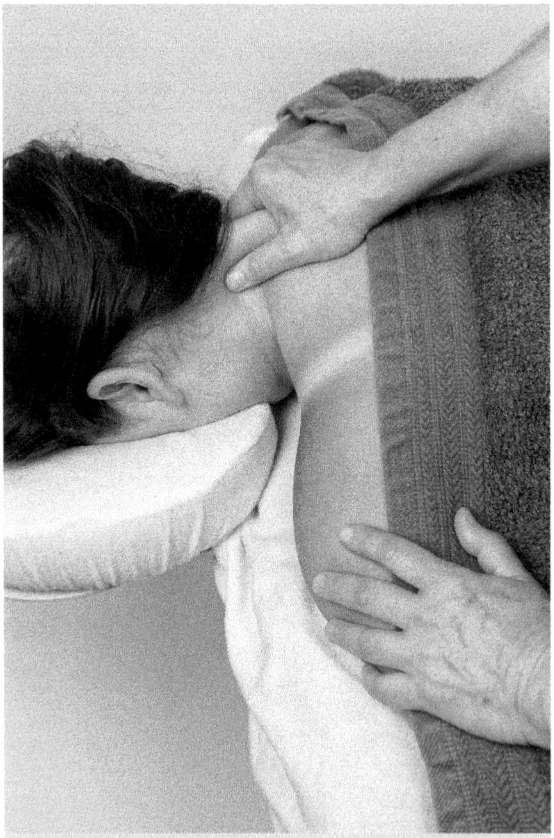

Figure 18.2
Kneading the posterior cervicals

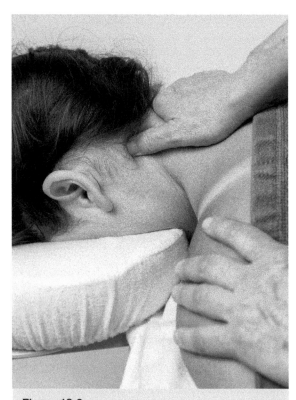

Figure 18.3
Treating the suboccipitals

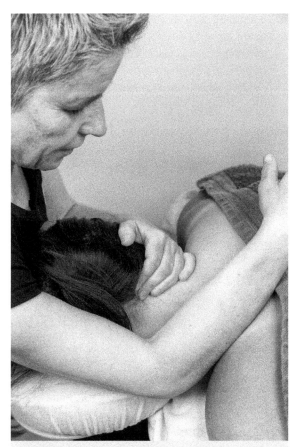

Figure 18.4
Broad work to the upper trapezius

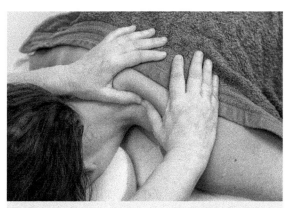

Figure 18.5
Stripping the upper trapezius

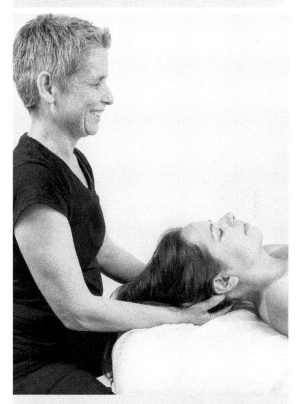

Figure 18.6
Holding the head and grounding

- **Trapezius**: using supported thumbs, muscle strip the upper trapezius. Stand or sit at the head of the table at the opposite corner to where you are working. Use body weight to apply deep muscle stripping from the occipital ridge to the acromioclavicular joint. Treat trigger points using thumb over thumb or supported fingers. **See Figure 18.5**

- Repeat on the other side and finish with forearm work to both trapezius muscles.

Holding the head and grounding

- Now turn your client so that they are in a supine position.

- In a seated stance, sit and hold your client's head for a few minutes. This is an incredibly relaxing experience. If you tune in with your listening touch you may also be able to feel the cranial rhythm which feels like a very subtle filling and emptying of fluid in a water filled balloon. **See Figure 18.6**

Sternocleidomastoid (SCM)

- Sit in a seated stance at the head of the table. To work the right SCM turn the client's head slightly to the right and bring it a little closer to their shoulder.

This puts the SCM on a slack and makes it easier to grasp for the trigger point work.

- Rest your right forearm on the table and have your left hand on the client's head. Use a pincer grasp to gently squeeze and compress the SCM starting up by the mastoid process. Work slowly as this muscle can be exquisitely tender. As you work down to the clavicular attachment, where the belly gets thinner, you can pronate your hand to grasp the muscle. Work with care as the carotid artery is in this region. 'Don't press on anything that presses back at you!' **See Figure 18.7**

- **Working the attachment points**: to work these points on the sternum and clavicle you can hook in with a downward pressure.

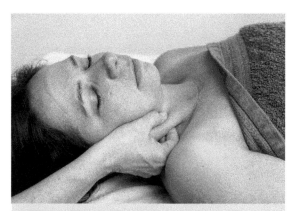

Figure 18.7
Working the SCM with pincer grasp

- To finish off use a claw-like hand and rake into the muscle above the point where the sternal and clavicular heads divide. Sweep upward to the occiput (the cranial fascia anchors around the ear). Use static pressure to work the attachment points around the mastoid process.

Platysma and clavicopectoral fascia

- Use myofascial release (MFR) cross hand stretch over the pectoral area to treat the superficial fascia and platysma muscle (i.e. the superficial muscle you see when you make a 'monster face').

- **Thoracic release**: place one hand under the head and the other on the client's chest. Put the fascia on a stretch and use your sense of listening touch to follow the tissues. Wait and hold for any releases that may occur. **See Figure 18.8**

- In addition, you can place your upper hand gently under the chin, which provides a more targeted fascial stretch of this area. **See Figure 18.9**

Intra-oral technique using gloves

The techniques below allow you to get to some of the attachment points of muscles inside the mouth. Explain to your client why you are doing this and ensure that they are comfortable with the techniques. Agree a signal so that you will come out of their mouth if they feel uncomfortable. Use fresh gloves on each client and always check for a latex allergy first. Vinyl gloves are an alternative. Although the techniques are very safe you

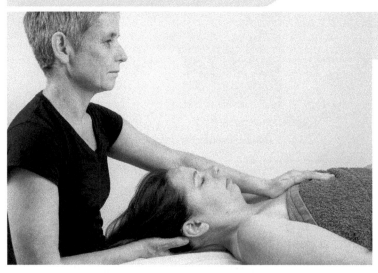

Figure 18.8
MFT thoracic release

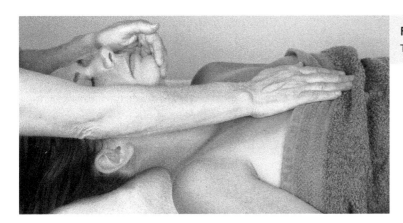

Figure 18.9
Thoracic release with hand under chin

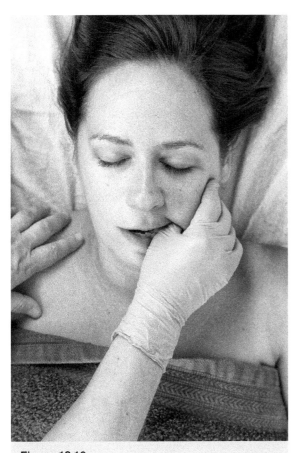

Figure 18.10
Treating the masseter

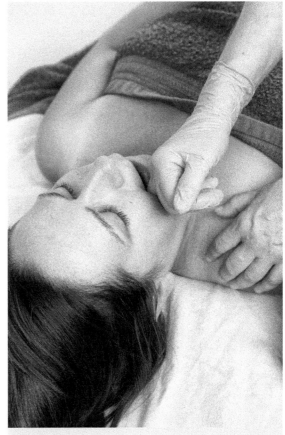

Figure 18.11
Treating the temporalis tendon

may also wish to check with your insurance provider that you are covered to carry out intra-oral work. If you do not wish to carry out these techniques yourself you can show the client how to self treat the muscles involved.

Masseter

- Sit at the side of the table on the opposite side to where you are working and ask the client to open their mouth.

- Wearing gloves, place your thumb against the buccal surface of the cheek and ask the client to half close their mouth. Move your thumb as far back between the cheek and the teeth as is comfortable. You should be able to feel the tip of your thumb touching the coronoid process, the fin shaped piece of bone rising from near the back of the mandible.

- Using the thumb and index finger, apply gentle compression to the masseter using a pincer grasp. Work slowly and carefully as the masseter trigger points can be very tender, so work with communication and keep an eye on your client's face. **See Figure 18.10, p. 349**

Temporalis tendon

- With the client's mouth open as far as possible without inducing pain, ask the client to shift their mandible towards the side being treated to allow more room to work. With the pad of your little finger of your right hand touching the inside cheek surface, glide your finger posteriorly very gently

until it runs into a fin shaped bony surface embedded in the cheek. This is the coronoid process.

- Place your little finger on the inside surface of the coronoid process and use gentle static pressure to examine where the temporalis tendon attaches. The tendon is very hard and will feel like a continuation of the coronoid process. Friction may be used if the tendon is not too tender. **See Figure 18.11, p. 349**

- Remove gloves.

External treatment of the temporalis

- With the client's mouth closed, work the temporalis tendon directly above the zygomatic arch (cheekbone) with transverse friction. Ask the client to clench their teeth and you will feel it move beneath your fingers. **See Figure 18.12**

- Repeat with the client's mouth open to stretch the tendon slightly. Less pressure is needed when the tendon is stretched.

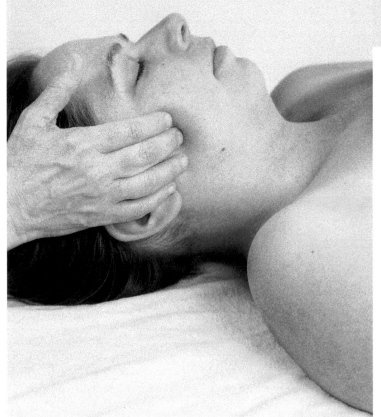

Figure 18.12
External treatment of the temporalis

- Use a 'shampoo' technique to relax the temporalis. Treat one side of the client's head at a time, working the muscle with soft relaxed fingers. You can also work the temporalis using deep thumb pressure by using the weight of the client's head to apply pressure to the muscle by gently turning their head onto a supported thumb. Work specifically and treat any trigger points you find.

Acupressure points

There are three points in front of the ear (at the side of the face) that are very effective for treating TMJ disorders. The middle point, SI 19, is the easiest to find and locating this one first will help you to orientate to the position of the other two.

Small Intestine 19 (SI 19): Auditory Palace

- **Location**: anterior to the tragus (the pointy bit in the middle of the ear) in a depression formed when the mouth is opened. **See Figure 18.13**

- Ask your client to open their mouth slightly and palpate for the small depression just in front of the

middle of their ear. Manipulate the point with thumbs or fingers and hold for 3–5 breaths.

San Jiao 21 (SJ 21): Ear Door

- **Location**: in another small depression just above SI 19.

- Manipulate the point in the same way as above.

Gall Bladder 2 (GB 2): Auditory Convergence

- **Location**: in another small depression just below SI 19 (located with the mouth open).

- Manipulate the point in the same way as above.

Stretches

Manual traction

- With the head in a neutral position, hook your fingers under the occiput. Gently traction the head back towards you with your fingers in the occiput and leaning backwards slightly. **See Figure 18.14**

SCM stretch

- Support the client's head on either side. Ask the client to breathe in and then on the out breath take them into a gentle rotation. Your upper hand

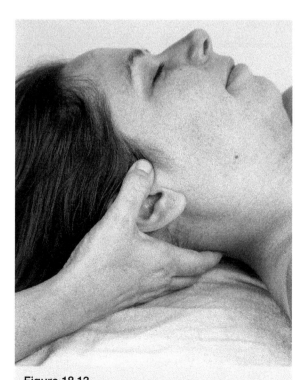

Figure 18.13
Location of acupressure point Small Intestine 19

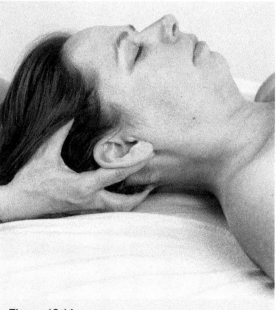

Figure 18.14
Manual traction

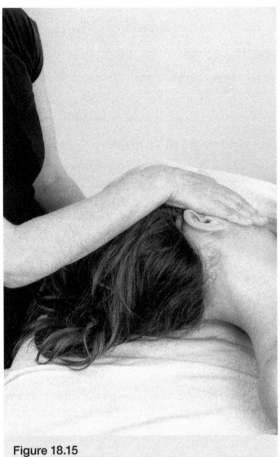

Figure 18.15
SCM stretch

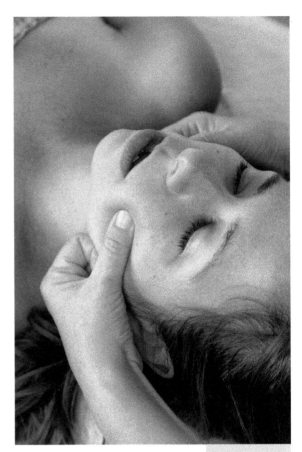

Figure 18.16

Figure 18.17

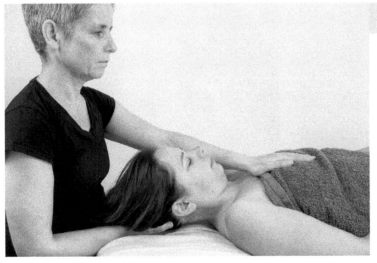

gently presses their head towards the table to encourage maximum range of motion (ROM). Both your hands are working – like rotating a ball in your hands. Work with client communication so that they tell you when they feel the stretch. Wait and hold for 10–30 seconds. **See Figure 18.15**

Stretch for the masticatory muscles

- Ask the client to open their mouth approximately 15 degrees. Place both of your thumbs on their chin. Ask the client to close their mouth while you provide resistance to the closure with your thumbs. Hold the masticatory muscles under isometric tension, for approximately 5 seconds. **See Figure 18.16**
- Finish the sequence with grounding and still work. **See Figure 18.17**

Teaching self-care suggestions

These can be found in the Self-Care Resourcess (available at uk.singingdragon.com/catalogue/book/9781909141230).

19
Stress and chronic pain protocol

Introduction

There are many times in treatment where a more overall stress reduction protocol is called for. This is particularly the case for conditions such as:

- Fibromyalgia
- Chronic fatigue
- Rheumatoid arthritis
- Irritable bowel syndrome (IBS)
- Musculoskeletal conditions where central sensitisation may be a strong component of the pain condition. (See Chapter 4 for an explanation of central sensitisation.)

The following are some ideas but be creative and adapt them as necessary. The protocol changes the mix of the HFMAST formula by using more heat, fascial work, acupressure and stretching and less trigger point work. Heavy trigger point work on clients who are sensitised with chronic pain issues, such as the above, can be counterproductive and on some occasions may lead to more pain. So trigger point work can be used, but start sparingly and build up if the client tolerates the work well.

Heat and preparatory work over drape

- Start with your client in a prone position.
- Begin with some deep grounding and relaxation work for your client. In horse stance, lie both of your forearms on either side of the client's spine. Lean your weight in gradually sinking down a bit deeper with each out breath of your client. Wait and hold the pressure as you feel your client gradually starting to relax and slow their breathing. **See Figure 19.1**
- **Double palming**: now work both erector spinae muscles at the same time by using a double palming technique while kneeling on the table in proposal stance. **See Figure 19.2, p. 356**

Acupressure points

- **Shu points**: now work the acupressure Back Shu points (also known as associated points). The Back Shu points are found 1.5 tsun lateral and level with

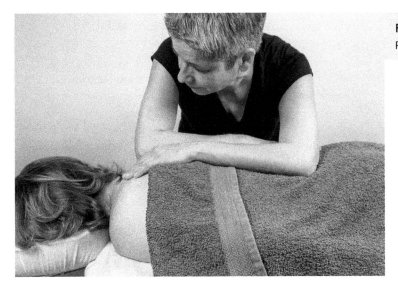

Figure 19.1
Preparatory work over the drape

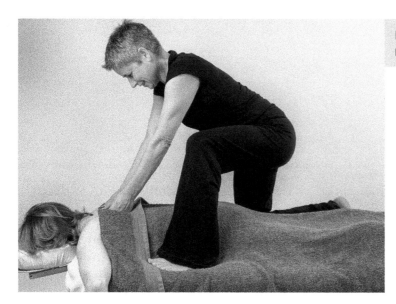

Figure 19.2
Double palming down erector spinae

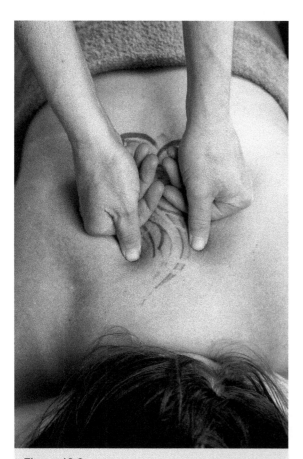

Figure 19.3
Working the shu points on the Bladder channel

the spinous processes of each vertebra (1 tsun = client's thumb width). Each Back Shu point corresponds to an organ in Chinese medicine and the points are used for treatment of chronic conditions. Start at the associated point for the Lung (BL 13), which is level with T3. (To find T3 come to the root of the spine of the scapula and draw a line back to the spine. Alternatively, count down three vertebrae from the prominent C7, which usually sticks out a bit on the back of the neck.)

- Using supported thumbs work bilaterally, coming down one vertebra at a time to work all the associated points. **See Figure 19.3**

Fascial work

- **Myofascial release (MFR) cross hand stretches**: these can be performed in many areas over the back. Place your crossed hands adjacent to one another in the area to be released; they should be a few inches apart at this point. Sink down until you have a sense of being on the deep fascial layers that run around and through the muscles. Then put a stretch on this tissue so you have a sense of tension between your hands – like a piece of material being stretched to a barrier. If you tune in with your sense of listening touch, after a while you will start to feel the sensation of the tissue starting to move beneath your hands. Make sure you maintain the stretch

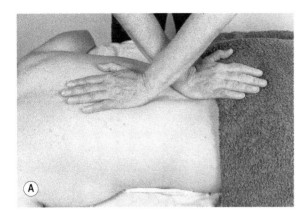

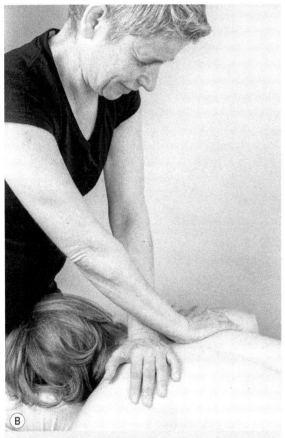

Figure 19.4A,B
Myofascial cross hand stretches

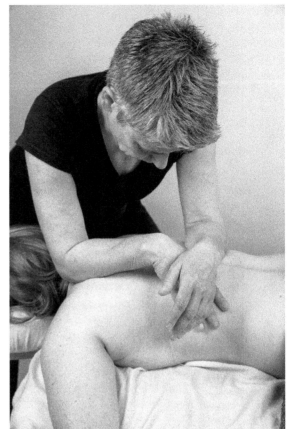

Figure 19.5
Leaning in with forearms

- **Leaning in with forearms**: in horse stance, use the medial side of your forearms to lean into the tissues in different places on the client's back. This can feel deeply relaxing for the client. **See Figure 19.5**

Recommended strokes to aid relaxation

- Apply wax or another medium. **See Figure 19.6, p. 358**

- **Single forearm effleurage**: stand in horse position at the side of the table, knees bent and spine relaxed but straight. Shift your weight onto your leg nearest the low back area. Use the soft medial part of your forearm to work into your client's low back, making sure your wrist is floppy and not tense. Shift your weight onto your upper leg for a light return stroke. Continue gradually working deeper into the musculature layer by layer. Cross to the opposite side of the table to work the other side. **See Figure 19.7A,B, p. 358**

and 'follow' the tissues until you feel the sense of tissue release described in the fascial chapter (see Chapter 7). This whole process takes around 3–5 minutes, so you will need to be patient. Repeat cross hand stretches on anywhere that is needed. **See Figure 19.4A,B**

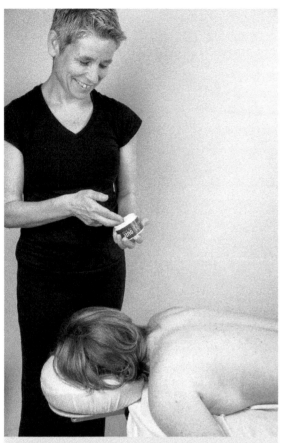

Figure 19.6
Applying wax

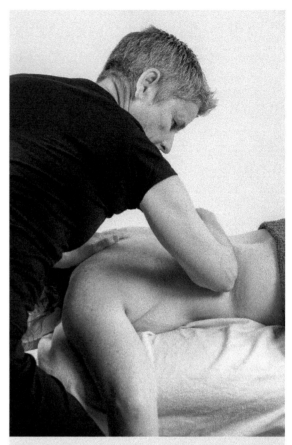

Figure 19.7B
Single forearm effleurage

Figure 19.7A
Single forearm effleurage

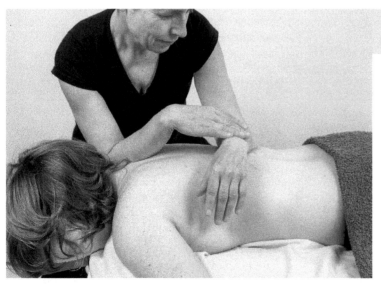

- **Power effleurage with hot stones**: heat is fantastic for most chronic conditions, such as fibromyalgia and rheumatoid arthritis. If you are trained and insured for hot stone work this is a great time to introduce some dynamic stone strokes. Stand at the head of the table in forward t'ai chi stance with a hot stone in each hand. Ask the client to take a breath in and let them know there will be heat coming and they should tell you if it is too much. Apply the stones with a few quick strokes to the top of the client's upper arms first as this is a less heat sensitive area. Then glide down either side of the spine using your body weight to work into the erector spinae muscles with the stones. Glide down to the low back with the stroke, working slowly and deeply, then come back up with a light return stroke and repeat. Breathe out as you work down the body and imagine qi flowing down your arms. **See Figure 19.8**

- **Deep forearm work from the head of the table**: this is a deeper technique, so make sure you start with the other strokes first to soften the area. From the head of the table in t'ai chi stance, start with the ulnar edge of your forearm next to the client's spine (do NOT use your elbow but make contact with a more broad surface). Keeping your wrist floppy, lean in and work slowly down the erectors. Keeping a comforting hand on the sacrum while working can also feel good for the client. **See Figure 19.9**

- **Trigger point work**: if the client has specific areas of pain (i.e. neck and shoulders) use the trigger point protocols outlined in Chapters 12–18 for treatment. However, be sparing with

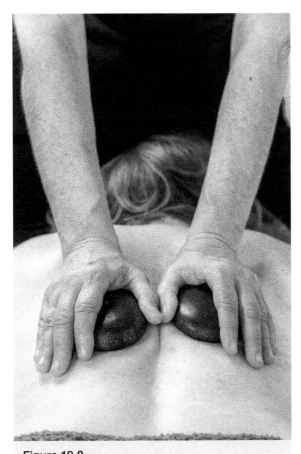

Figure 19.8
Power effleurage with hot stones

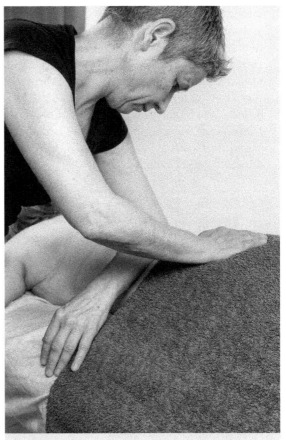

Figure 19.9
Deep forearm work from the head of the table

trigger point work as outlined earlier in this chapter.

- Now turn your client so that they are in a supine position.

- **Stone placement**: place large heated stones on the centre line of the body, i.e. on the breastbone, solar plexus and belly. These correspond energetically to major chakra points and also anatomically to areas of transverse fascial planes. Place your hands on the client's belly and heart stone and wait, tuning into the rise and fall of their breath. **See Figure 19.10**

- **MFR pelvic transverse plane release ('tummy sandwich')**: the majority of the myofasciae run vertically from head to toe but there are places where there are transverse continuities – rather like the hoops of a barrel. One such place is found at the pelvic diaphragm. Place one hand under the sacrum and your top hand between the umbilicus and the pubic bone. Make sure the upper hand has the little finger side towards the pubic bone to prevent your thumb straying into the groin area inadvertently. Press your hands towards each other very slightly as if you are holding a water filled balloon. Wait for the signs of yielding and tissue release before following the tissue to the next barrier. This whole process could take up to 5 minutes or longer in some cases.

If you feel confident and sensitive with your listening touch, you can carry out this technique with the hot stones still in place. If not remove it and replace afterwards. **See Figure 19.11**

- **MFR solar plexus transverse fascial plane release**: repeat the above technique, this time with your hands sandwiching the solar plexus area found just at the base of the ribs. **See Figure 19.12**

- **Fascial leg pulls**: take the weight of the client's leg in your hand and make sure you have a soft grip. Lean back until you feel the tiniest bit of traction. Wait and hold and follow any movement that is initiated as a result of the stretch. Continue until you feel a softening and a fascial release that will almost feel like the limb is lengthening towards you.

- Wait for several releases, until there is no more movement.

- If at first you do not get a sense of where the limb wants to move, try initiating a very small movement, e.g. giving the leg a little lateral rotation, internal rotation or compression and seeing where it seems to go more easily. It's like you are saying to the leg 'Do you want to go this way? Yes or no?' **See Figure 19.13, p. 362**

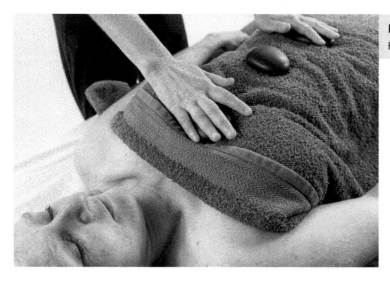

Figure 19.10
Hot stone placement

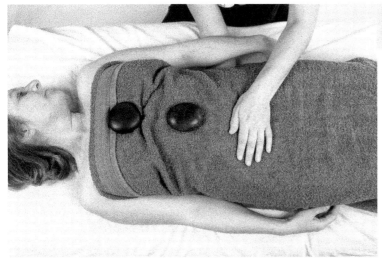

Figure 19.11
Pelvic transverse fascial plane release

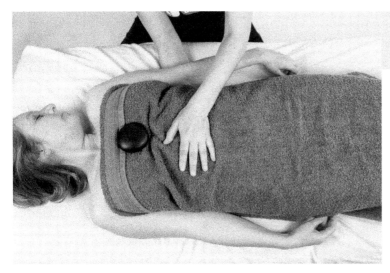

Figure 19.12
Solar plexus transverse fascial plane release

- **Arm pull**: take the client's hand in both your hands and grasp at the base of their palm whilst spreading the palmar fascia slightly. Place their arm on a slight traction. Now wait until you feel the client's arm start to move as if of its own accord. Make sure you are not consciously initiating a movement. Once you feel the response in the tissues, then you can follow the movements whilst making sure to keep their arm on a slight stretch. Watch out for still points where the movement ceases as these are places

you need to hold on a stretch until you feel the sensation of tissue release. Follow the client's arm into several barriers and releases until you feel the whole fascial chain has softened and let go. **See Figure 19.14A,B, pp. 362, 363**

- **Working the conception vessel**: the conception vessel in Chinese medicine runs down the midline of the body and is related to emotional issues. Working the area of the conception vessel in the chest region will help to disperse emotional tension

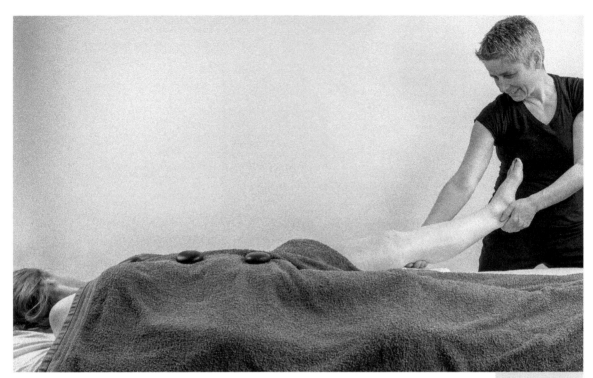

Figure 19.13
MFR leg pull

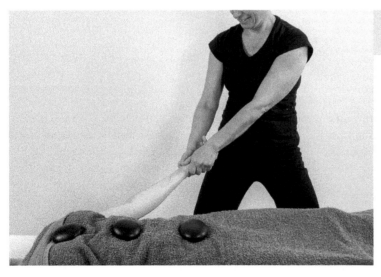

Figure 19.14A
MFR arm pull

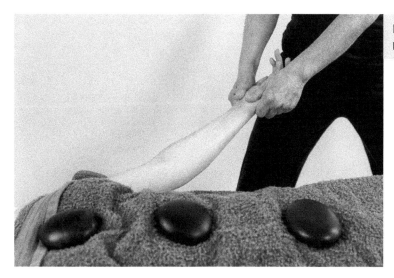

Figure 19.14B
MFR arm pull

that is held in the chest. Put your hands together in prayer position and work down the centre of the sternum in a rocking motion with the ulnar edge of your hand. **See Figure 19.15**

Working with the breath

The breath is often restricted in chronic health problems and releasing trigger points and adhesions in the muscles for breathing can be very helpful for the client.

- **Working the diaphragm**: with thumbs working bilaterally, work up and under the rib with static compressions to help release the diaphragm. Work with the client's breath; as they breathe out sink deeper into the tissues and treat any trigger points you find by waiting and holding for a release. Work laterally outwards, moving a thumb width further each time. See Figure 19.16, p. 364

- **Stripping the intercostal muscles**: standing on the opposite side of the table in t'ai chi stance, use supported fingers to strip in between the ribs to treat the intercostal muscles. Make sure you also work the lateral portion of the ribs, so carry your stroke around the body as far as you can. Continue to the pectoral area, working around breast tissue appropriately. **See Figure 19.17A,B, pp. 364, 365**

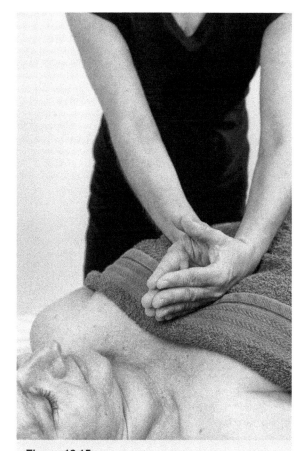

Figure 19.15
Working the conception vessel

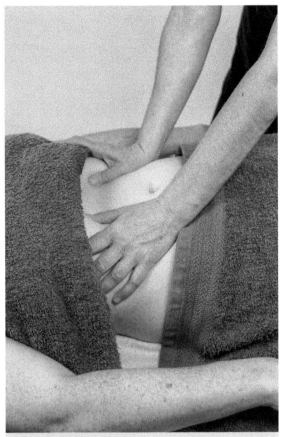

Figure 19.16
Working the diaphragm

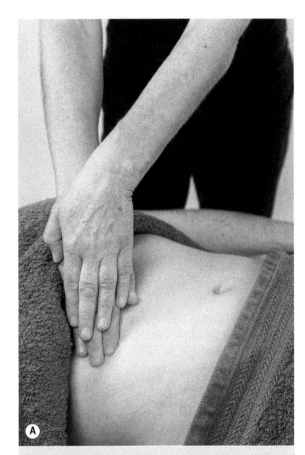

Ⓐ

Figure 19.17A
Stripping the intercostals

Neck work

- **Deep work to the posterior neck**: working the back of the neck deeply is a great way to bring the client into their parasympathetic nervous system. Slide your fingers under their neck and work slowly from distal to proximal, pressing up into the posterior cervical muscles as you do so. **See Figure 19.18**

- **Cervical mobilisation**: gently move the client's head in a figure-of-eight movement. Work slowly encouraging the client to let you take the weight of their head. **See Figure 19.19**

- **Face massage**: finish with a good old fashioned soothing face massage. Still the ultimate in relaxation! **See Figure 19.20, p. 366**

- **Holding the head and grounding**: finish the session by gently holding the client's head,

grounding yourself and simply 'being' with your client. **See Figure 19.21, p. 366**

Acupressure points

The following are several acupressure points that can be useful in treating the emotional component of chronic pain issues. These can be integrated into the sequence at any point.

Governing Vessel 20 (GV 20): Hundred Convergences

- **Location**: follow the line from the tips of both ears upwards. Where the two lines meet at the top of the head there is a depression: this is GV 20. With your hands cupping the client's head, hold the point for 3–5 breaths.

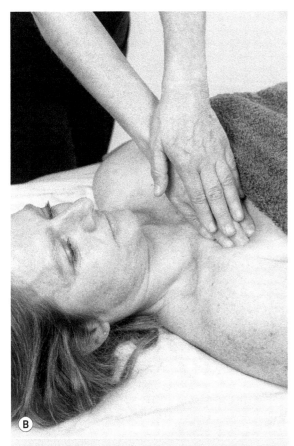

Figure 19.17B
Stripping the intercostals

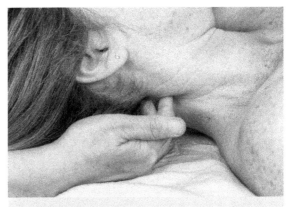

Figure 19.18
Deep work to the posterior neck

- GV 20 is a powerful point for promoting calmness and bringing clear energy to the head. Traditionally it is believed to help open up the crown chakra for connection to greater spiritual experiences. Great for the beginning or end of a treatment. **See Figure 19.22, p. 366**

Conception Vessel 17 (CV 17): Chest Centre

- **Location:** on the sternum, level with the fourth intercostal space and between the nipples. A wonderful calming point.

- Use your third finger to hold the point for 3–5 breaths. It feels nice to have your other hand under the client's head as you do this. **See Figure 19.23, p. 367**

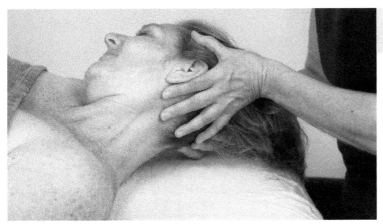

Figure 19.19
Cervical mobilisation

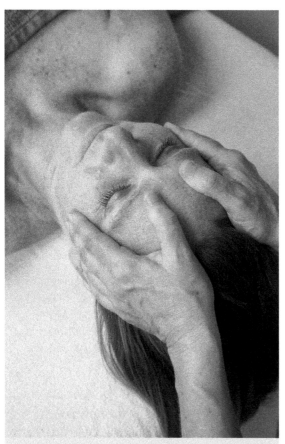

Figure 19.20
Face massage

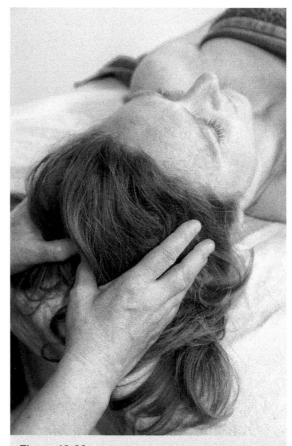

Figure 19.22
Acupressure point GV 20

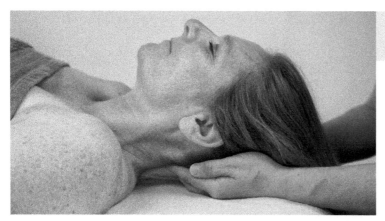

Figure 19.21
Holding the head and grounding

Heart 8 (Ht 8): Lesser Mansion

- **Location**: ask your client to make a loose fist. Heart 8 is found where the tip of the little finger rests between the 4th and 5th metacarpal bones. A good point for calming the emotions and you can also teach your client this one as a self-help technique.

- Hold with your thumb in position for 3–5 breaths. **See Figure 19.24**

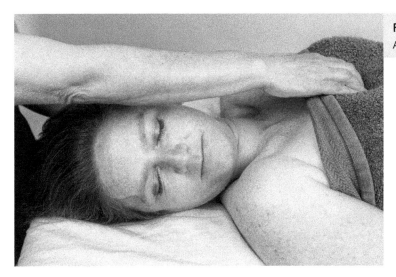

Figure 19.23
Acupressure point CV 17

Stretches

Any stretches you know will feel great for chronic pain issues. Listed below are a few good ones.

Gluteal stretch

- Take the corner of the drape and pull it under the client's thigh so that they can hold the end of it for security. Get into kneeling t'ai chi stance on the table with your outside leg up at right angles and your foot flat on the table. Flex the client's leg at the knee and hip and place it into the fold of your thigh with your outside hand on their knee. Use your inside hand to hold down the client's other leg and press their flexed leg towards their belly by leaning forward with your pelvis into a lunge. As always, work with client communication and breath. **See Figure 19.25, p. 368**

Piriformis stretch

- From the last position you can flow straight into a piriformis stretch. This time take the client's leg across the centre line, again leaning forward into a lunge. **See Figure 19.26, p. 368**

Spinal twist

- Finish with a fabulous spinal twist. Place your client's bent left leg over their right. Standing side on to the table, anchor down the client's shoulder in the pectoral region with your right hand. Use your left hand on the thigh to take your client

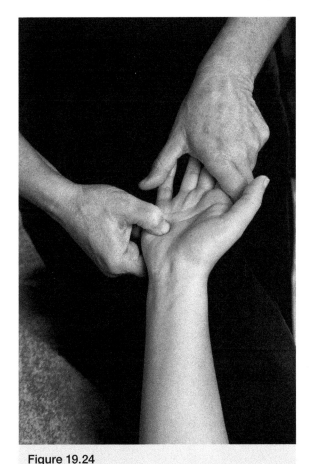

Figure 19.24
Acupressure point Ht 8

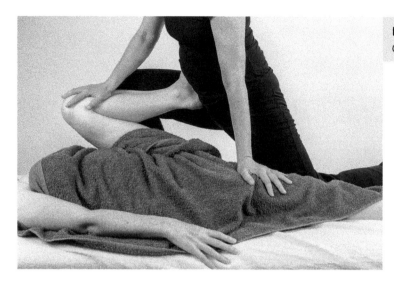

Figure 19.25
Gluteal stretch

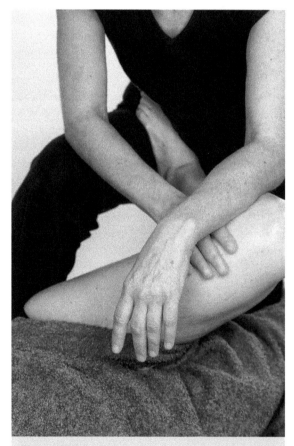

Figure 19.26
Piriformis stretch

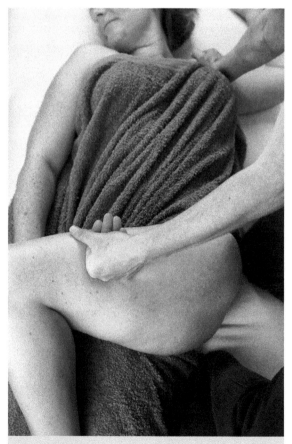

Figure 19.27
Spinal twist

into a gentle spinal twist, working with their breath and communication. Feels amazing!

See Figure 19.27, p. 368

Teaching self-care suggestions

Self-care suggestions are extremely important in cases where stress and central sensitisation may be a strong component of the client's pain issue. Make sure you are aware of the issues discussed in Chapter 4 and use education and appropriate self-care suggestions to help reduce unhelpful thoughts and behaviours that may be contributing to the pain condition.

A

ABCDEFW mnemonic   64, 66
abdomen/belly
  client's, undraping/exposing   13–14, 218
  muscles *see* oblique abdominals; rectus
        abdominis therapist's   15, 15–16
abductors, hip, side-lying stretch   218, 312
Achilles tendon   327
  soft tissue release   329
acromioclavicular (AC) joint   229, 232, 236,
        241, 247, 347
actin   122–3
active elongation in myofascial
        stretching   171
active isolated stretching (AIS)   160, 166,
        167–8, 168–70, 174
active range of motion tests   68, 69, 70
active stretching
  dynamic   161, 162–3
  static   161
active trigger points   126
activities (functional/physical)
  assessing   66
  of daily living   60, 66, 70
  gradual exposure *see* graded exposure
  pacing   191
acupressure points (acupuncture
        points; A)   6, 141–55
  back pain   154, 221–2
  East–West fusion   144–6
  forearm/wrist/hand pain   287–8
  hip and pelvis pain   310–11
  leg/knee/foot pain   339–41
  neck pain   153, 241–2
  research   153–4
  shoulder girdle pain   267
  shoulder pain   221–2
  stress-reducing effects   355–6, 364–6
  temporomandibular joint pain   351
  trigger points and   127–9, 151, 152
acupuncture needles *see* needles
adductors, hip   305–6, 309, 333, 337
  stretches   312
adhesions, trigger points causing   121
adhesive capsulitis (frozen shoulder)
        56, 78, 122
aerobic exercise   185
aesthetics *see* beauty and aesthetics
agenda setting   180
ah shi (`ouch') points   127–9, 130, 144, 145,
        148, 151
allodynia   44, 124
American Organization for Bodywork
        Therapies of Asia (AOBTA)   141, 144
Amma   141
amputees, phantom limb pain   39

anaesthetics in trigger point therapy
        116, 130
anatomy trains   90–1, 106, 127
  meridians and   146, 147, 148, 152
ankle
  decompression   330
  mobilisation   339
  retinaculum, fascial release   338
ankylosing spondylitis, exercise   186
arms
  client's
    pull   271–2, 361
    range of motion tests   69
  therapist's   19
aromatherapy, stones   81
art
  of listening touch   18–20
  massage as   5
arteries and acupuncture points   151
arthritis *see* osteoarthritis; rheumatoid
        arthritis
Asian bodywork *see* bodywork
asking questions   63
assessment   55–71
  diagnosis vs   55
  HOPRS approach   60–70
  initial client enquiry   58–9
  what and how of   59
  why of doing an   55–6, 59
assisting active isolated stretching   169
athletic events *see* events
attachment trigger points   125
attention, paying   62
attitude (client's)   64
Auditory Convergence   351
Auditory Palace   351
autonomic effects, trigger points   120, 121
axillary border of scapula   257–8

B

back
  low
    broad work to   293
    cross hand stretch to   291–2
  upper, fascial finger work   227
back pain (mainly low/lumbar)   201–24
  acupressure   154, 221–2
  cases   73
  exercise   186
  heat application   73, 76–8, 201
  MRI, 38
  self-care   224
  stretching   160, 204–5, 212–13, 216,
        216–17, 217, 219, 222
  tissue damage without   38

Back Shu points   355–6
ballistic stretching   161, 162
Barnes, John F, 100, 106, 108, 164, 171
beauty and aesthetics
  linens   11
  table   10
bee venom injecting of trigger
        points   130
behavioural change strategies   179, 180
beliefs (client's)   64
  about pain   35, 64
  unhelpful *see* unhelpful thoughts and
        beliefs
belly *see* abdomen
benchmarking   69–70
Benjamin, Ben   168, 295
bent knee hamstring stretch   342
best research evidence   58
biceps   265
bicycling   185
biological component of pain   35
biopsychosocial model (BPS) of pain,
        35–7, 49
biotensegrity   92–7
Bladder 13 (BL 13)   356
Bladder 31–34 (BL 31–34)   221
Bladder 36 (BL 36): Support   221, 320
Bladder 60 (BL 60): Kunlun Mountains   221
Bladder channel
  in leg work   317
  in low back pain   202
  shu points   356
Bladder tendinomuscular channel   147
blood flow *see* circulation
blood vessels
  acupuncture points and   151
  compression with trigger points   121
bodywork   141–53
  Eastern/Asian   144, 145, 148, 149
    fascially-based explanation   152–3
    modalities   141–2
  emotions in   25–31
  fascia as bodyworker's Holy Grail
        86–7
  outcome-based approach to   59–60
bolsters and bolstering   11, 12–14
  leg/knee/foot pain   317, 333
bone, tendon insert onto   91
Bone Holes
  Squatting   311–12
  upper/second/central/lower   221
botulinum (Botox) injecting of trigger
        points   130
boundaries   27
  energetic *see* energetic boundaries
brachioradialis   276, 280

brain
    injury, acupressure   153
    pain and   35, 37–46, 190
    see also neuroscience
breast draping   13–14
breath
    client's
        in meditation and mindfulness   181,
            182, 183
        in stretching   166
        working with   363
    therapist's   15, 15–16
bursitis, trigger point misdiagnosed
        as   122
butterfly press on iliotibial band and vastus
        lateralis   331

C

cancer   21
    acupressure for symptoms of   153
cardiac... *see* heart
carpal bones, palm press   287
carpal ligament
    dorsal   279
    transverse   280–2
carpal tunnel   281, 339
    disorders/symptoms/syndrome   121,
        225, 238, 271, 272
catastrophising with pain   35–6
    reducing   47, 190, 191–2, 194
Celestial Gathering   242, 267
cells
    connective tissue, stretching
        stimulating   171
    fascial   88
    ice slowing metabolic activity   75
    as tensegrity tent   95–6
Central Bone Hole   221
central sensitisation   43, 48, 49, 55, 70
    fascia and   103
    stress and   355
    trigger points and   124–5
central trigger points   125
cervical muscles, posterior   228–9, 346
cervical spine
    flexion   243–4
    lamina groove   237–8
    lateral flexion   244–5
    mobilisation   245, 364
    transverse process   229, 238, 239
chest (therapist's)   16
Chest Centre   365
chronic fatigue syndrome   143
chronic obstructive pulmonary disease,
        acupressure   153
circulation (blood flow)
    heat increasing   74
    ice decreasing   75
circumduction of shoulder,
        supported   236, 257

clavicle   229, 230, 231
    sternocleidomastoid attachment
        points   240, 348
    subclavius and pectoralis major
        attachments underneath   260
clavicopectoral fascia   348
closed questions   63
cognitive behaviour therapy (CBT)   179,
        191–2
cold (cryotherapy)   6, 73–84
    application principles   80–1
    cautions   81
    contrast bathing with hot and   75–6, 81
    evidence   78–80
    forearm/wrist pain   271
    ice *see* ice
    leg/knee/foot pain   317
    self-administered   193
    stones *see* stones
    trigger point   78, 130–1
collagen, fascial   88, 150–1
Colon 16 (Large Intestine 16)   241
combinations of ideas in fascial work   111
common extensor tendon attachment,
        friction   275–6
common flexor tendon attachment,
        friction   277–8
common sense
    self-care   192, 193–4
    therapist's   48–9
communication with client   26–7
    confident   57
    self-care   187, 190
    stretching   165–6, 169
    trigger point work   133–4
    see also information
compensation ·64
competitive sports events *see* events
complementary therapy and self-care   177
compression techniques *see* pressure/
        compression
conception vessel   361–3
Conception Vessel 17 (CV 17)   365
confidence, communication of   57
connective tissue   87–8
    stretching stimulating cells in   171
    thixotrophy   108
consultation form   64–5
continuing training and education   58
contraction
    fascial   92
    muscle
        contract–relax and contract–
            relax agonist contract (in PNF
            stretching)   166
        crowd surfing theory   122–3
        see also pre-contraction stretching
contractures
    stretching in prevention and treatment
        of   174
    trigger points causing   121

contraindications   20–2
contrast (hot and cold bathing)   75–6, 81
control
    health locus of   178–9, 184
    letting client know they are in
        control   27
coordination, centres of   152
coracobrachialis   265
costal surface of scapula, attachments
        on   230–1
countertransference, body-centred   28
covers, table and face cradle   11
craniosacral therapy   3, 106, 107–8
creams/ointments/unguents   193
critical thinking about
        contraindications   22
cross-fibre friction *see* friction
cross hand stretches
    forearm/wrist/hand pain   271
    hip and pelvis pain   291–2, 302, 307
    leg/knee/foot pain   318
    low back pain   204–5, 219
    neck/shoulder pain   225–6
    shoulder girdle pain   249
    stress-reducing effects   356–7
    temporomandibular joint pain   348
crowd surfing theory of muscle
        contraction   122–3
cryotherapy *see* cold
Cubit Marsh   287
cultural sensitivity towards clients   58
cushions   11
cycling   185

D

daily living, activities of   60, 66, 70
de qi   149–50
de Quervain's tenosynovitis   46
decompression
    ankle   330
    fingers (digits of hand)   284
    toe joints   339
deep fascia   89
    work   102, 247–8
        knowing you are in the deep
            fascia   110
        neck/upper back   227, 364
        shoulder   227
        shoulder girdle   247–8
deep flexor compartment (leg)   327–8
deep spinal muscles in low back
        pain   208–9
deep work
    fascia *see* deep fascia
    in low back pain   213
        with forearms   207, 213
        with palms   211–12
    stress-reducing effects   359
    t'ai chi and   15
delayed onset muscle soreness *see* muscles

deltoids 250–3
  anterior fibres 252, 264
  posterior and middle fibres 250
  stripping 253
depression and pain 45
Descartes 37, 39
diagnosis 64
  assessment vs 55
  of medical condition, mistaking trigger
    points for 121–2
diamond draping of gluteals 12
diaphragm, working the 363
digits
  foot see toes
  hand, decompression 284
disc (intervertebral), herniated 22
  trigger point misdiagnosed as 122
do no harm principle 26–7
dorsal carpal ligament 279
dorsal surface
  foot 338
  hand 279–80
double palming
  erector spinae 203, 355
  gastrocnemius 318
downward dog, fascial stretching 172
draping 12–14, 27
  in active isolated stretching 170
  hip and pelvis pain 291
  low back pain 201
dry needling, trigger/ah shi points 129,
  130
duration of treatment, estimating 59
dynaments 92
dynamic stretching 160, 161–3
  pre-workout or pre-event 159
  technique 161–3
dysmenorrhoea see menstrual pain

E

Ear Door 351
Eastern (traditional) medicine
  bodywork see bodywork
  fascial stretching 172
  Western and, fusion/integration 5–6
    meridians and acupressure work
      and 144–6, 152–3
    self-care and 180, 183
education
  of client see information
  of therapist, continuing 58
effleurage
  back
    with hot stones 359
    in low back pain 206, 208, 209,
      211–12, 213
    stress-reducing effects 357–9
  palmar see palming
  pectoralis major 261
elastin, fascial 88

elderly, acupressure in care of 154
electricity 109, 150–1
  resulting from pressure
    (piezoelectricity) 108, 150
emotions 25–31
  assessment and 58, 61, 64, 65–6
  bodywork and 25–31
  pain and 25–6, 35, 49
  see also stress; trauma
employment see work
ending a session, explaining what will
    happen 27
energetic boundaries and distances, 28–30
  fascial work 110
energy crisis, metabolic 125
epicondylitis
  lateral (tennis elbow) 187, 271
  medial (golfer's elbow) 187, 271, 277–9
equipment 9–14
erector spinae 207–9
  double fists down onto 203–4
  in low back pain 202–3, 203–4, 207–9,
    225
  in neck/shoulder pain 227–8
  palming 202–3, 225, 355
events (competitive sports performance),
    stretching
  stretching immediately prior to
    performance 159, 174
  stretching improving performance 159
evidence (research), best 58
exercise/workout/training 185–9
  evidence for 186–7
  stretching after 158
  stretching as regular part of routine 159
  stretching before 158, 159, 160
  see also events (sports)
extension
  toes 339
  wrist 285
extensor(s)
  forearm/wrist 275–6, 279
    stretch 288–9
  lower leg 335
  neck, stretch 243–4
extensor digitorum longus 335
extensor hallucis longus 335
extensor retinaculum 279
external locus of control 178

F

face cradle 9
  cover 11
face massage 364
family and assessment 64
fascia 85–113
  as bodyworker's Holy Grail 86–7
  constituents 87–8
  deep see deep fascia
  definition 85–6

  Eastern bodywork and 152–3
  fluid dynamics and 103–4, 109
  heat increasing pliability 74, 78
  hip and pelvis pain 291–2
  lateral line 302
  manipulation (of Stecco) 104, 151–2
  muscle see myofascia
  pain and 101–3
  palmar 283
  sandwich see sandwich
  stretching 170–2
  structure/anatomy 89–90
    newer understanding 90–1
  superficial see superficial fascia
  techniques/work (F) 6, 99–111, 132, 171
    direct and indirect fascial release 105
    forearm/wrist/hand pain 271–2, 283
    hip and pelvis pain 291–3
    leg/knee/foot pain 317–18
    low back pain 203–5
    neck/shoulder pain 225–7
    practical principles 109–10
    shoulder girdle pain 247–9
    stress-reducing effects 356–7
    toolbox 104–5
    why it works 108–9
  trigger points and 129–30, 132
fascial fitness routines 172
fascial stretch therapy 172
fatigue, acupressure 153
  see also chronic fatigue syndrome
fear avoidance 35
feedback from client 27
feeling see palpation
feet (therapist's) 15–16
Feldenkrais method of somatic
    education 99
femoral triangle 309–10
fibres, fascial 88, 186
fibromyalgia
  exercise, yoga 184
  shiatsu 154
  stretching in treatment of 174
  thermal therapy 77
fibula, release of hamstring attachments
    at 320–1
fight, flight and freeze 25–6
Finando, Steven and Donna 118, 145, 150,
    151, 152
finger(s) and/or thumb pressure 145, 152
  in low back pain 204, 208–9, 213–14, 292
  in neck/shoulder pain 228–9, 236–7,
    238–9
    upper back fascia 227
  posterior cervical muscles 228
    masseter 350
  sacrum 204, 213–15, 292
  shoulder girdle fascia 248
  temporalis 351
  see also digits; fists and knuckles; paddy
    pawing

finger pull   286–7
fists and knuckles
    adductors   333
    erector spinae   203–4
    gluteals and lateral rotators   213
    hamstrings   317
    pectorals   263
    plantar surface of foot   330
    quadratus lumborum   293
    rhomboids   226
    scalenes   234, 273
    shoulder girdle   247
    trapezius   226, 234
flexibility
    stretching to improve   157–8
    in treatment plan   58
flexion
    cervical   243–4
    toes   339
    wrist   285
flexor(s), forearm/wrist   277–9, 280
    stretch   289
flexor digitorum longus   327, 328
flexor hallucis longus   327, 328
flexor retinaculum   280–2
fluid dynamics and fascia   103–4, 109
focus   19
foot pain   317–44
    acupressure points   339–41
    fascial release   317–18
    muscle and trigger point work   320–39
    self-care   344
    stretches   342–4
forearm work
    gastrocnemius   325
    low back pain   206–7
    stress-reducing effects   357, 359
    trapezius/scalenes   234
forearm/wrist/hand pain
    acupressure points   287–8
    case   34
    fascial work   271–2
    muscular and trigger point work,
        272–87
    self-care   289
    stretches   271, 274, 279, 281, 288–9
    thermal therapy   77, 271
forward t'ai chi stance   16–17
friction work (cross-fibre)
    deltoid anterior fibres   252–3
    forearm
        common extensor tendon
            attachment   275–6
        common flexor tendon
            attachment   277–8
        extensor retinaculum   279
    patella   336
    patellar tendon and ligament   335
    piriformis and lateral rotators   215–16
    supraspinatus/infraspinatus/teres minor/
        subscapularis attachments   254

frozen shoulder   56, 78, 122
Fuller, Buckminster   92, 93, 94
functional activities see activities
fusion, centres of   152

G

Gall Bladder 2 (GB 2)   351
Gall Bladder 20 (GB 20)   241–2
Gall Bladder 21 (GB 21)   241
Gall Bladder 29 (GB 29)   311–12
Gall Bladder 30 (GB 30)   310–11
gastrocnemius   324, 325, 328
    soft tissue release   329
    stretches   343–4
        cross hand   318
gels
    gel-to-sol theory   108
    water in gel-like state   109
geodesic domes   93, 94
Gestalt psychology   4
Gifford's (Louis) 'hassles', 192–4
glenohumeral joint range of motion   265
gliding (fascial), loss   102
    therapy   102–3
gloves for intraoral work   348–9
gluteal muscles (gluteus minimus and
        medius)   213–15, 218, 295–6,
        300–2
    broad work   295–6
    diamond draping   12
    skin rolling over   292–3
    stretches   222, 367
glycosaminoglycans (GAGs)   88, 89, 102
goal
    follow up   180
    setting   179, 180, 187
golfer's elbow (medial epicondylitis)   187,
        271, 277–9
Golgi receptors   97
Governing Vessel 20 (GV 20)   364–5
graded (gradual) exposure to
        activities   191
    exercises   187, 191
Great Bone   241
Great Ravine   339–41
ground substance   88–9, 103–8, 171
grounding   19, 28
    neck/shoulder work   225, 237, 364
    power of   15
    temporomandibular joint pain   347
    traumatised patients and   28, 29–30
Gushing Spring (Kidney 1)   317, 319, 341

H

hamstrings   317
    release work   299
    stretching   318, 342–3
        with strains   172–4

hand pain see forearm/wrist/hand pain
hands (therapist's)   19
    see also cross hand stretch; fingers and/or
        thumb pressure; fists and knuckles;
        paddy pawing; palming
Hara   15
`hassles' (Louis Gifford's)   192–4
head
    grounding and holding the   346, 364
    manual traction   243, 351
headaches and migraines
    self-care   179
    trigger points and   115, 120, 124, 131, 241
        suboccipital   228, 239
    vicious cycle   44
health
    history-taking   60–6
    locus of control and   178–9, 184
heart (client's)
    problems, trigger points misdiagnosed
        as   121–2
    workout, in active isolated
        stretching   168
heart (therapist's)   16
Heart 8 (Ht 8)   366
heat see hot
height of table   11
herbal remedies   193
HFMAST approach   6, 7, 199
    acupressure points and   143
    fascial work in   110
    low back pain   201
    in planning of treatment   70–1
    trigger point therapy and   136
    see also individual components
hip (and hip joint)
    abductors, side-lying stretch   218, 312
    adductors see adductors
    mobilisation   337
    rotators, lateral   213, 215–16, 297
hip and pelvis pain   291–315
    acupressure points   310–11
    fascial work   291–3
    heat   291
    muscular and trigger point work   293–
        310
    self-care   315
    stretches   291–2, 296, 312–15
    tissue damage without   38
history-taking   60–6
hold–relax (in PNF stretching)   166
holism   92, 97, 177
homunculus   43
hope, inspiring   58
HOPRS approach to assessment   60–70
horse stance   17
hot (H; thermotherapy)   73–84, 74
    application principles   80
    back pain   73, 76–8, 201
    cautions   80
    contrast bathing with cold and   75–6, 81

evidence base 76–8
  forearm/wrist pain 77, 271
  hip and pelvis pain 291
  leg/knee/foot pain 317
  neck pain 77, 225
  self-administered 193
  shoulder girdle pain 247
  shoulder pain 73, 225
  stones see stones
  stress-reducing effects 355, 359, 360
  temporomandibular joint pain
      78, 345–6
  trigger points 74, 77–8, 132
Hundred Convergences 364–5
hyaluronic acid (HA) 74, 89, 102–3
hydration of tissues during stretching 171
hyperalgesia 44, 124
hypothenar eminence 283

I

ice (for injury etc.) 74–5, 80–1
  evidence for 78–9
iliac crest
  attachments to quadratus
      lumborum 211
  cleaning 302
iliac scissors 212
iliacus 218–19, 302, 307
  see also iliopsoas stretch
iliolumbar ligament 295
iliopsoas stretch 315
iliotibial (IT) band 305, 321, 330–3
imaging
  brain, in chronic pain 43–4
  tissue damage and levels of pain 38–9
inflammation (inflammatory response)
  fascial 101–2
  ice and 78
information for client (incl. teaching and
      education)
  pain and 45, 48
    neuroscience of 125, 184–90, 194
  self-care see self-care
  see also communication
infraspinatus 259
Ingber, Donald 95–6
injecting trigger points 130
injury (physical trauma)
  brain, acupressure 153
  ice see ice
  stretching (pre-/post-exercise) in
      prevention of 158, 160
  see also strains
insomnia, acupressure 153
integration work
  low back pain 205, 208
  to pectorals 263–4
  to trapezius 232
  see also structure
integrins 95, 96

intercostals 260–1, 363
internal locus of control 178, 179
interoception 100–1
interpersonal skills 57
intervertebral disc see disc
intraoral techniques 348–50
intrinsic musculature of foot, soft tissue
      release 329
ischaemic pressure in trigger point
      therapy 132
ischial ramus, adductor magnus
      attachments to 306
ischial tuberosity 215, 297, 299, 315, 320

J

jaw disorders 345
  see also temporomandibular joint
      disorder/pain
Jing multi-modal approach/method 3–4,
      5, 6
  HFMAST see HFMAST
  trigger point therapy and 132
Jing triangle 236
jingjin (tendinomuscular channels) 147–8
joints
  patients
    inflammation see osteoarthritis;
        rheumatoid arthritis
    range of motion see range of motion
  therapist's 15
Jumping Round 310–11

K

key trigger points 125–6
  treatment 133
Kidney 1 (Ki 1) 317, 319, 341
Kidney 3 (Ki 3) 339–41
Kiernan, Tracey 115, 345
kinesio taping 192–3
kinesis myofascial integration (KMI) 106,
      152
kneading, posterior cervicals 228, 346
knee
  indirect fascial work around 336
  meniscal damage see meniscal damage
  pain 317–44
    acupressure points 339–41
    case 46
    fascial release 317–18
    muscle and trigger point work 320–
        39
    self-care 344
  replacement surgery, stretching
      following 174
  see also bent knee hamstring stretch
kneeling t'ai chi stance 17
knuckles see fists and knuckles
Kunlun Mountains (Bladder 60; BL 60) 221

L

labour pain, acupressure 153
Langevin, Helene 102, 103, 148, 149–50
language used (with client) 190
  stretching 165
Large Intestine 4 (LI 4) 288
Large Intestine 11 (LI 11) 287–8
Large Intestine 16 (Colon 16) 241–2
latent trigger points 126
lateral epicondylitis (tennis elbow) 187, 271
lateral flexion, cervical spine 244–5
lateral hip rotators 213, 215–16, 297
lateral line, fascial 302
latissimus dorsi 257–8
  stretch 255
    side-lying 258
Lederman, Eyal 163–4, 165
leg(s) 317–44
  draping 13
  pain 317–44
    acupressure points 339–41
    fascial release 317–18
    muscle and trigger point work,
        320–39
    self-care 344
    stretches 318, 338, 339, 342–4
  pulls 310, 318, 360
  see also phantom limb pain; straight leg
      hamstring stretch
lengthening/elongation of fascia during
      stretching 171
Lesser Mansion 366
levator scapula 230, 233
Levin, Stephen 93, 94, 95
ligaments 92
listening, in assessment 59, 61–2
listening (transformative) touch 18–20,
      109
  in fascial work 97, 104, 106, 109
  in stretching 166
location (site) of pain 65
lock and stretch
  dorsum of foot 339
  tibialis anterior 338
locus of control, health 178–9, 184
longitudinal friction see Z stroke
loving kindness (metta) 62
Lower Bone Hole 221
lubrication (little or none) 109
  dorsal foot stripping 338
  forearm and wrist pain 279
  hamstring stripping 321
  hip and pelvis pain 293
  low back pain 205, 208
  neck and shoulder pain 237
lumbar pain see back pain
Lung, Back Shu point 356
Lung 5 (Lu 5) 287
lung disease, chronic obstructive,
      acupressure 153

M

magnetic resonance imaging (MRI), pain experience and findings on 38–9
makko Ho stretches 172
manual therapy 101, 104
 meridians and acupressure points 144, 150
 self-care and 178
  neck pain 187
  osteoarthritis 186
 trigger points 115, 116, 130, 131–2, 132–3
manual traction see traction
masseter 349–50
masticatory muscle stretches 353
 see also masseter; temporalis
Mattes' method (of active isolated stretching) 167–8
mechanical lengthening of fascia during stretching 171
mechanics (patient and therapist) 15–20
 fascial work 110
 stretching 165
mechanoreceptors, fascial 97–101, 109
medial epicondylitis (golfer's elbow) 187, 271, 277–9
medical conditions
 concurrent
  asking about/assessing 65
  contraindicating 21–2
 exercise effects 186
 stress reduction 355
 stretching in treatment of 172–4
 thermal therapy 77
 trigger points caused by 123
 trigger points misdiagnosed as 121–2
meditation 180–3
 definition 180–1
meniscal damage/tears/injury 46
 pain absent 38
menstrual pain (dysmenorrhoea)
 acupressure 153
 heat therapy 78
mental health problems see psychological problems
meridians 141–55
 East–West fusion 144–6
 myofascia and 146–51
 research 153–4
metabolism
 cellular, ice slowing 75
 energy crisis 125
metacarpals, working between 283
metatarsals, working between 330
metta 62
MICE (Movement, Ice, Compression and Elevation) 79
microtearing, fascial 101–2
microtensegrity 95–6

migraines see headaches and migraines
mindfulness 180–3
 client 180–3
 definition 181
 therapist 29
  bodywork mantra for 19
mind–body
 interventions 100–1, 184
 pain model 33–4
mirror neurones 28
mirroring 62–3
misdiagnosis with trigger points 121–2
mobilisation (by therapist)
 ankle 339
 cervical 245, 364
 foot 339
 hip joint 337
 lower back 201–2
 shoulder girdle 266–7
  scapula 250, 255–7
 see also range of motion
mobilisation exercises in self-care 187, 194–5
money sign 229
monitoring progress 57–8
morning sickness 143
Moseley, Lorimer 40, 42, 45, 189
motion see movement
motivation for self-care 179
 exercises 165, 187
mouth, working within 348–50
movement (motion) 91–2
 range of see range of motion
 trigger points causing restrictions in 121
movement therapy 101
MRI (magnetic resonance imaging), pain experience and findings on 38–9
Müller, Divo 162, 164, 172
multi-modal approach see Jing multi-modal approach
muscle(s)
 adhesions and contractures 121
 chains and slings 90, 91
 contraction see contraction; pre-contraction stretching
 fascia see myofascia
 movement and 91–2
 single unit muscle theory or idea 90–1, 170
 soreness
  delayed onset (DOMS) 75, 79, 197
  ice reducing 75
  stretching reducing 158–9
 strength (therapist) 15
 stretching see stretching
 stripping see stripping
 techniques and treatment 6
  forearm/wrist/hand pain 272–87
  hip and pelvis pain 293–310
  leg/knee/foot pain 320–39

 low back pain 206–19
 neck/shoulder pain 227–41
 shoulder girdle pain 249–67
 temporomandibular joint pain 346–51
 tight, heat effects 74
 trigger points see trigger points
muscle energy technique (MET) 163, 165, 166, 167
myalgic encephalomyelitis (chronic fatigue syndrome) 143
Myers, Tom 12, 90–1, 106, 127, 146–7, 171, 320
myofascia
 meridians and 146–51
 work on (incl. release/MFR and stretches) 102, 106, 132, 171–2
  hip and pelvis 291–2, 302, 306–7, 360
  stones 81
  stress-reducing effects 356–7
  temporomandibular joint pain 348
  in trigger point deactivation, indirect 131
 see also cross hand stretches
myofibroblasts and pain 103
myosin 122–3

N

nausea and vomiting 153
 in pregnancy (morning sickness) 143
neck
 extensor stretch 243–4
 pain 225–45
  acupressure 153, 241–2
  exercise 186–7
  fascial techniques 225–7
  grounding 225, 237, 364
  muscular and trigger points techniques 227–41
  self-care 245
  stretches 234, 243–5
  stretching in treatment of 174
  thermal therapy 77, 225
  see also whiplash
 stress-reducing work 364
needle(s) (acupuncture)
 dry needling of trigger/ah shi points 129, 130
 grasp phenomenon 149–50
needle tower structure 95
nerves
 acupuncture points and 151
 compression with trigger points 121
nervous (neural) system
 fascial connections 97–101, 109
 pain pathways 44–5
 plasticity 190
 see also autonomic effects; brain
neuroimaging (brain imaging) in chronic pain 43–4

neuromatrix model of pain 40–1
neuroscience of pain 39–45
  education 125, 184–90, 194
  placebo effect 47
neurovascular bundle in femoral triangle 310
Nimmo, Raymond 132
No! (client saying) 27
nocebo effect 48
nociceptors and nociception 39–42
  fascia and 101, 103
nutritional factors, trigger points 123

O

oblique abdominals, internal and external 302
observation 60, 66
obturator internus 207
occupation see work
oedema, ice reducing 75
oil 12
ointments/creams/unguents 193
older persons (the elderly), acupressure in care of 154
open questions 63
optimism, inspiring 58
oral cavity, working within 348–50
orthopaedic tests, special 60, 69
Oschman, James 100, 108, 150
osteoarthritis
  exercise 186
  heat 77
  stretching 174
  trigger point misdiagnosed as 122
osteoporosis 21–2
  exercise 186
'ouch' (ah shi) points 127–9, 130, 144, 145, 148, 151
outcome-based approach to bodywork 59–60

P

pacing of activities 191
Pacini's receptors 97
paddy pawing
  gluteals 203
  pectorals 263–4
  trapezius 225, 345, 346
pain (emotional) see emotions; trauma
pain (physical - in general) 33–51
  acupressure in relief of 153
  assessment 69–70
    current pain condition 65
    past or concurrent pain conditions 65
  beliefs about 35, 64
  biopsychosocial model (BPS) 35–7, 49
  chronic 33–51
    progression from acute to 45

complex puzzle of 33–4
fascia and 101–3
gate control theory 40
ice reducing 75
implications for treatment 48–9
indicating threat (rather than damage) 46, 190
ingredients of combined creative approach to treatment of 53
outcome-based approach to 60
perception see perception
placebo and nocebo effects 47–8
radiating see referred pain
self-care see self-care
sensitisation see sensitisation
stretching and its effects on 160
trigger point-related 121, 127
  therapy 133–4
vicious cycle 44–5
what it tells us 46–7
pain scales 69–70
  trigger point 134
palm press (palmar compression)
  carpal bones 287
  tensor fasciae latae 331
palmar surface (client's) 282–4
palmaris longus 280
palming (incl. effleurage) 141, 152
  back of body 291
    gastrocnemius 218
  erector spinae 202–3, 225, 355
  gluteus medius and minimus and tensor fasciae latae 218
  in hip and pelvis pain 291
  leg/knee/foot pain 317
  in low back pain 202–3, 211–12, 218
palpation/feeling (of soft tissues) 60, 67
  trigger points 133, 135
paraphrasing 62–3
passion for massage 3
passive range of motion tests 68–9
passive static stretching 161
patella 335–6
patellar tendon and ligament 335
patience in fascial work 109
pectineus 310
pectoral muscles 260–3, 274, 275–6
  pectoralis major 260–2
    stretch 267
  pectoralis minor 262–3, 274–5
  prone stretch 234
  side-lying 'Devil' stretch 269
pelvis
  pain see hip and pelvis pain
  transverse plane of pelvis, myofascial release 306–7, 360
perception (of symptoms)
  centers of 152
  of pain 4, 39–40
    heat decreasing 74
performance in sports events see events
peripheral sensitisation 42–3, 49

peroneals 334
  working the groove between the tibialis anterior and 335
pes anserinus region, cleaning 305
phantom limb pain 39
physical activities see activities; exercise
physical sensations see sensations
piezoelectricity 108, 150
pillows and pillowcase 11
pin and stretch
  gluteus minimus 300–2
  psoas 219
pincer techniques 135
  brachioradialis 276, 277
  masseter 350
  sternocleidomastoid 240, 348
  trapezius (upper) 229
piriformis 215–17, 296–7
  release 216, 296–7
  stretch 222, 297, 367
  trigger point 120
placebo effect 47–8
plan (treatment) 57
  HFMAST approach 70–1
  trigger points and 124–5
plantar surface of foot, soft tissue release 329–30
plantaris 324
platysma 348
POLICE (Protection, Optimal Loading, Ice, Compression and Elevation) 79
Pollack, Gerald 90, 109
Pool at the Bend 287–8
popliteal fossa 320, 324
popliteus 324
positional releases of psoas 219–20, 307
positioning
  low back pain 201
  for static stretching 166
positive regard, unconditional 61–2
post-facilitation stretch 167
post-isometric relaxation 167
post-traumatic stress disorder (PTSD) 25, 26
postures (stances) 16–18
power effleurage
  with hot stones 359
  in low back pain 206, 208, 209, 213
  stress-reducing effects 359
practice 20
practitioners see therapists
pre-contraction stretching 163, 166–7
  see also muscle energy technique; proprioceptive neuromuscular facilitation
pregnancy 22
  acupressure point avoidance 241, 288
  heat application 80
  labour pain, acupressure 153
  morning sickness 143
  psoas work contraindicated in 218
presenting symptoms, shiatsu 154

pressure/compression in trigger point
  therapy   135
  release   132, 135
  trapezius (upper)   229
  see also decompression
PRICE (Protect, Rest, Ice, Compression and
  Elevation)   79
progress monitoring   57–8
prone work
  draping for   12–13
  low back pain   201–18
  neck/shoulder pain   225–34
  shoulder girdle acupressure points   267
proposal stance   17
proprioception   100, 101
  stretching stimulating   171
proprioceptive neuromuscular facilitation
  (PNF) stretching   160, 163, 165, 166,
  167–8, 174
  piriformis   297
protection (therapist) in
  retraumatising   28–30
provocation of pain   65
psoas   218–19
  side-lying stretch   312
  see also iliopsoas stretch
psychological (mental health) problems
  and distress   21
  pain and   35, 45, 65
  support and strategies to help with   194
  trigger points and   123
  see also stress; trauma
psychological wellbeing (effects on)
  heat   84
  meditation and mindfulness   181–2
  stretching   160
psychology   4
PTSD (post-traumatic stress disorder)   25, 26
pubic bone   307–8, 360
  ramus   337
pulmonary disease, chronic obstructive,
  acupressure   153

Q

qi   141, 145, 146, 148, 152
  blockage and restoration   152
  definition   151
  obtaining   149–50
qi gong   172, 177, 184
quadratus femoris   297
quadratus lumborum   209–13
  cross hand stretches   292
  release   213, 293
  stones   82
  trigger point   115, 117, 120
    treatment   209–11, 293
quadriceps   335–7
  stretches   342
quality of pain   65
questions, asking   63

R

radial deviation   285
radiating pain see referred pain
range of motion (ROM)   60
  active   68, 69, 70
  assessment   60, 67–9, 70
  hand/wrist   284–5
  heat improving   78
  hip joint   337
  passive   68–9
  pectineus   310
  shoulder girdle   265
  stretching and   157, 162, 163, 164, 165,
  166, 167, 169
  see also mobilisation
receptor-tonus technique   132
rectus abdominis   308
rectus femoris   312, 337
red flags   20, 27, 63
referred (radiating) pain   65
  trigger points causing   127, 133
reflecting back   62–3
reflexology, stones   81
refresher session for home exercises   187
rehabilitation time, heat reducing   74
relaxation, strokes aiding   357–63
release (soft tissue incl. fascia)
  direct and indirect   105
  in hip and pelvis pain   292, 293, 295,
  296, 297, 299, 302, 305, 306–7, 307–8,
  310
  in leg/knee/foot pain   317–19, 320–1,
  323, 324, 329–30, 338–9
  in low back pain   203, 204–5, 207, 216,
  218–19, 219, 219–20
  myofascial see myofascial work
  in neck/shoulder pain   228, 235–6
  sensations of see sensations
  in shoulder girdle pain   261–2
  in temporomandibular joint pain   348
repetitive strain injury (RSI)   33, 39, 271
  case of   46
research evidence, best   58
resistive tests   69
reticulin, fascial   88
retinacula cutis fibres   89
retraumatisation in session   27–8
rheumatoid arthritis
  exercise   186
  heat   77
rhomboids   232, 249
  fist work   226
rib (12th) attachments of quadratus
  lumborum   211, 293
RICE (Rest, Ice, Compression and
  Elevation)   79
rocking, low back pain   201–2
Rolf, Ida   5, 15, 66, 105, 106, 108, 146
Rolfing (structural integration)   66, 87,
  105–6

rotation
  foot   339
  shoulder girdle   250
rotator(s) (hip), lateral   213, 215–16, 297
rotator cuff tears, pain absent   38
Ruffini's receptors   97

S

sacrotuberous ligament   297–9, 320
sacrum
  cross hand stretch to   291–2
  work over   212, 213–15
    finger work   204, 213–15, 292
safe space (for client)   26–7
San Jiao (SJ 21)   351
sandwich (fascial/myofascial)   89
  tummy   306–7, 360
sarcomere   122, 123, 125
satellite trigger points   125–6
sawing, scapula   250
scalenes   238–9, 272–4
  side-lying work   234–6
  stretch   244–5, 274
scanning palpation, trigger points   135
scapula
  attachments on costal surface of   230–1
  axillary border   257–8
  mobilisation   250, 255–7
  skin rolling over   248
  vertebral border   236–7, 257
scapulothoracic joint range of
  motion   265
scars   22
Schleip, Robert   85, 87, 97–8, 101, 104, 108,
  109, 151, 162, 164, 171, 172
sciatica   66, 221
  MRI, 38
science, massage as   5
seated position (therapist)   17–18
Second Bone Hole   221
self-care (and its teaching)   4, 177–97
  acupressure points   143
  components of successful
    strategies   179–80
  exploring various strategies   180–92
  forearm/wrist/hand pain   289
  hip and pelvis pain   315
  leg/knee/foot pain   344
  low pain back   224
  motivation see motivation
  neck/shoulder pain   245
  resources   7
  shoulder girdle pain   269
  stress reduction   369
  stretching   164–5, 169–70, 194–5
  temporomandibular joint pain   353
self-insight   58
sensations (physical)
  receiver's, of tissue release in fascial
    work   108

therapists
   of tissue release in fascial work   107
   unusual   30
sensitisation   42–3
   central *see* central sensitisation
   fascia and   103
   peripheral   42–3, 49
   stress and   355
   trigger points and   124–5
sensory receptors, fascial   97–101, 109
serratus anterior   258
shearing of middle trapezius   230
shiatsu   141, 144, 149
   fibromyalgia   154
   presenting symptoms   154
   self-care   178
   stretches   172
shoulder(s), clients   225–45
   frozen   56, 78, 122
   pain   225–45
      exercise   187
      fascial techniques   225–7
      heat   73, 225
      muscular and trigger points
         techniques   227–41
      self-care   245
   supported circumduction   236, 257
shoulder(s), therapist's   19
shoulder girdle pain   247–9
   acupressure points   267
   fascial work   247–9
   heat   247
      stretches   255, 258, 267–9
   muscular and trigger point work
      249–67
   self-care   269
Shoulder Well   241
Shu points, Back   355–6
side-lying work
   draping for   13
   hip abductor stretch   218, 312
   iliacus release   302
   latissimus dorsi stretch   258
   pectoral stretch   269
   psoas stretch   312
   scalenes   234–6
   subscapularis   258
   trapezius   234–6, 255–7
site of pain   65
sitting position (therapist)   17–18
six, magic or power of   6–7
skin
   fascia and   89
   rolling
      gluteal area   292–3
      low back pain   205
      neck (back of)   227
      shoulder girdle   248
sleeplessness (insomnia), acupressure   153
sliding (fascial), loss   102
   therapy   102–3
sliding filaments   122–3

slowness (in massage work)   19
   fascial work   110
Small Intestine 11 (SI 11)   242, 267
Small Intestine 19 (SI 19)   351
SMART mnemonic   60
smudging in brain map   43–4
Snelson, Kenneth   92, 94–5
social/socioeconomic factors
   assessment   65–6
   pain and   36–7
   sensitivity towards client's social
      background   58
soft tissues
   injury, ice *see* ice
   palpation *see* palpation
   release *see* release
solar plexus transverse fascial plane
      release   360
soleus   327
somatic eduction, Feldenkrais method
   of   99
somatization of pain   45
soreness *see* muscles
spinal muscles, deeper, in low back
      pain   208–9
spine
   herniated disc *see* disc
   twist   367–9
Spleen 6 (Sp 6)   341
sports events *see* events
spray (with vapocoolant) and stretch   78,
      130–1
Squatting Bone Hole   311–12
stances   16–18
static friction, piriformis and lateral
      rotators   215–16
static stretching   160, 161, 165–6, 166
   post-workout   158
   pre-workout or pre-event   158, 159
   technique   161
Stecco family   100, 102, 152
Stecco fascial manipulation   104, 151–2
Stecco points   151–2
sternal attachments
   pectoralis   260
   sternocleidomastoid   240, 348
sternocleidomastoid   240–1, 347–8
   stretch   351–3
   trigger points   120
Still, Andrew Taylor   99
still work   20
stones (hot or cold)   12, 81
   back pain   73, 201
   case   73
   power effleurage with   359
   in stress reduction   359, 360
straight leg hamstring stretch   342–3
strains, stretching treatment   172–4
strength, muscle
   stretching and its effects on   168, 172
   therapist   15
stress (emotional)   26, 65–6, 355–69

assessment   55, 64, 65–6
fascial stiffness and   103
reduction   355–69
   mindfulness or meditation-based
      (MBSR)   180, 181, 182
   see also trauma
stretch reflex   168–9
stretching (S)   6, 157–76
   common wisdom and evidence for or
      against   157–61
   details of methods   166–72
   myofascial *see* myofascial work
   PNF *see* proprioceptive neuromuscular
      facilitation
   principles (with all methods)   165–6
   self-care   164–5, 169–70, 194–5
   spraying (with vapocoolant) and   78,
      130–1
   techniques   161–4
   therapeutic/in treatment   163–4, 164–5
      back pain   160, 204–5, 212–13, 216,
         216–17, 217, 219, 222
      forearm/wrist/hand pain   271, 274,
         279, 281, 288–9
      hip and pelvis pain   291–2, 296,
         312–15
      leg/knee/foot pain   318, 338, 339,
         342–4
      neck/shoulder pain   234, 243–5
      recommendations   174
      research   172–4
      shoulder girdle pain   255, 258, 267–9
      stress-reducing effects   367–9
      temporomandibular joint pain   348,
         351–3
   see also cross hand stretches; lock and
      stretch; pin and stretch
stripping
   adductors   333
   deltoid   253
   dorsal surface of foot   338, 339
   dorsal surface of hand   280
   extensor retinaculum   279
   extensors of forearm   275, 279
   flexor hallucis longus   328
   flexor retinaculum   281
   flexors of forearm   277
   gastrocnemius   325
   gluteals and lateral rotators   213
   hamstrings   321, 323
   infraspinatus   249
   intercostals   363
   levator scapulae   232
   oblique abdominals   302
   palmaris longus   280
   quadratus lumborum   211
   quadriceps   336–7
   rectus abdominis   308
   rhomboids   249
   scalenes   234, 238, 272
   soleus   327
   supraspinatus   249

stripping (*Continued*)
  tibialis anterior   338
  trapezius   234, 347
  triceps   254
stroke, acupressure   153
structure (body) and biotensegrity   92–7
  considerations in assessment   61
  integration (SI)
    approaches   106
    Rolfing   66, 87, 105–6
subclavius   260
suboccipitals   346
  posterior   239–40
subscapularis   264–5
  side-lying work   258
  stretch   268
superficial fascia   89, 151
  acupuncture points   151
  work
    knowing you are in the superficial
      fascia   110
    low back pain   204
    sacrum (in hip and pelvic pain)   292
supervision of exercises   187
supinator   276–7, 280
supine position
  draping   13–14
  stretches   222
    hip adductors   312
Support (Bladder 36; BL 36)   221, 320
supraspinatus   247, 249
surgery
  knee replacement, stretching
    following   174
  placebo effect   47
swelling, ice reducing   75
symptoms
  perception *see* perception
  presenting, shiatsu   154
  providing an acceptable explanation   57

T

T draping   13
table   9–12
t'ai chi   15–19
  biotensegirity and   97
taping, kinesio   192–3
teaching (T)   6
templates, fascial techniques as   110
temporalis   126, 350–1
  tendon   350
temporalis trigger points   126
temporomandibular joint disorder/
    pain   345–53
  acupressure   351
  hot or cold therapy   78, 345–6
  muscular and trigger point work   346–
    51
  self-care   353
  stretches   348, 351–3
  trigger point misdiagnosed as   122

tendinomuscular channels   147–8
tendinosis
  exercise   187
  ice   80
tendon insert onto bone   91
tennis elbow (lateral epicondylitis)   187, 271
tenosynovitis, de Quervain's   46
tensegrity   92–7
tensor fasciae latae   300, 330–3
teres major   254
teres minor   254
  stretch   268
terminology   125–6
Thai massage   141, 144, 161, 269
thenar eminence   282–3
therapists (practitioners)
  assisting of active isolated
      stretching   169
  mechanics *see* mechanics
  physical sensations *see* sensations
  relationship with client (alliance)   4, 28,
      56–7, 58, 59, 70, 180, 187
  successful, individual qualities   57–8
  t'ai chi   15–19
  trigger points as best friend of   115–17
thermotherapy *see* hot
thixotrophy, connective tissue   108
thoracic release   348
thoughts, unhelpful *see* unhelpful thoughts
    and beliefs
Three Yin Junction   341
thumbs *see* fingers and/or thumb pressure;
    thenar eminence
tibia, release of hamstring attachments
    at   320–1
tibialis anterior   334
  stretch   344
tibialis posterior   327, 328
  working the groove between the
    peroneals and   335
tightness *see* muscles
time line in treatment   60
  estimating duration   59
  heat reducing rehabilitation time   74
tissues
  following, in fascial work   110
  hydration during stretching   171
  pain and   34, 37–43, 45
    pain absent with tissue damage   38
    pain without tissue damage   39
toes
  decompression of joints of   339
  flexion and extension   339
topical remedies   193
touch
  receptors (mechanoreceptors),
    fascial   97–101, 109
  transformative *see* listening touch
towels   11
traction (manual)
  hand/wrist   286
  head   243, 351

training
  bodyworkers, continuing   58
  sports *see* exercise/workout/training
transformative touch *see* listening touch
transverse carpal ligament   280–2
transverse fascial plane release
  pelvis   306–7, 360
  solar plexus   360
transverse process (and attachments)
  cervical   229, 238, 239
  quadratus lumborum and   209–11, 293
trapezius   229–30, 232, 234–6, 247, 255–7,
    346–7
  broad work   232
  fist work   226, 235
  middle   230
  paddy pawing   225, 345, 346
  side-lying work   234–6, 255–7
  trigger points   126
  upper   128, 129, 225, 227, 229–30, 346,
    346–7
    spasm   77
trauma
  emotional (clients with)   25–31
    contraindications   21
    retraumatisation in session   27–8
    see also stress
  physical *see* injury
Travell, Janet   5, 78, 115, 116–19, 121, 123,
    125, 127, 130–1, 152, 229
triceps   254
  stretch   267
trigger points   115–39
  acupressure points and   127–9,
    151, 152
  causes and perpetuation   123–4
  central sensitisation and   124–5
  composition   125
  definition   119–20
  effects   121
  fascia and   129–30, 132
  misdiagnosis and myths attributed
    60, 121–2
  as therapist's friend   115–17
  therapy   130–7
    cold   78, 130–1
    forearm/wrist/hand pain   272–87
    heat   74, 77–8, 132
    hip and pelvis pain   293–310
    incorporation into massage
      treatments   132–4
    leg/knee/foot pain   320–39
    low back pain   206–19
    neck/shoulder pain   227–41
    planning   124–5
    research   131–2
    self-administered   193
    shoulder girdle pain   249–67
    stress-reducing effects   359–60
    temporomandibular joint pain
      346–51
trochanteric notch   297

trust in therapeutic relationship   57
tuina   141
tummy sandwich   306–7, 360

U

ulnar deviation   285
uncoiling the trapezius   229–30
unconditional positive regard   61–2
unguents/ointments/creams   193
unhelpful thoughts and beliefs   35–6, 64,
      189, 191–2
   reducing   70–1, 179, 191–2
Union Valley   288
Upledger, John   3, 107
Upper Bone Hole   221

V

vapocoolant spray and stretch   78, 130–1
vastus intermedius   337
vastus lateralis   331, 333
veins and acupuncture points   151

vertebral border of scapula   236–7, 257
visceral manipulation   106
visual assessment (=observation)   60, 66
vomiting see nausea and vomiting

W

warm-up, stretching   159, 160, 174
water in gel-like state   109
wax   12
webbing, thumb–forefinger   280
weight, body (therapist)   15
Western medicine
   fusion with Eastern medicine see Eastern
      medicine
   trigger points in   127, 129
whiplash   37, 45
   case   73
   self-care   188
width of table   10
Wind Pool   241–2
windscreen wiper stroke,
      gastrocnemius   325

work/occupation/employment
      (client's)   64
   trigger points and   124
wrist pain see forearm/wrist/hand pain

X

X-rays, pain experience and findings
      on   38

Y

yellow flags   63–4
yoga   183–5
   fascial stretching   172
   psychological benefits   160
   as self-care   183–5

Z

Z stroke (longitudinal friction)
   extensor retinaculum   279
   flexor retinaculum   282